Principles of Esthetic Integration
Claude R. Rufenacht

CLAUDE R.
RUFENACHT
Geneva,
Switzerland

Principles of Esthetic Integration

quintessence books

Quintessence Publishing Co, Inc
Chicago, Berlin, London, Tokyo, Paris, Barcelona,
São Paulo, Moscow, Prague and Warsaw

Library of Congress Cataloging-in-Publication Data

Rufenacht, Claude R.
Principles of esthetic integration / Claude R. Rufenacht.
p. cm.
Includes bibliographical references and index.
ISBN 0-86715-369 5
1. Dentistry—Aesthetic aspects. I. Title.
[DNLM: 1. Esthetics, Dental 2. Dentistry—methods WU 100 R922p 2000]
RK54 .R843 2000
617.6—dc21
00-027819

Printing and Binding: Bosch-Druck, Landshut, Germany
Printed in Germany

ISBN 0-86715-369-5

Dedication

To my family
for their support,
encouragement,
and understanding.

Table of Contents

Preface

In the field of dentistry, the esthetic approach has always been based on the imitative elaboration of forms, colors, and structures whose intrinsic beauty is supposed to enhance the patient's appearance. However, the mental perception of an object and its concrete realization based on this perception must be considered purely static. Walter Armstrong's dictum, "Beauty is fitness expressed," suggests that esthetics results from both a subconscious feeling of accomplishment and a perfect adaptation to function; that is, the static characteristics of an object can only generate beauty through their dynamic interaction. As Mondrian states, "Beauty does not arise from the particular character of a form but from the dynamic relationships existing between forms." Neither forms in themselves nor the relationships between them should take precedence; each deserves particular attention.

However, when the technical criteria for the restoration of dental or periodontal forms and structures are reevaluated and new theories and modalities of treatment proposed, both the dynamic relations between objects and their static particularities have been neglected. This has occurred inadvertently because the principles ruling esthetics, eluding Cartesian logic, have been accessible only through irrational, intuitive, and emotional knowledge.

The purpose of this book is to help practitioners develop their own individual conscious knowledge of these esthetic principles—not only of forms, but of a conception of the nature of forms resulting from this relation. This esthetic knowledge constitutes a prerequisite to harmoniously integrating dental elements into the particulars of the facial design, to responding to functional requirements, and to detecting, explaining, and providing corrections to the multiplicity of esthetic failures and disharmonies.

I would like to acknowledge the invaluable assistance provided by M. Rafael Contreras, head of my laboratory, and to express my gratitude to the staff members, friends, and colleagues who have participated in this endeavor.

CHAPTER 1

Morphological Integration

Function and Form

In dentistry, dentofacial morphological characteristics have always been understood according to the concept, shared by the ancient Greeks, the European Renaissance, and the modern era, that the main objective of art is the imitation of reality.

But in addition to this apparently simple concept, the application of which actually requires unusual perceptive and manual capabilities, Greek art has always assumed also that perfect corporal beauty requires the application of strange mathematical formulas based on absolute physical norms involving all parts of the body. According to Pythagorean theory, corporal beauty is necessarily based on the mathematical notion of the proportionate body. Unfortunately, however, the metric grids and organic forms have never been brought into complete concordance, and the dream of form as the expression of mathematical order—that is to say, unique, perfect, and repeatable—has totally vanished.

Though mathematical formulas may or may not determine formal beauty, function certainly determines form. Morphological reality necessarily results from adaptive relational conditions, and these conditions have been extremely well defined: "function creates the organ," and "necessity creates shapes." That is, a tooth should look like a tooth to function like a tooth (Fig 1-1).

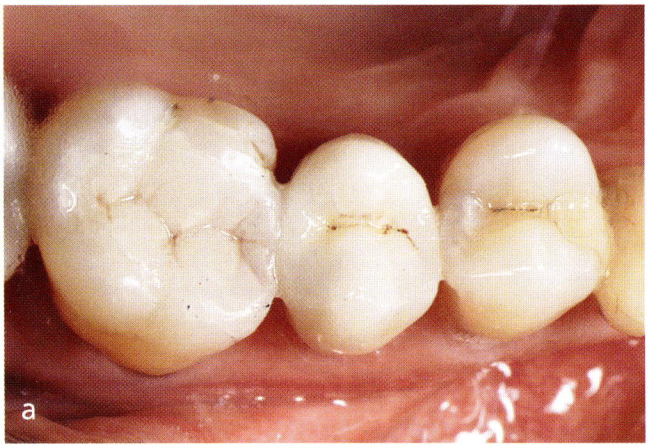

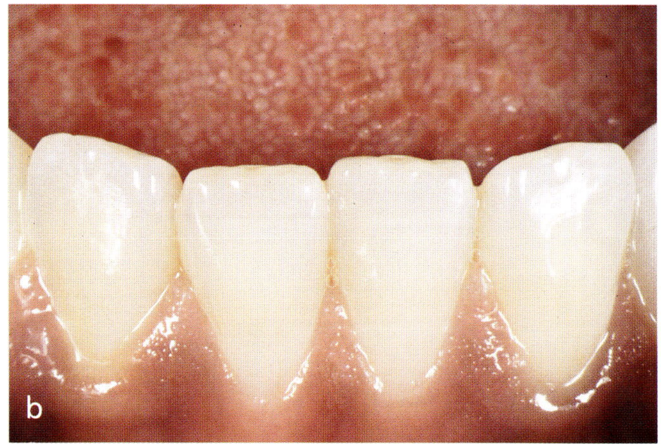

Figs 1-1a and 1-1b The morphological design of a tooth, the characteristics of its shape, result not from chance but from adaptative relational conditions, from precise function. The shape and characteristics of a molar (a), bulky, solid, and rounded, or an incisor (b), flat and sharp-edged, are determined by their different functions.

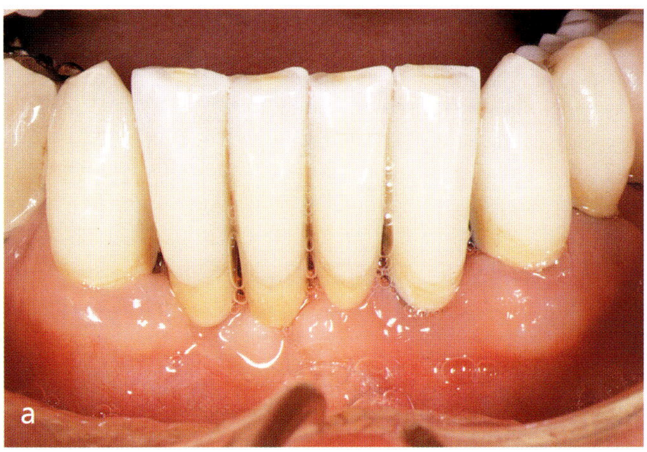

Fig 1-2a The imitation of reality, an artistic concept promoted by the ancient Greeks and the European Renaissance, has maintained its influence to the present day. But in the field of clinical dentistry this influence often remains difficult to demonstrate. This implant-supported fixed prosthesis perfectly illustrates one of the various aspects of technical morphological deviations.

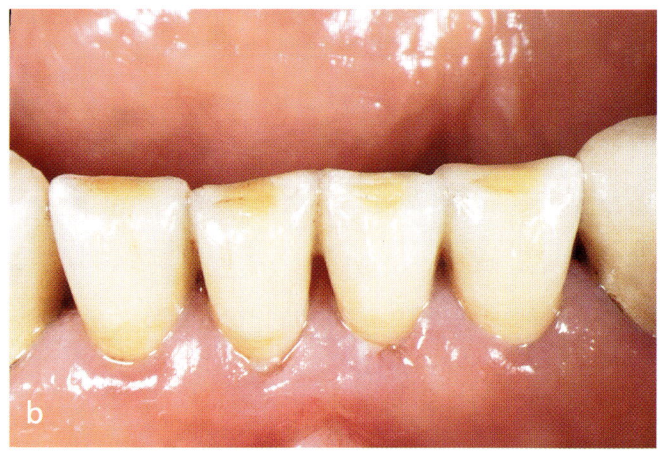

Fig 1-2b The imitation of reality involves the natural duplication of a tooth color and shape, excluding, however, the imitation of the various impacts of the aging process, which renders it unable to satisfy functional requirements.

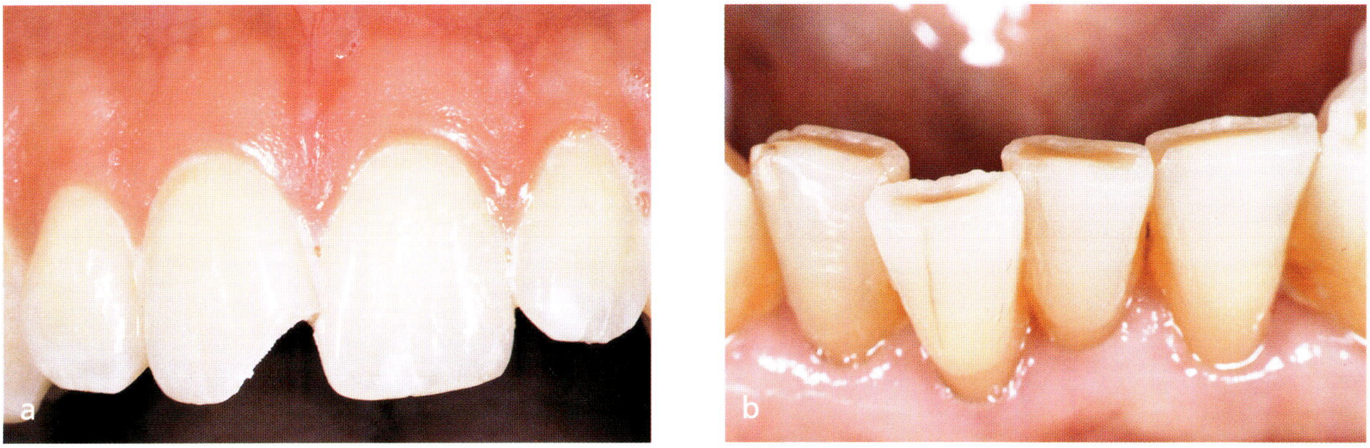

Figs 1-3a and 1-3b Compromises in the stomatognathic system of traumatic origin, (a) accidental or (b) functional, always display more or less marked morphological deviations.

However, in average clinical practice, it appears that dentistry has never totally recovered from the collapse of Pythagorean theory; abnormal, grotesque, artificial dentate forms, flat, oversized, or undersized, seem to be the rule. They may well offend the patient's innate sense of anatomical normality, yet professionals tolerate them (Fig 1-2). It seems that daily contact with compromised dentitions, reinforced by their reading of the literature, has made dentists the victims of a visual distortion of morphological reality. When publications dedicated to dental anatomy present as standard dental elements that have already undergone some stages of wear, one understands why defects are rather eradicated than restored and why artificial elements are systematically built up to conform to already existing antagonistic deformities. The art of perception, a basic requirement for the imitation of nature, is all too often lacking. As a result, habits, preconceived ideas, and symbols, all products of faulty perception, invade the mind and obscure the vision.

Further, this critical statement of clinical reality calls in question not only the morphological nature of the restorative process but also the various occlusal concepts and materials used and abandoned in an endless fervor of updating enthusiasm. It is most unlikely that a morphological utopia created by imagination and habits could ever produce beneficial treatment when clinical reality daily shows that defects in the stomatognathic system from trauma or dysfunction are always materialized through morphological alterations, affecting both tooth and supporting structures (Figs 1-3 and 1-4).

"Morphology is destiny" (H. Shavell), and so the criteria and characteristics of dentofacial morphological norms are strictly defined according to their

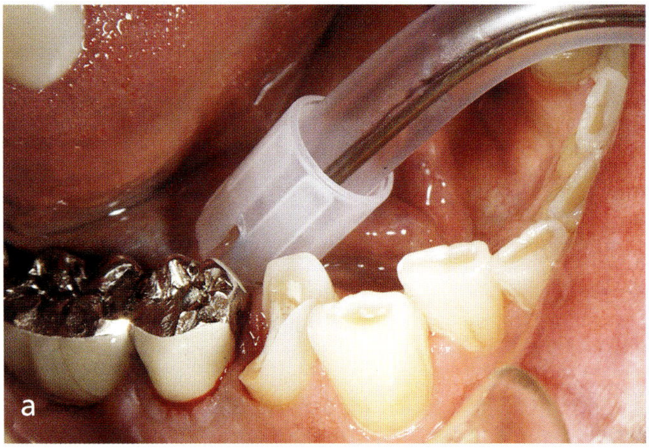

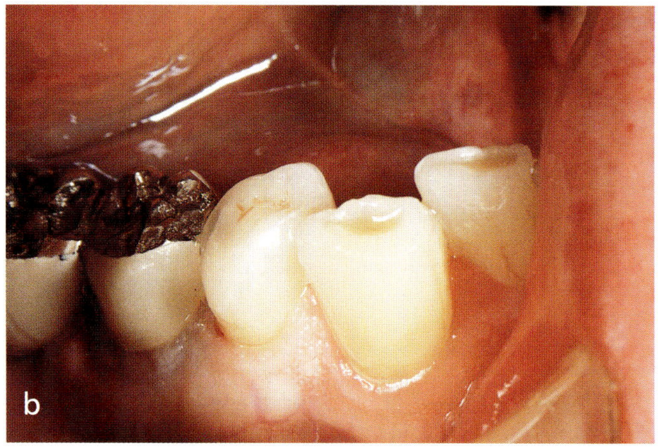

Figs 1-4a and 1-4b It is unrealistic to think that morphological deviations or alterations will not interfere with the original function. The introduction of a bonded restoration in an occlusal scheme showing evident manifestations of functional trauma from incisors to the posterior area may satisfy patient's and dentist's inclination for updated tooth-colored restorations. Yet, poorly shaped and simply adapted to antagonist deformities, it can neither restore function nor resist the existing traumatic conditions.

ability to fulfill specific functional requirements. In medicine and dentistry, that is, discrimination between function and dysfunction or between health and disease stands as fundamental and common practice. But the use of these same scientific criteria, which habit has progressively and insidiously instituted, in the discriminating evaluation between the ugly and the beautiful (Figs 1-5 and Fig 1-6) can only result in a confusion of genres.

The functional and esthetic qualities of a form may seem related, but they are far from being based on identical parameters. Functional normality has nothing to do with formal normality, a notion that has always resisted clear definition.

On observation, dentofacial morphology normally consists of constants and variations, all able to fulfill functional requirements. Subtle variations and differences of form, in contrast, fulfill esthetic requirements (Fig 1-7).

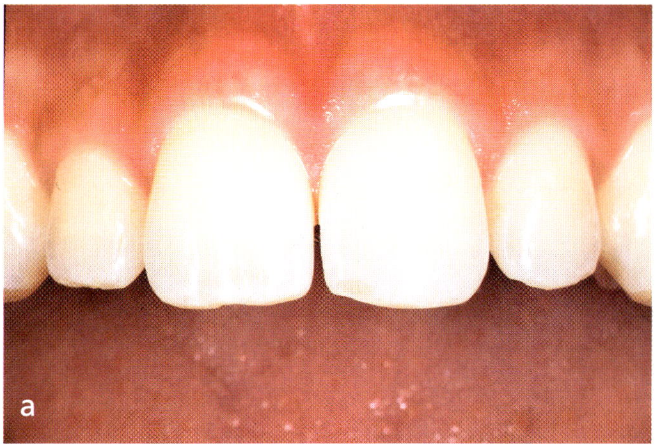

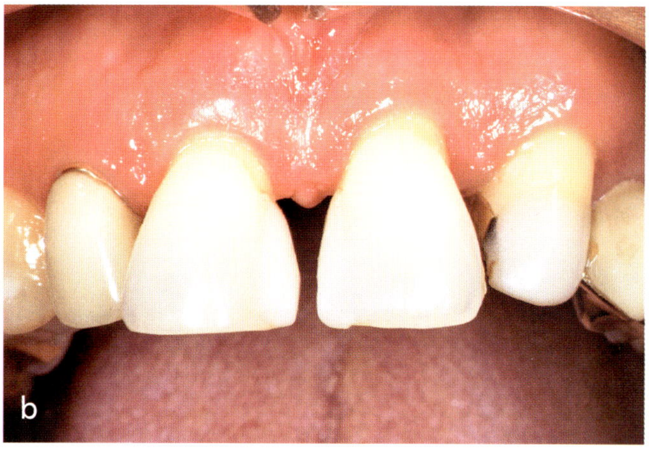

Figs 1-5a and 1-5b The view of a composition as beautiful or ugly is partly subjective, whereas objective scientific criteria discriminate strictly between (a) health and (b) disease. In these compositions the association of health with beauty and disease with ugliness can be considered as casual and at the same time as the result of reasoning and subjective perception.

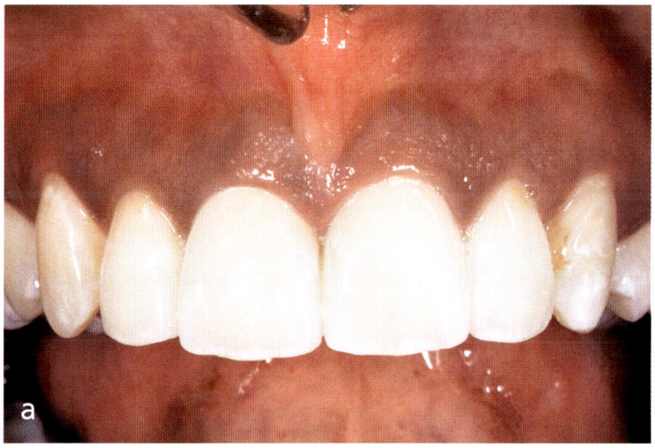

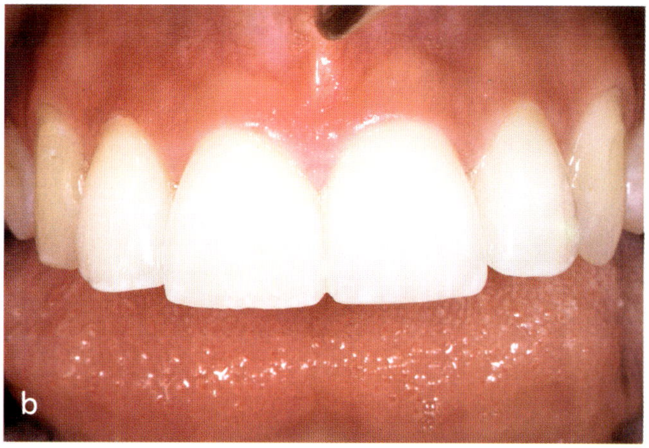

Figs 1-6a and 1-6b In these compositions, which have each received four porcelain veneers, the presence of tissue pigmentation may subjectively impair the esthetic appearance of the first (a), whereas the second (b), presenting tissue conditions more compatible to Western standards, may appear beautiful. Yet this esthetic judgment is not only totally subjective but also opposes reason by ignoring the wear affecting the morphology of the maxillary right canine. This contradicts the assumption that esthetics and function are naturally associated.

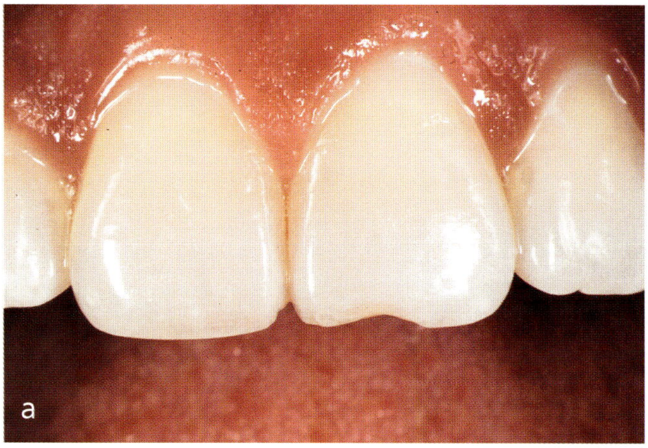

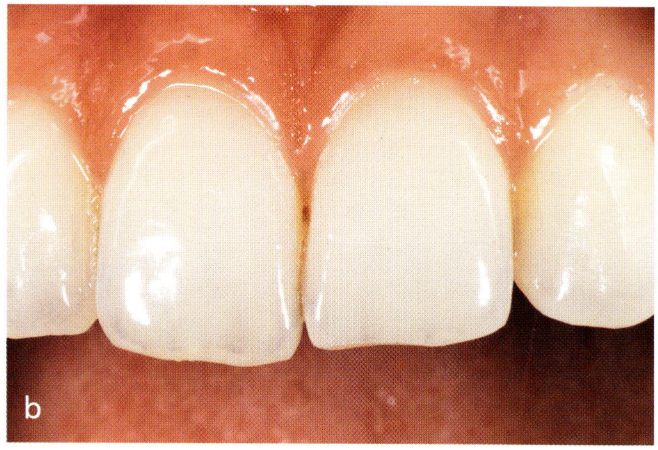

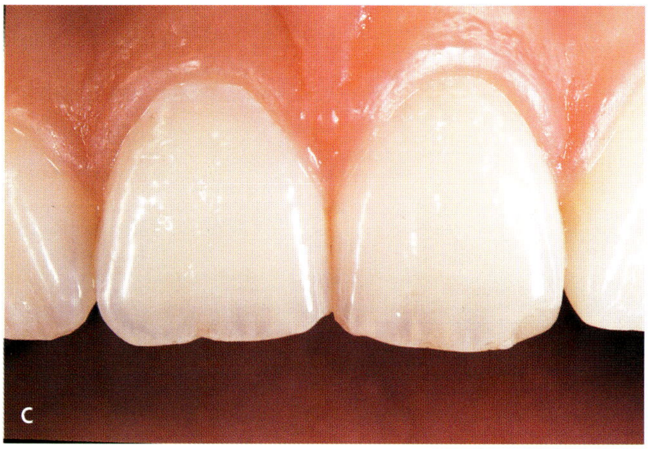

Figs 1-7a to 1-7c The design of these dental entities presents the standard morphological characteristics of maxillary central incisors, which reflect their specific function. These entities also differ more or less markedly in tooth shape. It can be stated that dental entities (a) and (c) can only be differentiated by means of the impacts of the functional or accidental traumas that have affected the right or left central incisors. Closer observation, however, shows that (c) has been given a more rounded incisal edge and (a) a more pronounced distal curvature and more rounded angle. All these variations, evident or subtle, respond to the requirements not of function but of esthetics.

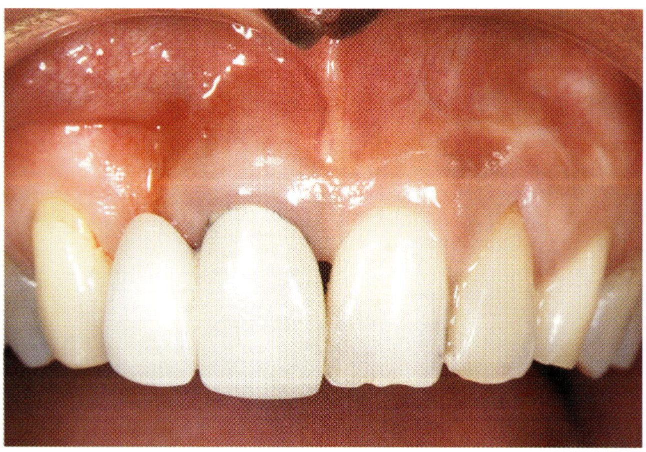

Fig 1-8 The dynamic forces that generate beauty are not born of chance but of the esthetic nature of the relations between different shapes or elements. The absence of correlation between the fixed partial denture prosthesis, supporting tissue, and adjacent teeth testifies to the rupture of esthetic relations that has taken place in this composition.

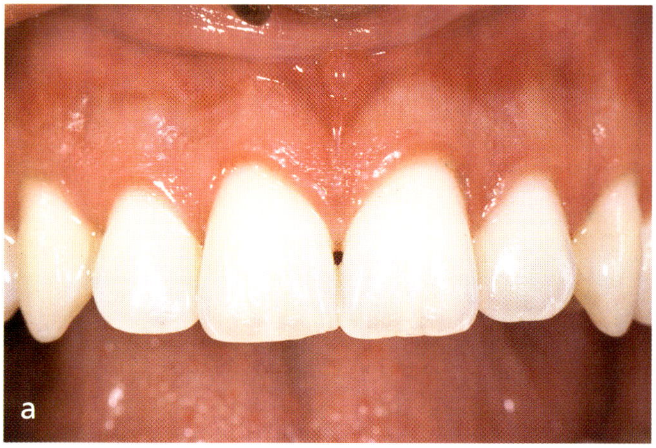

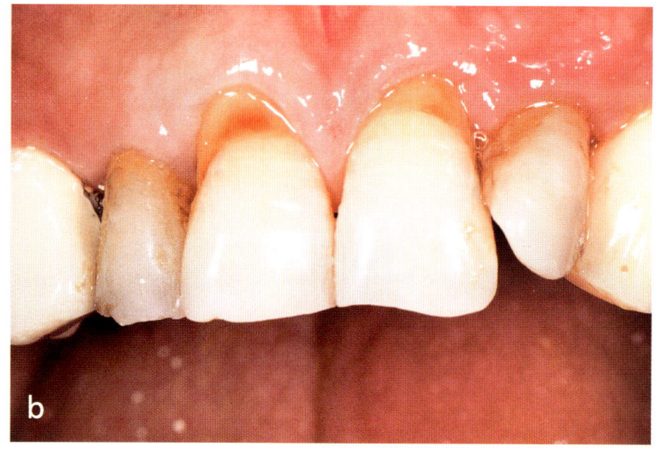

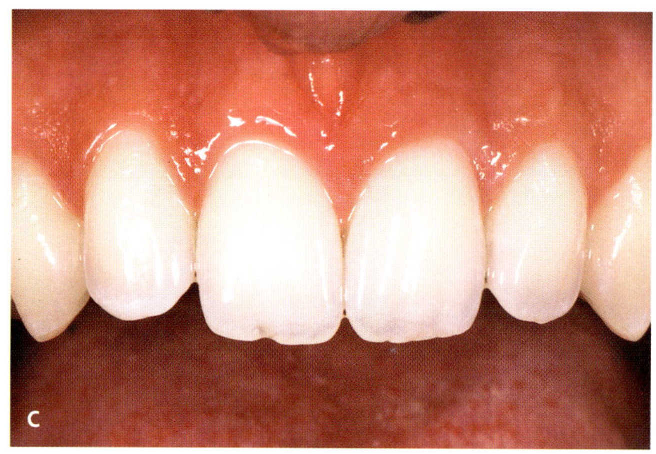

Figs 1-9a to 1-9c The factors that participate in the esthetic quality of a composition still await clear definition. It can be noted that the tooth-gingival relationships displayed in (a) and (c) present marked dissimilarities both in the design of the marginal papilla and the location of the gingival zenith. The hypothesis that morphological variations—differences in the amplitude of concavities and convexities in the transitional zone connecting crown to root—may dictate variations in tooth-gingival relational design is supported by the axiom, "shapes create relations as relations create shapes" (b).

From an esthetic point of view every element of a composition represents in itself an exclusively static entity that will only have esthetic effect in dynamic interaction with other elements. This means that the nature of the relations between two elements dictates the shape of the related elements, which in turn dictates the nature of other relations according to the axiom, "shapes create relations as relations create shapes."

With regard to preexisting environmental structures in expectation of association with new dental elements, esthetic dentistry can be defined as relational. It determines relations and creates forms accordingly, but excludes the creation of self-imagined autonomous entities. In the puzzle of a composition, the introduction of an improper element can rarely fool the discerning eye or satisfy the mind (Fig 1-8). In the restorative process, the misperception of the interdependence of elements invariably results in the application of laws of hazard. Esthetics rests on other laws (Fig 1-9).

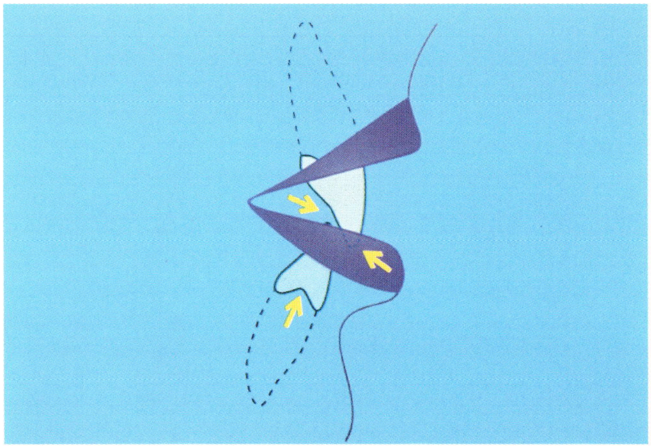

Fig 1-10 In our field of interest it can be stated that there are only three esthetic relational elements. While interocclusal and periodontal relations have long engrossed the attention of the profession, the esthetic nature of the relations between dental, perioral, and facial structures on the contrary has never really received objective and correct definition.

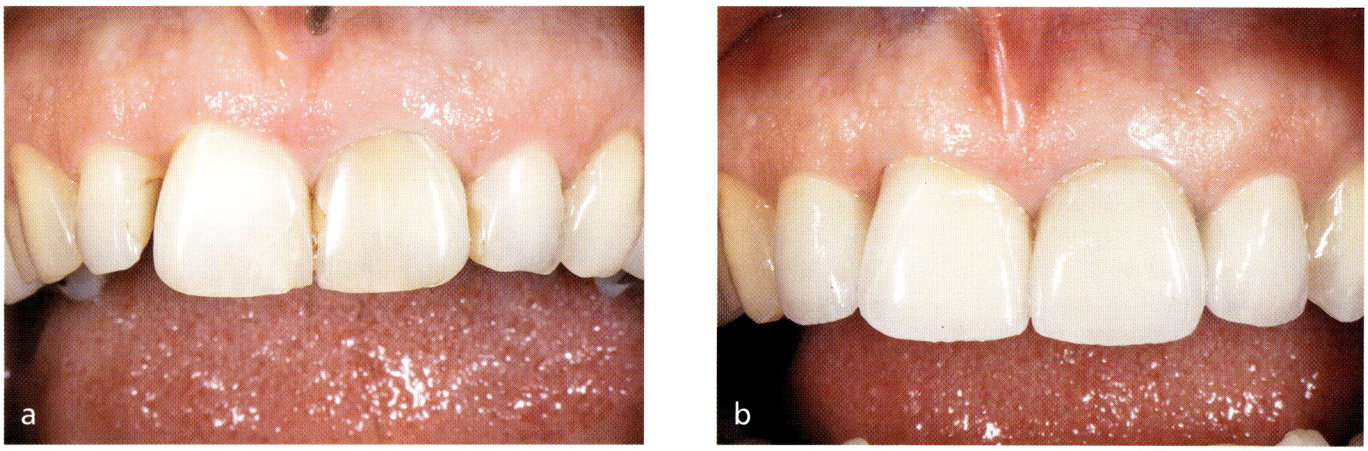

Figs 1-11a and 1-11b The reconstitution of the original tooth shape is easy when original relational elements or elements of reference are present. In this example the deterioration of oral conditions due to the progression of wear has not only affected the maxillary (a) left anterior area but has also led to migratory movements of the maxillary right anterior segment. The original esthetic conditions are easily restored by duplicating the shape and position of the original existing elements of the maxillary anterior segment (b).

Nonetheless, in modern dentistry, dental elements are usually conceived and realized as autonomous entities, without regard to the relational requirements of esthetics. Clinicians deal not only with the restored tooth but also with its esthetic integration into environmental conditions involving not only periodontal support and interocclusal relationships but also perioral structures (Fig 1-10).

All these elements are part of the chain of relations between face and lips, lips and teeth, and teeth and periodontal support. These are crucial to dentofacial esthetics, while perioral structures serve as basic reference points in the reconstitution of original dentofacial harmony. The imitation of nature, while remaining an unalterable conceptual principle, only makes sense when understood as an enhanced du-

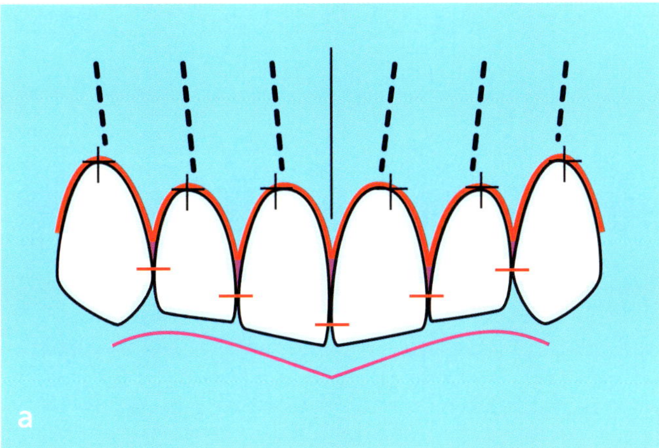

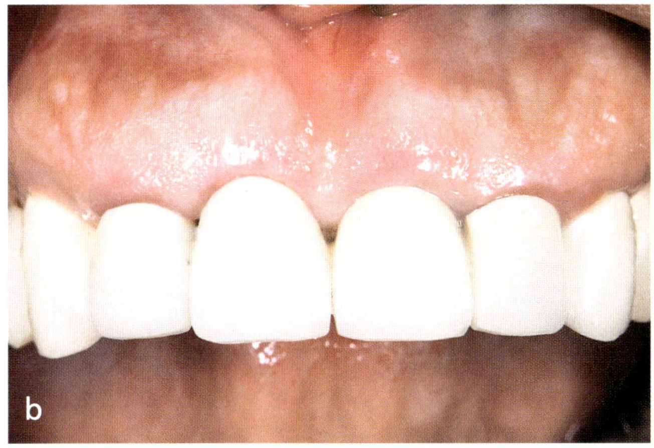

Figs 1-12a to 1-12c To overcome the problem arising from the absence of any elements of reference in the rehabilitative process, such as can be observed in (b) and (c), a group from Zürich two decades ago published a sketch fixing the parameters necessary to perfect the esthetic appearance of the anterior segment. These parameters involve a specific inclination of tooth axial direction, a location of contact points, gingival level and gingival zenith, and a specific design of the incisal line (a). This sketch must be used with extreme caution as it not only involves objective parameters resulting from pertinent clinical observations but also introduces subjective preferential parameters and totally ignores individual differences (see Fig 1-13).

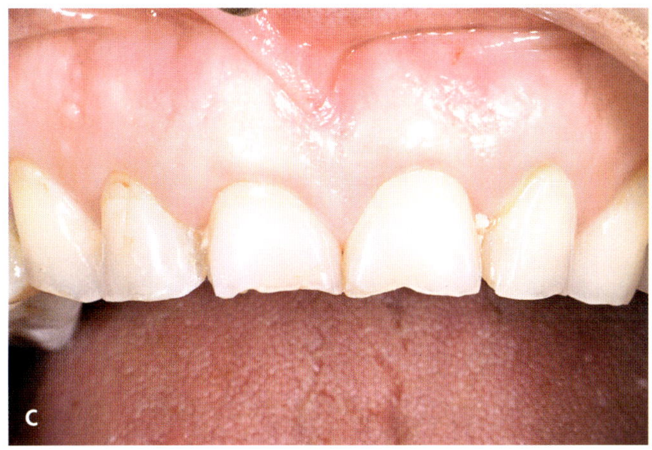

plication of original elements within the framework of the existing dentofacial composition, which will reconstitute the chain of relations affected by the loss of a specific connective link. Again, "shapes create relations as relations create shapes" (Fig 1-11).

Contrary to what has been written, no fixed characteristics can dictate the esthetic form of a dentofacial composition (Fig 1-12). Only basic morphological characteristics and individual morphological variables adapted to specific relational conditions exist (Fig 1-13). In a restorative process the reconstitution of compromised elements should always conform to a morphological normality by including variables that can with related environmental elements harmoniously realize the esthetic appearance of the whole.

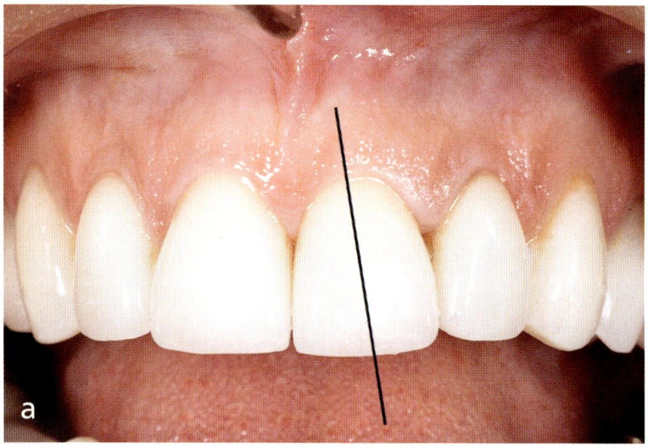
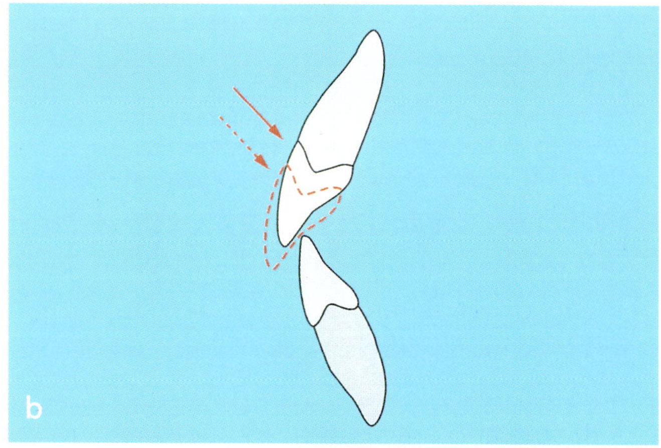

Figs 1-13a and 1-13b This patient, who has been treated for a high lip-line smile presumably corrected by surgical tooth elongation and the insertion at a higher level of porcelain veneers, complains of functional discomfort and poor esthetics. (b) Functional comfort can be provided by restoring vertical anterior relationships or anterior guidance lost in the previous treatment. It has to be noted that this type of therapeutic approach in the treatment of high lip-line smiles, though favored by periodontists, systematically ends up impairing the anterior guidance, neglecting a basic functional requirement. (a) Esthetically, the location of tooth-gingival zenith on the left central incisor in a position central to the long axis of the tooth and the location of the gingival level on the lateral incisors higher than that of the central incisors, even though not conforming to the parameters for perfecting the esthetic appearance of the anterior segment, does not seem to be responsible for the esthetic failure of this composition. Rather, the imbalance of tooth-axial direction mainly caused by the distal inclination of the left central incisor appears most disturbing.

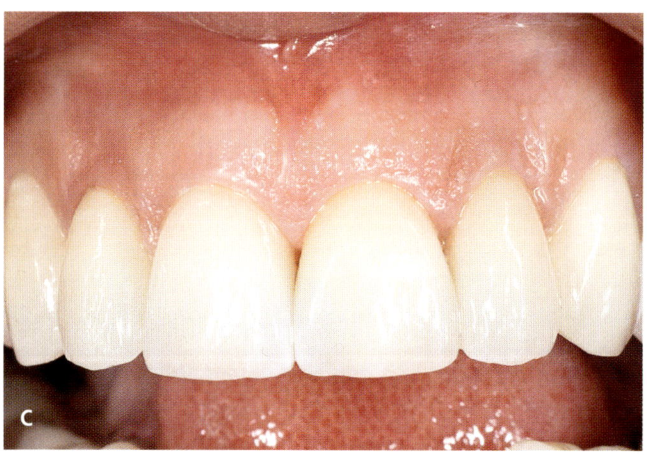

Fig 1-13c The insertion of new veneers slightly increased in length and the correction of tooth axial balance, finalized with the accumulation of ceramic on the buccal and distal cervical aspect of the left central incisor, have succeeded in restoring tooth axial equilibrium and esthetic appeal. Surprisingly, and without any modification of the periodontal support, this accumulation of material on the distal cervical aspect of the left central incisor has succeeded in creating in visual perception an illusory optical displacement of tooth zenith that from an esthetic point of view confirms the axiom, "Shapes create relations as relations create shapes."

It is the absence of existing elements of reference that generates confusion by leaving the imagination unrestrained in the conception of forms. What is needed in such cases is an appreciative visual reading of specific relational conditions that can allow for a correct reconstitution of related elements. Even in the most compromised situations it is unlikely that all the elements of the dentofacial composition have undergone severe alterations. Usually at least perioral and facial structures have maintained their original morphological characteristics and need only to recover the esthetic dynamic generated by their meeting with appropriate elements. The conceptual restoration of compromised dentofacial entities, limited in our field of interest to dental elements and periodontal support, should always be undertaken with a view at the same time both to function and esthetic arrangement.

Dental Components

The restorative reproduction of the dental element has gradually reached an extremely high level of authenticity thanks to the competence of prominent dental technicians, the improved quality of the materials, and the sophistication of technology. Yet the esthetic variability of the average laboratory production is far from demonstrating that technical knowledge and artistic sense are universal (Fig 1-14).

The color and constitutive material of the dental element have been emphasized at the expense of form, which has usually been left to personal taste, selected samples, or the laws of hazard. The profession needs to rethink this narrow focus on material and appreciate that dental esthetics also requires a

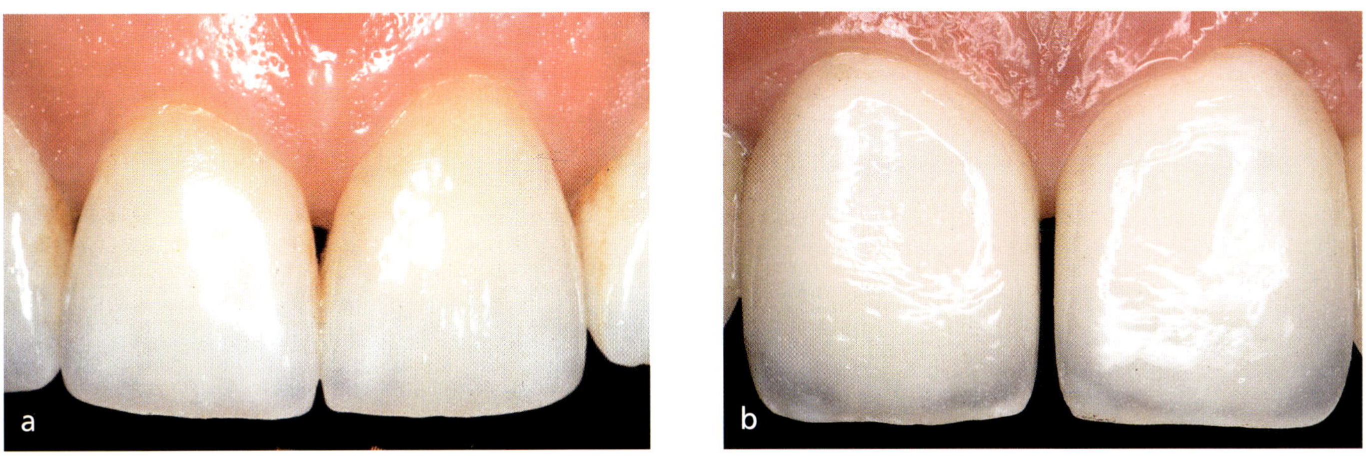

Figs 1-14a and 1-14b Two different technical and individual approaches to producing a tooth's structural authenticity testify to variations in perceptive capabilities and demonstrate the difficulty of totally avoiding the forces of habit, preconceived ideas, or preferential inclinations. The beauty of a tooth as an isolated entity makes no sense if it cannot be evaluated in its confrontation with environmental conditions that include perioral structures. ([a] Courtesy of Dr Bozzi, Comacchio, Italy, [b] courtesy of Dr Fornararo, Firenze, Italy.)

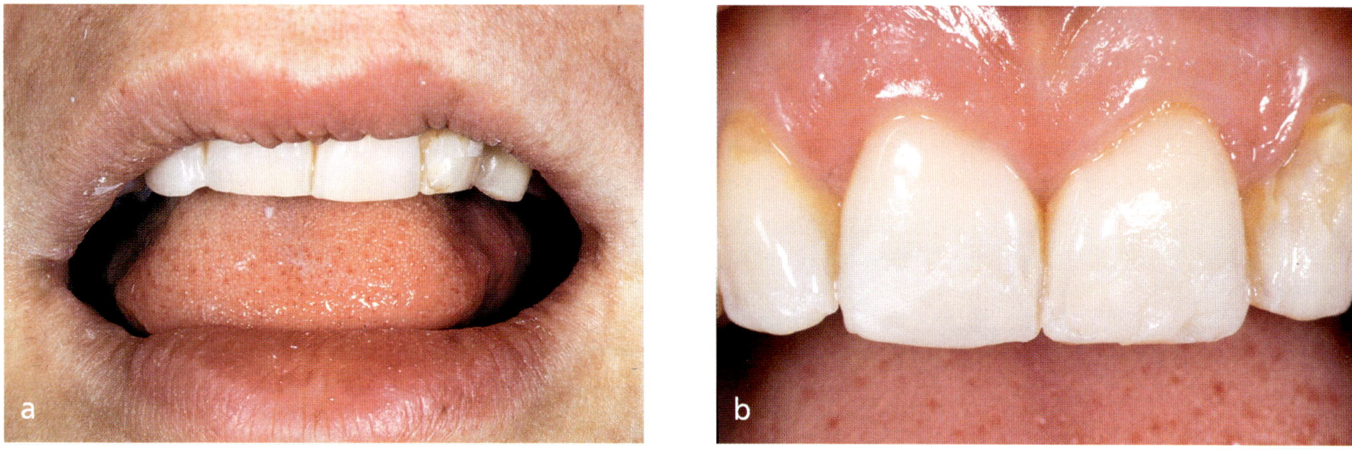

Figs 1-15a and 1-15b (a) Initial dentofacial situation or confrontation of worn-out dental elements with perioral environmental conditions. (b) Close view of a diagnostic tooth restoration (composite).

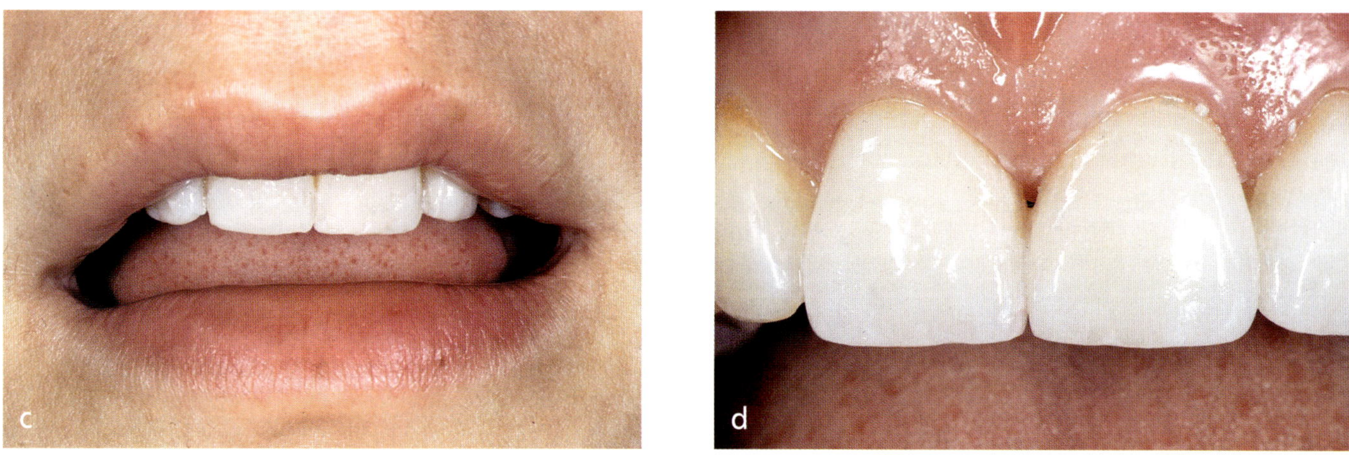

Figs 1-15c and 1-15d (c) Confrontation of the diagnostic tooth restoration with environmental conditions. (d) Technical restoration of the anterior segment extending from the right central incisor to the left canine. The imitation of nature requires duplication of the diagnostic setup, and is frustrated here by an evident reduction of central incisor width at the gingival third.

visual confrontation with environmental elements (Fig 1-15).

In other words, the clinician's perception of esthetics remains too intimate, too technically oriented. The dental element is never appreciated in its strategic position, that is to say, in a common visual relationship between periodontal support and perioral and facial structures.

Periodontal Components

From an esthetic point of view, the characteristics of tooth morphology and tooth location are directly dictated by the structural design of related periodontal and perioral structures. The collapse of periodontal structures following tooth loss or periodontal pathologies, a situation which can be considered one of the hallmarks of dental pathologies, obscures the nature of the relational tooth-periodontal support. However, the elements of the perioral structures that create tooth-lip or tooth-face relationships do not usually take part in this degradating phenomenon. In the

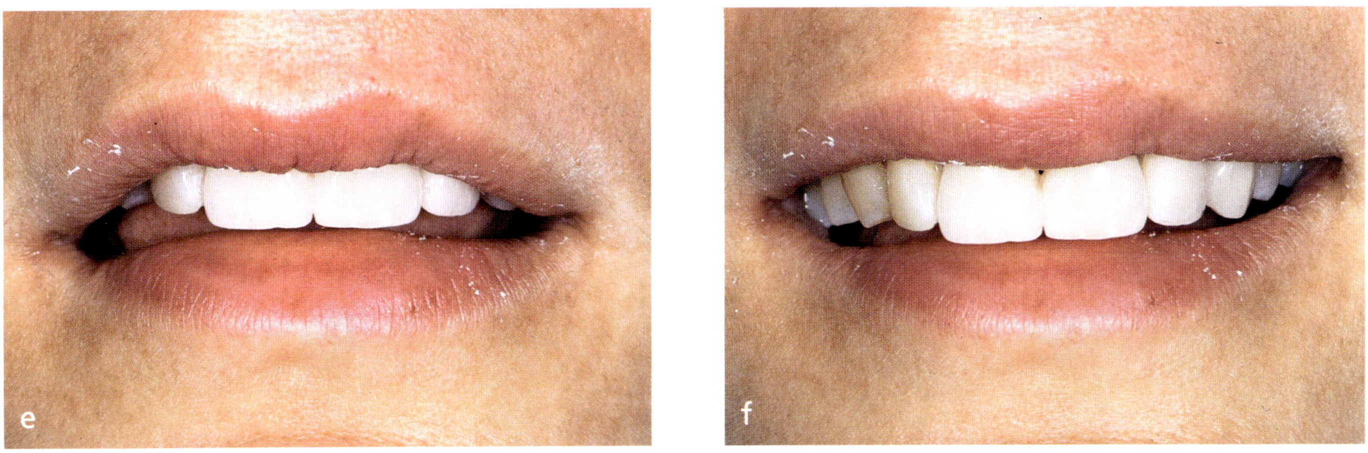

Figs 1-15e and 1-15f (e) Appealing confrontation with environmental conditions, underlining the accuracy of tooth-length extension. (f) In smiling, however, one cannot help noticing both the faulty duplication of the maxillary central incisors' shape, displaying a too-rounded proximal curvature that was described as a reduction of tooth width at the gingival third, and the faulty design of the incisal edge in its confrontation with lower lip design. At one place or another the failure to follow the axiom, "shapes create relations as relations create shapes" will lead to esthetic failure.

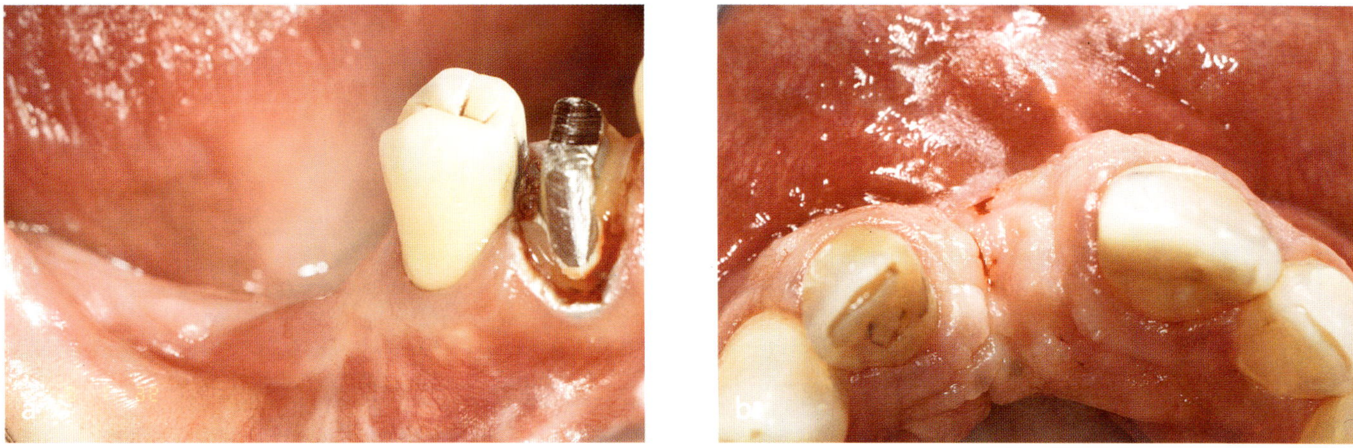

Figs 1-16a and 1-16b (a) Vertical and (b) horizontal ridge collapse as defined in the literature. In clinical reality, combined manifestations of these two types of defects are most common. (Courtesy of Dr Cornellini, Rimini, Italy.)

comprehensive esthetic conception of the restorative process there remains no other alternative than to understand the nature and particularities of these structures, since they represent the only available frame of reference indicating the original tooth morphological design and the nature of the dental arrangement.

An esthetic understanding of the spatial position of the dental elements as fixed by the relational characteristics of tooth-perioral structures, completed and refined in conformity with functional and phonetic requirements, is crucial to the restoration of a collapsed periodontal support, which has to be assessed not only according to the osseous availability but also according to the overlying tooth location and tooth morphological normality.

The restoration of the collapsed ridge, which the literature has described as vertical, horizontal, or complex according to its spatial extension (Fig 1-16), has long engrossed the attention of periodontists to such an extent that in modern dentistry not only are crest deformities systematically corrected but the prevention of ridge collapse is usually made part of the process of tooth extraction (Figs 1-17 to 1-19). In the treatment of deformities, professionals have successively selected two different therapeutic approaches, which can be classified as replacement materials and periodontal regeneration.

The use of replacement materials or fillers that can perfectly meet all the requirements in the restoration of the collapsed ridge is compromised not only by the expansion of implant therapy (Figs 1-20 and

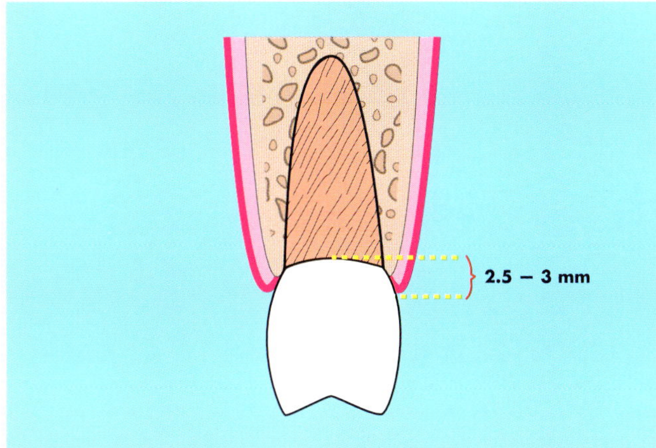

Fig 1-17 Ideal tissue conditioning of fresh extraction sites requires from an ovate pontic an intrusion into socket's depth extending no more than 2.5 mm to 3.0 mm from gingival tissue margin.

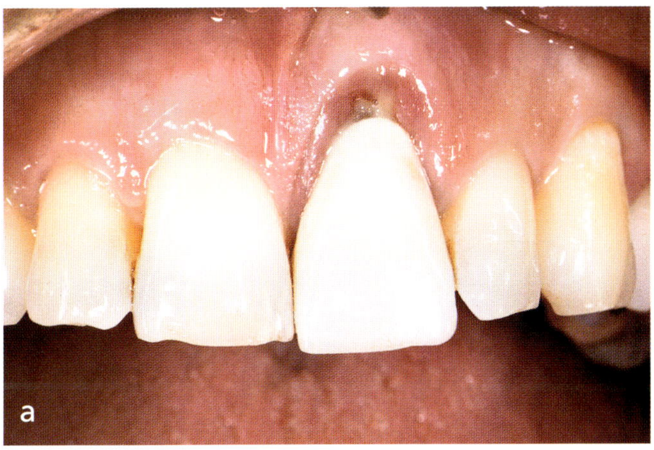

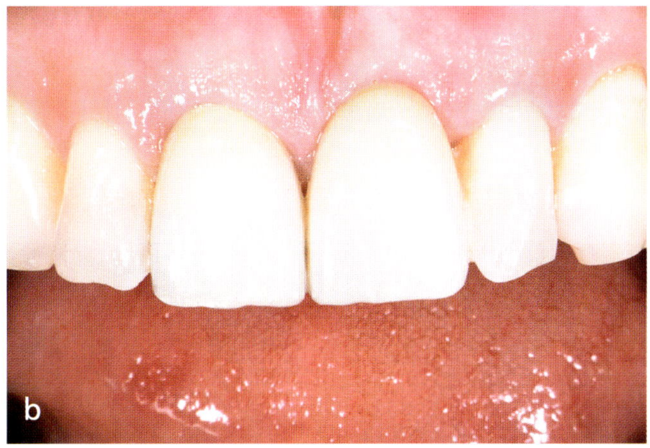

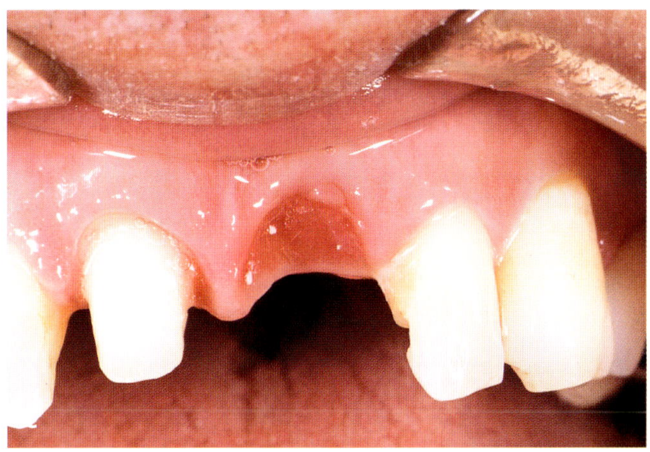

Figs 1-18a to 1-18c The use of fillers, such as hydroxyapatite (HA) particles, continues to be a perfectly valuable therapy for the correction of deformed ridges or crest maintenance as long as no implant use is foreseen. However, the approach is incompatible with regenerative techniques. (a) Clinical situation before extraction, (b) provisionalization at 8 weeks, (c) clinical situation at provisional removal with still-visible HA particles.

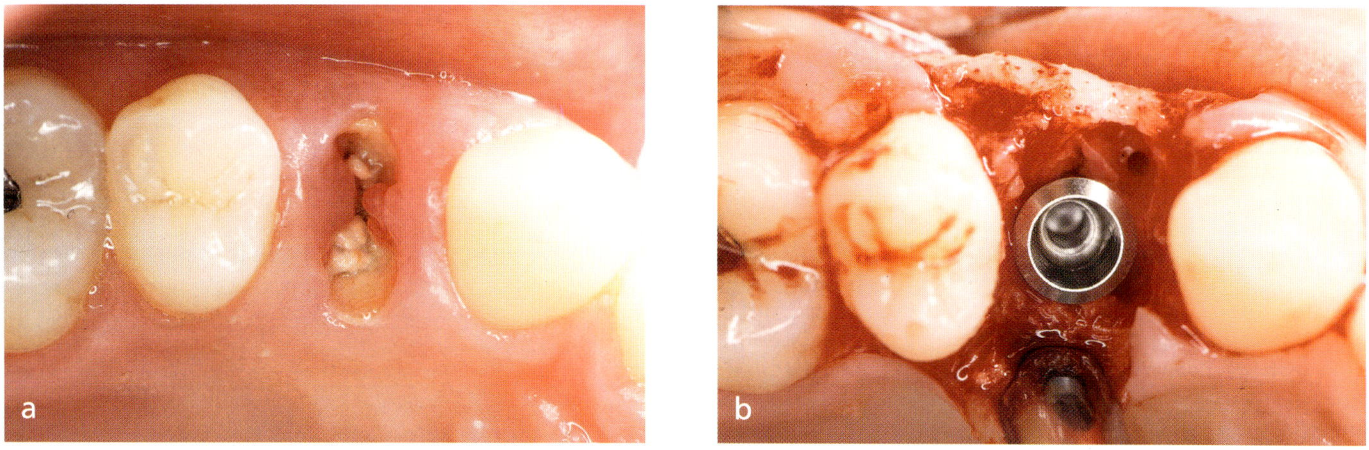

Figs 1-19a and 1-19b The prevention of ridge collapse following extraction is best achieved with immediate implant placement when sufficient soft tissue availability is present for site coverage. (a) Clinical situation before extraction and (b) at first-stage implant surgery. (Courtesy of Dr Cornellini, Rimini, Italy.)

1-21) in demand of osseous tissue for integration but also by the fact that today periodontal regeneration has become a clinical and biological reality. As a result, replacement materials, though far from outmoded, must present specific qualifications of resorption, safety, and osseoinduction to be part of the periodontal regenerative arsenal.

Osseoinduction requires the potential differentiation of mesenchymal cells into osteoblasts with subsequent formation of new bone, a process that is thought to be induced by a protein termed *bone morphogenic protein.* Histologically, osseoinduction is positive when cartilage differentiation takes place after 10 days, lamellar bone formation after 20 days, and bone marrow formation after 30 days.

Now that the basic requisites for periodontal regeneration have been identified, however, we need further research to identify factors that could enhance the efficiency and predictability of this thera-

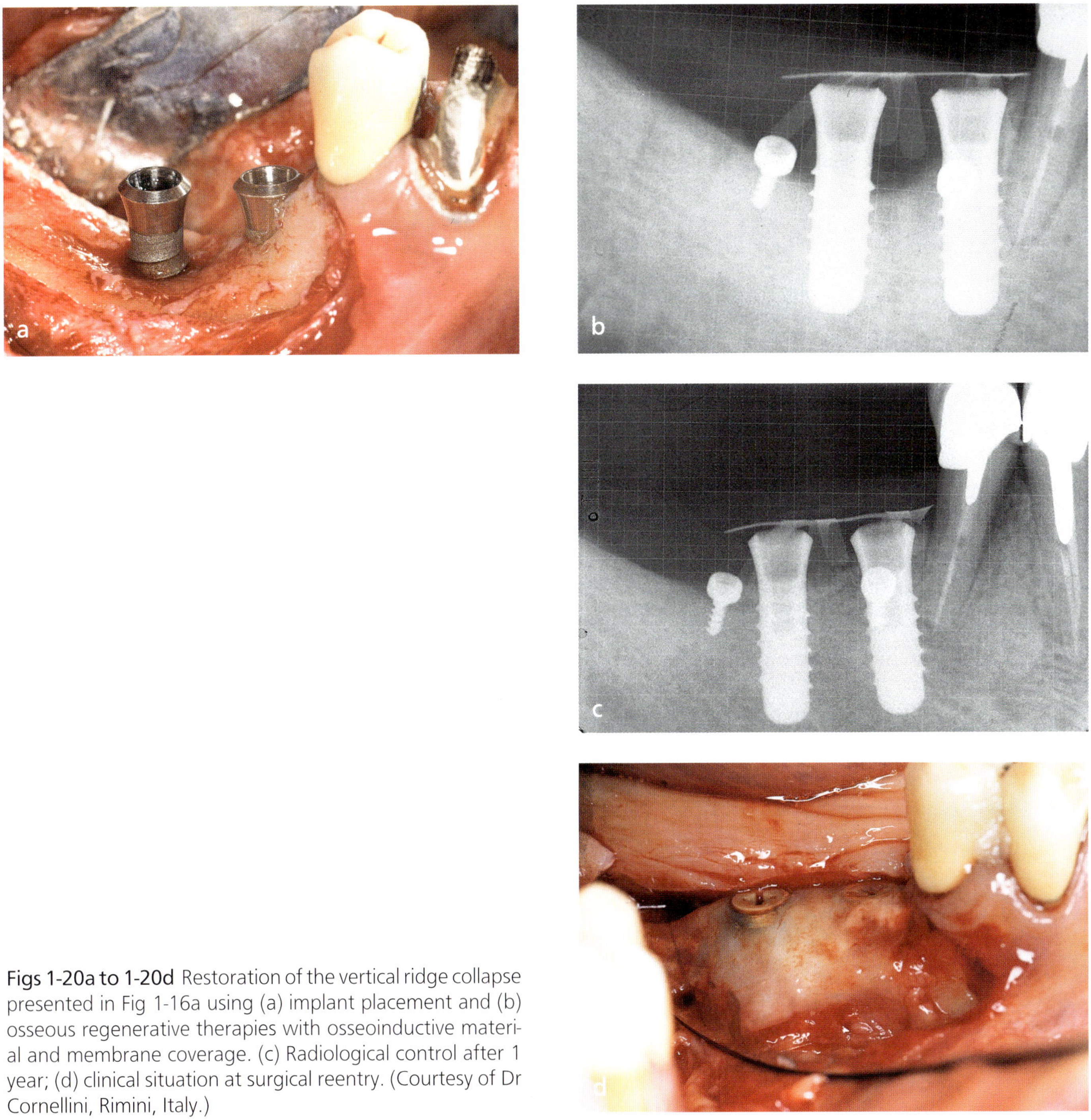

Figs 1-20a to 1-20d Restoration of the vertical ridge collapse presented in Fig 1-16a using (a) implant placement and (b) osseous regenerative therapies with osseoinductive material and membrane coverage. (c) Radiological control after 1 year; (d) clinical situation at surgical reentry. (Courtesy of Dr Cornellini, Rimini, Italy.)

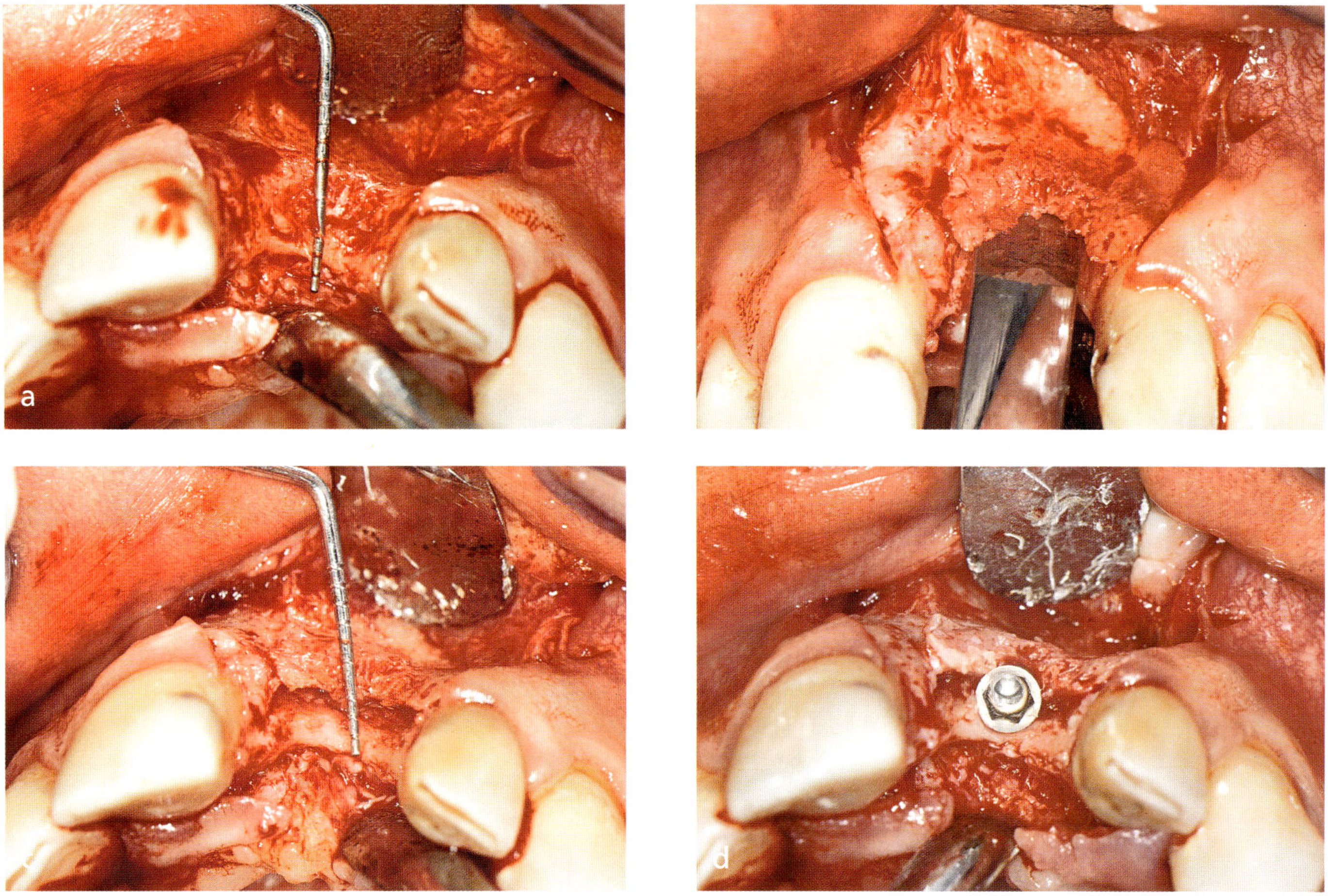

Figs 1-21a to 1-21d (a) Clinical view of the horizontal ridge collapse seen in Fig 1-16b, following flap elevation, corrected by means of a vertical osseous splitting using a diamond drill and elevator (b) with careful separation of osseous walls, taking advantage of bone elasticity (c) and implant placement (d). (Courtesy of Dr Cornellini, Rimini, Italy.)

py. In today's state of research the clinician is left to interpret data from clinical trials and from personal clinical experiences. Practically, this means an ongoing evaluation of observed and reported results leading to a sense of the advantages and limitations of each periodontal regenerative technique.

Regenerative techniques are many and are all worthy of study. While the complex regulated series of events in tissue regeneration is being unraveled, affording new inroads in biotechnology in future therapy, continuous updating will be necessary.

Now that clinical philosophy requires not only the restoration but also the prevention of ridge collapse, and the therapeutic approach for crest restoration, thanks to osseous regenerative therapies, remains identical whether for implant or pontic support, final treatment decisions are based on "what works best in the clinician's hands."

Perioral Components

For the esthetic dentist and the prosthodontist, the morphological appreciation of perioral and facial components has always been a hazardous process since this appreciation has never conformed to a well-defined methodology but rather proceeds from a farrago of imperatives of a clinical, esthetic, biometric, anthropometric, or morphopsychological nature. This confusion is naturally sustained by the reading of the literature, which is replete with elements of investigations, validated or unvalidated, that finally are never of any practical use.

One should add that we have no impact on existing facial morphological conditions, whether beautiful or ugly, square or round, young or old, whatever type of volumes or depressions they display, with the

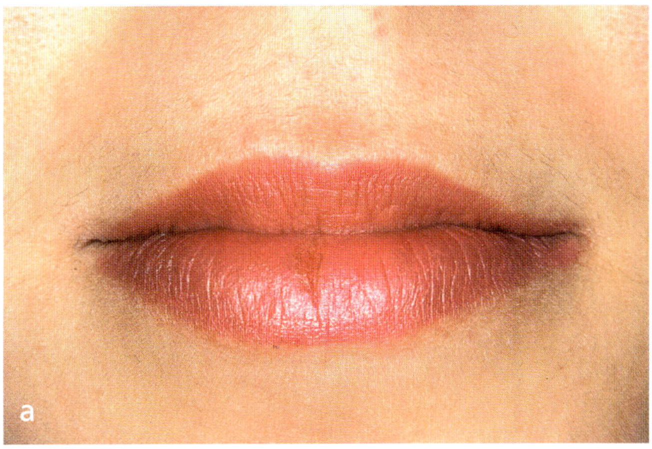

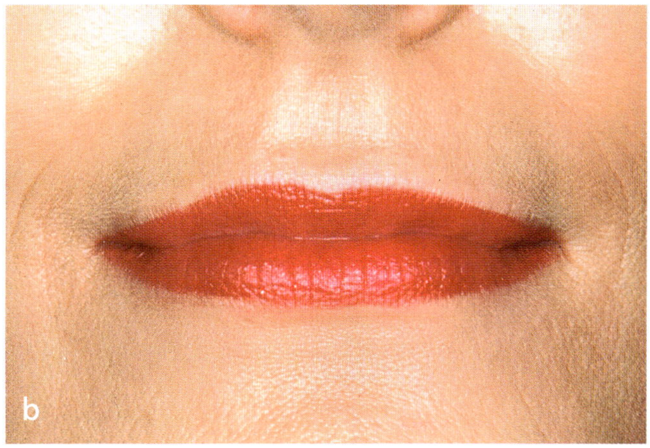

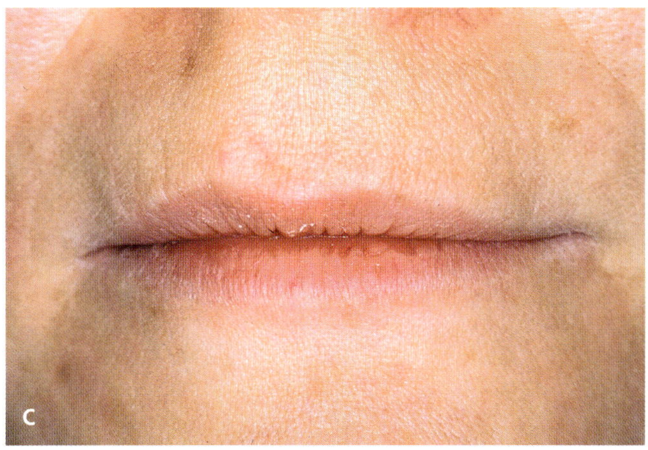

Figs 1-22a to 1-22c A description of lip design, despite its esthetic appeal, remains of little value if its particularities are not correlated with the specific esthetic characteristics of related structures. The evaluation of lip design may be disturbed by various elements, such as the presence of makeup, the impact of the aging process and loss of collagenous tissue, and the impact of plastic surgery. (a) Nicely contoured lip design of a woman in her 30s with minimal cosmetic layering. (b) Thin upper and lower lips of a woman in her 50s strongly colored to promote an illusory visual expansion of the dentofacial composition and thereby mask the impact of aging stressed by related short dental elements. (c) Thin lips as a result of collagenous loss. This does not even raise the question whether the related tooth should be made short or long. A basic principle in human esthetics that results from an adaptation to deficiencies does not constitute a basic principle in human esthetics best achieved with a full correction of deficiencies.

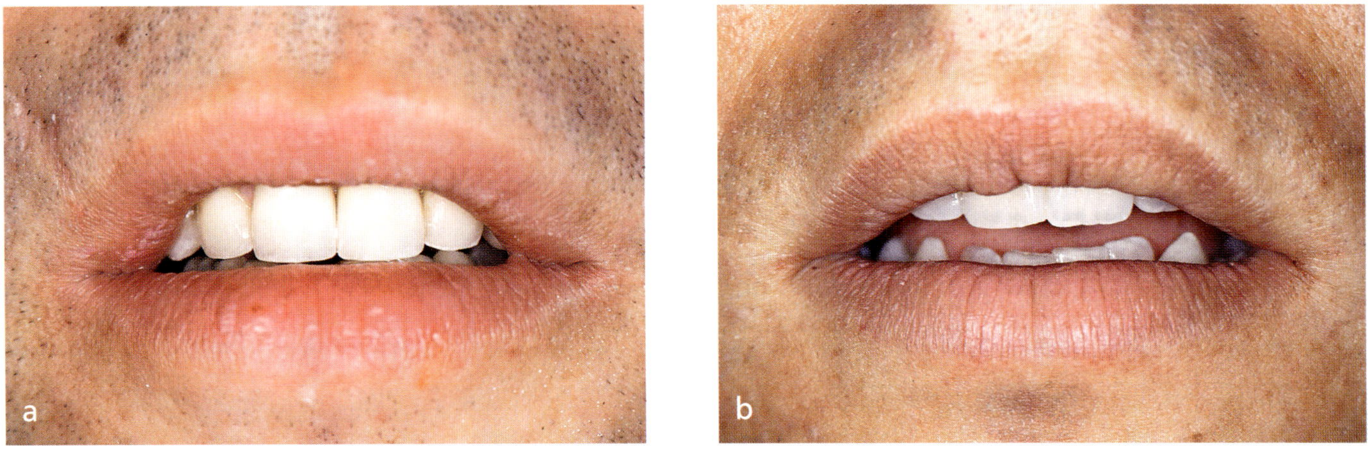

Figs 1-23a and 1-23b (a) Lower lip design showing a decreasing width from center to mouth corners. The upper border line is flat and slightly raised in its center. (b) The lower lip presents in its structure two raised "bumps," or a width increase more elongated on the left side, while its upper border line nicely undulates from each part of the central depression. The presumption that such particulars may be related to determining tooth shaping and position is supported by the axiom, "shapes create relations as relations create shapes."

exception of the lower facial third when treatment planning includes the removal of the various manifestations of bite collapse. Yet the facial composition remains the only framework in which we can find elements of anchorage with which to integrate our restorations harmoniously.

The principles of harmony involving a visual relationship between elements of a different nature, such as those between tooth and lip, will naturally be the focus of our attention. The most common appreciative approach to lip design poses a simple question—thin or thick? (Fig 1-22)—which leads to another involving related dental elements—short or long?

Systematic clinical observation and evaluation have reinforced a feeling, as yet lacking scientific validation, that lower lip width or thickness could depend upon related upper tooth length or tooth inclination according to a rule of order: "The thinner the lip, the shorter the tooth or the more lingualized in

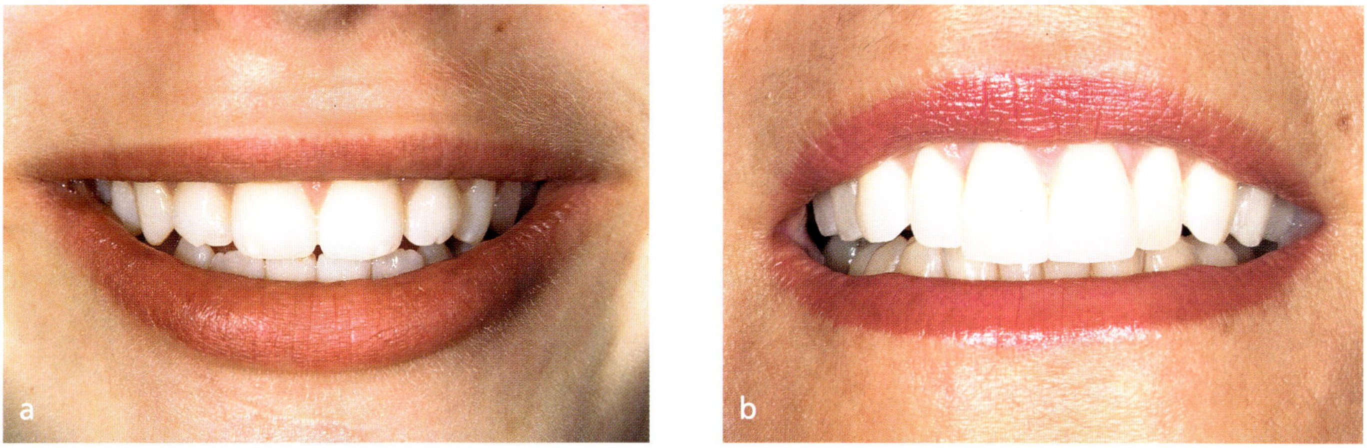

Figs 1-24a and 1-24b (a) Thin upper lip structure with straight linear design, correlated with an upper segmental arrangement characterized by small rounded dental elements in regular alignment. (b) Upraised upper lip design with elongated antagonist artificial maxillary incisors providing appropriate elements of counterbalance.

its axial inclination," or "The thicker the lip, the longer the tooth or the more buccal its sagittal axial inclination." A sharper reading of the lower lip's formal particulars will reveal not only subtle individual variations affecting its general design or the tracing of its upper border line but also various and numerous morphological width variations, which can be observed when the lip is subjected to repetitive interrogations at rest position (Fig 1-23).

Unlike that of the lower lip, upper lip design presents few morphological particulars of relational interest. Upper lip design, raised or flat, is best appreciated in the dynamic that takes place between the rest position and half the width of the smile and is usually correlated with long or short dental elements that seem to work as contrary tensional strengths, generating esthetic appeal (Fig 1-24). The nature of the development of the smile and the amount of tooth display will give any practitioner good indica-

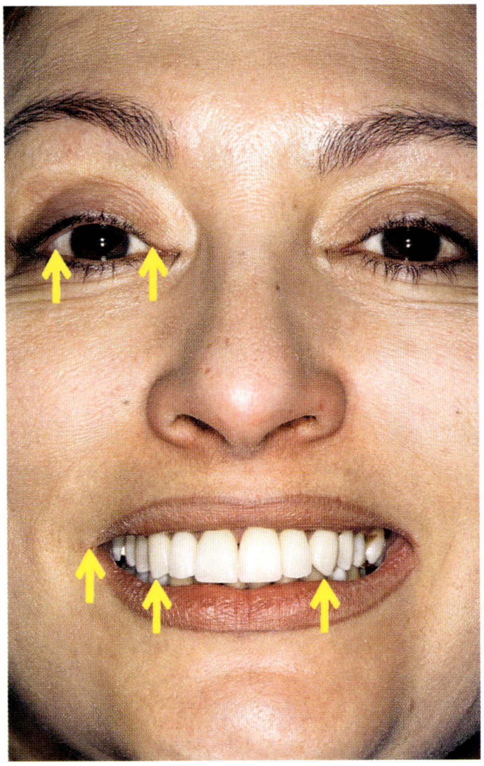

Fig 1-25 The following points of contrast will be of interest in the eye: the outside limit of the white part of the eye, the inside limit of the white part of the eye, the middle point of the pupilla; in the mouth: the outside point of the commissural angle, the tip of the maxillary and mandibular canines, the tip and mesial angle of the canine.

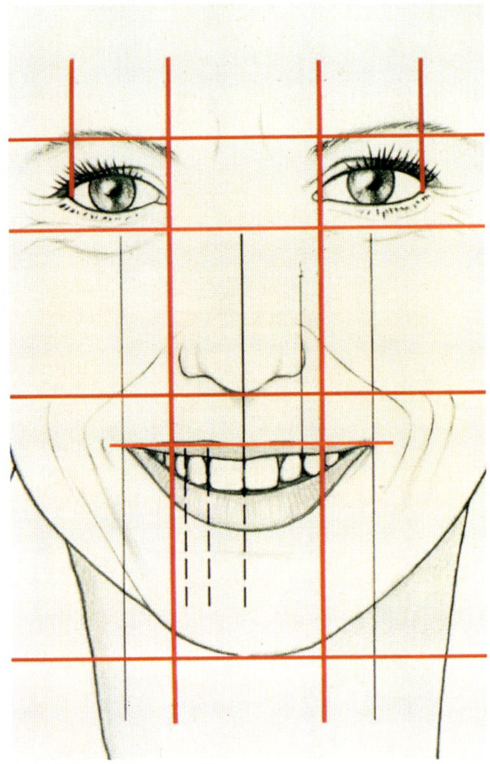

Fig 1-26 Schematic linear tracing connecting facial points or points of contrast that will serve as elements of support for rehabilitation.

tions whether morphological deviations in tooth-gingival relationships will be displayed or remain hidden.

Though the dream of a mouth design with a perfect mechanical alignment of white and identical dental elements, duplicating the stereotype in every fashion magazine, may very well stimulate the imagination and represent for many a restorative objective, its full esthetic value can only be attained if it is correlated with appropriate environmental conditions, which require from professionals a sensitive appreciation of relational elements. In this search for facial harmony, elements of contrast (Fig 1-25)—that is, closed morphological angles or light spots like mouth corners or inner and outer eye angles—have to be carefully evaluated while a visual and progressive mental definition of logical linear tracings connecting these elements is instituted, in the manner of Italian Renaissance attempts to coordinate the nature of

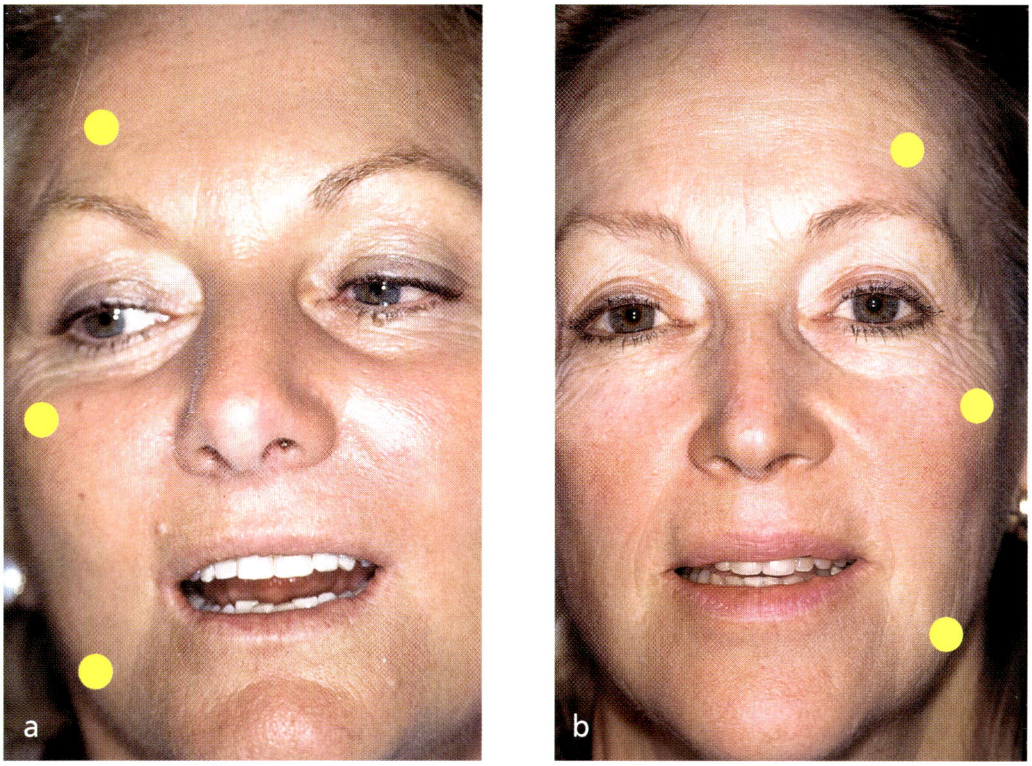

Figs 1-27a and 1-27b Determination of the external part of the frontal protuberance can be rendered difficult with a depressed frontal transitional zone, whereas determination of the osseous landmarks, such as the outside part of the zygomatic process or the mandibular angle, can be rendered similarly difficult in the presence of a good amount of fatty tissue.

things by application of a "mathematical" order or self-constraining architectural system (Fig 1-26). Though naturally this does not presuppose an ideal in the outcome of dentofacial esthetics, it will at least permit prosthodontists to use elements of support that have long proved their efficiency in other architectural fields.

Furthermore, the basic elements of anatomical knowledge may also help in the dentofacial restorative process, in that some osseous volumes, like the protuberance of the forehead, the zygomatic process, and the mandibular angle (Fig 1-27), become significant in the individualization of the restorations. This enumeration of indispensable anatomic elements may seem somehow restrictive, but it shows that solid relational elements are extremely difficult to apprehend.

Bibliography

Abrams L. Augmentation of the deformed, residual edentulous ridge, for fixed prosthesis. Compend Continue Educ Dent 1980;1:205–213.

Blunt A. Artistic Theory in Italy. New York: Rykwert J Ed, 1940.

Charbonneaux J, Martin R, Villard F. Grèce Classique: L'Univers des Formes. Paris: Gallimard, 1972.

Ciancaglini R. Riabilitazione Orale. Milan: Masson, 1999.

Evangelidis DE. L'Art Grec. Athens: A Theodom Ed, 1980.

Garber DA, Rosenberg ES. The edentulous ridge in fixed prosthodontics. Compend Contin Educ Dent 1981; 2:212–223.

Geller W, Kwiatkowski SJ. The Willi's glass crown: A new solution in the dark and shadowed zone of esthetic porcelain restorations. Quintessence Dent Technol 1987;11: 233–242.

Hautecoeur L. Histoire de l'Art. Vol 3: De la nature à l'abstraction. Paris: Hammarion, 1959.

Huyghe R. Histoire de l'Art Contemporain. New York: Arno Press, 1968

Jovanovic SA, Schenk PK, Orsini M, Kenney FB. Supracrestal bone formation around dental implants: An experimental dog study. Int J Oral Maxillofac Implants 1995;10: 23–31.

Langer B, Calanga L. The subepithelial connective tissue graft: A new approach to the enhancement of anterior cosmetic. Int J Periodontics Restorative Dent 1982;2:22–33.

Lawrence AW. Greek Architecture: The Pelikan History of Art. London: Penguin, 1957.

Lazzara RJ. Immediate implant placement into extraction sites. surgical and restorative advantages. Int J Periodontics Restorative Dent 1989;9:332–343.

McDowell A. Realism: A Study in Art and Thought. London: Constable, 1918.

Misch CE. Division of available bone in implant dentistry. Int J Oral Implantol 1990;7:9–17.

Pincus CR. Building mouth personality. J S Calif Dent Assoc 1938;14:125–129.

Renner RP. An Introduction to Dental Anatomy and Esthetics. Chicago: Quintessence, 1985.

Schärer P, Rinn La, Kopp FR. Aestetische Richtlinien. Berlin: Quintessence, 1980.

Seibert J. Reconstruction of deformed, partially edentulous ridges using full thickness onlay grafts. Part I. Technique and wound healing. Compend Contin Educ Dent 1983;4:537–553.

Seibert J. Reconstruction of deformed, partially edentulous ridges using full thickness onlay grafts. Part II. Prosthetic periodontal interrelationships. Compend Contin Educ Dent 1983;4:549–562.

Simion M, Baldoni M, Zaffe D. Jawbone enlargement using immediate implant placement associated with a split-crest technique and guided tissue regeneration. Int J Periodontics Restorative Dent 1992;12:462–473.

Simion M, Trisi P, Piattelli A. Vertical ridge augmentation using a membrane technique associated with osseointegrated implants. Int J Periodontics Restorative Dent 1994;14:496–511.

Toscani O. Faces. Rome: Castelvecchi, 1997.

Wheeler RC. Dental Anatomy, Physiology and Occlusion, ed 5. Philadelphia: Saunders, 1974.

Winter R. Achieving esthetic ceramic restoration. J Calif Dent Assoc 1990;18:21–24.

CHAPTER 2

Biological Integration

Biological Conditions

All the elements of oral structures present at the same time both esthetic and biological interconnective particulars. In clinical practice, the respectful restoration of healthy biological relational conditions should always take precedence over esthetic relationships. As a matter of fact, a loss of control of biological relationships whose fragility may lead to structural breakdown will invariably generate disease.

Etiologic factors that may lead to biological rupture of the relational conditions include not only inflammatory and systemic diseases but also iatrogenic factors. Faulty margins or rough, oversized, or undersized restorations that ignore biological relational integrity promote bacterial colonization and inflammation. Such inflammation commonly causes irreversible damage to tissues, which will reform at another level in another form. Every rupture of biological relational conditions invariably leads to esthetic structural alterations, which may impair the appearance of morphological normality.

Esthetically, forms only exist through and for the creation of relationships. Yet, it must be stressed that the biological connection ruling tooth-to-periodontal support, unlike esthetic relations, presents consistent and collective characteristics.

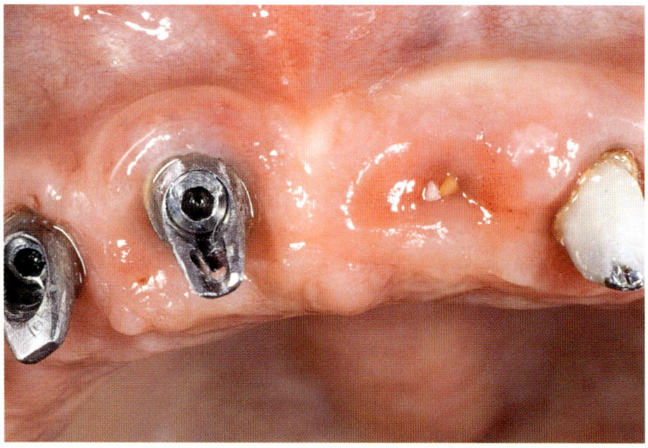

Fig 2-1 The dentogingival unit and the implant-mucosal unit are both elements of the body that penetrate the lining epithelium, yet they have important morphological, histological, and physiological differences. Along with the pontic-gingival unit, they constitute the key relational elements whose biological and esthetic integration will depend on the technical expertise of the restorative dentist.

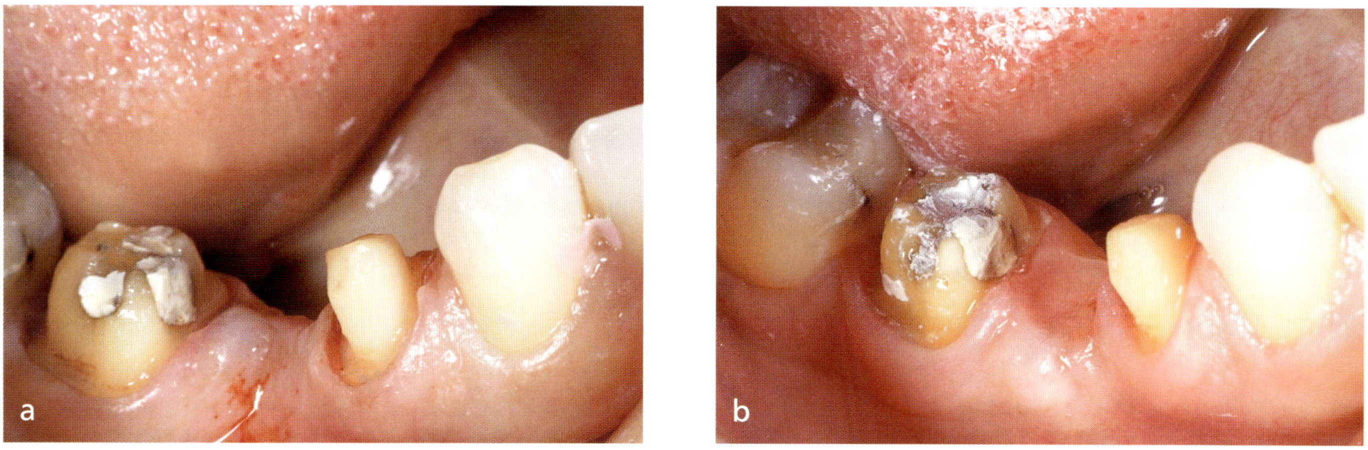

Figs 2-2a and 2-2b Unlike the dentogingival and implant-mucosal units, the pontic-gingival unit has contact only with the epithelium of the edentulous area. As shapes only exist by and for the creation of relationships, esthetic requirements demand a systematic preparation of this area to design and integrate a dental element duplicating the morphological particulars of an original tooth-gingival unit.

In modern dentistry, both the dentogingival unit and the fixture-mucosal unit can be considered unique elements of the body that penetrate the lining epithelium (Figs 2-1 to 2-3). They represent the two poles of the collective biological relational elements whose histological particulars should remain fixed in the visual memory of the restorative dentist. He or she alone will have to face the challenge of substituting another dental element for the original tooth while keeping intact specific histological relational conditions.

However, in the clinical approach to the edentulous ridge, attention will be focused on esthetic considerations since the morphological design of the

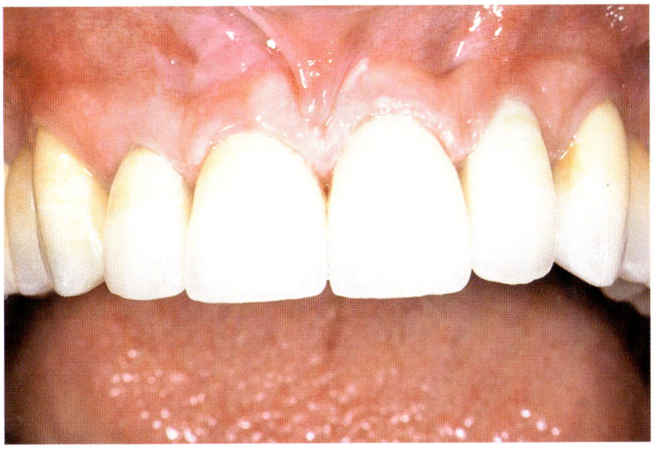

Fig 2-3 In good clinical conditions showing little vertical resorption, the morphological imitation of nature in its shapes and relations remains a perfectly valid objective whatever the type of units used: dentogingival, implant, or pontic-mucosal. In this 12-unit fixed-denture prosthesis, 2 years postinsertion, both canines and left central incisor are dentogingival units, the right lateral incisor is supported by an implant, and the right central incisor and left lateral incisor (replacing a failing implant) are pontic-gingival units. Five implant-mucosal units provide support for the posterior segment.

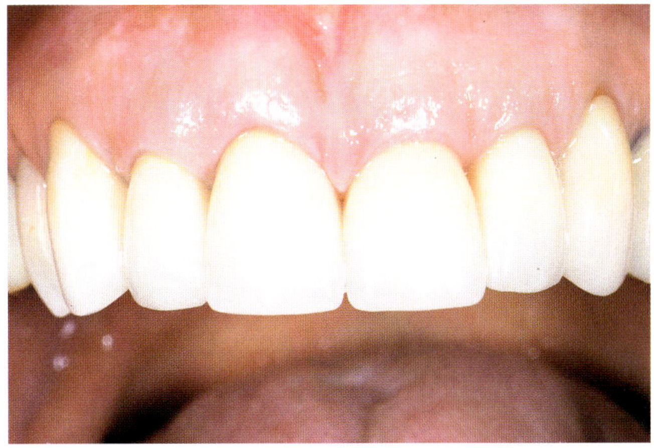

Fig 2-4 An identical therapeutic approach has been used for this fixed-denture prosthesis maintained in the anterior area by two implant-mucosal units located on both lateral incisors. Three years postinsertion, tissue stability seems to be harder to maintain around tooth-supported elements.

dental elements related to this area (Fig 2-2) is directly dictated by the specific morphological design displayed by this relation. It can be said that the biological integration and maintenance of dental elements in oral structures, whatever the nature of their support—tooth, fixture, or alveolar crest—represent both a fundamental objective in restorative dentistry and a prerequisite in esthetic dentistry (Figs 2-3 and 2-4).

The Dentogingival Unit

The histological characteristics of the dentogingival unit determine the relationships between connective tissue, epithelium, and dental element. Studies have shown that the combined dimension of the junctional epithelium and the connective tissue attachment to the tooth, referred to as the biological width, presents a dimensional width of 2.04 mm,[1–4] which appears to be consistent among all individuals. However, the sulcus depth, measured from the top of the margin-

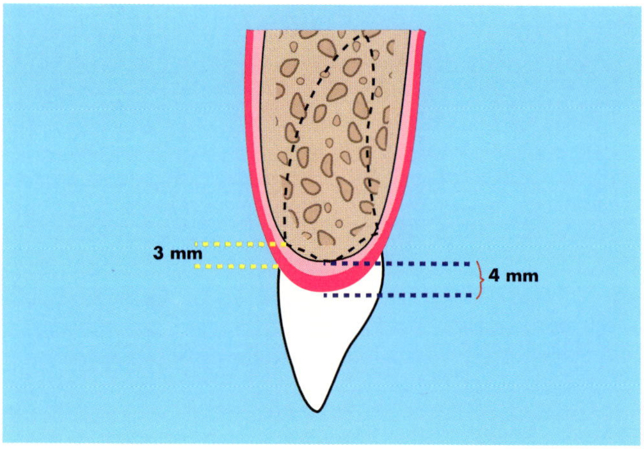

Fig 2-5 It has been established that tissue stability is best achieved when the distance between the marginal papilla and the osseous crest reaches 3 mm on the buccal side of the tooth and 4 mm on the proximal areas.

al papilla to the highest level of the junctional epithelium, shows no such consistency. Statistically, the sulcus depth averages 0.69 mm, a measure that habit has arbitrarily extended to 1 mm, according to recent scientific investigations.

Research has demonstrated that marginal tissue was made most stable when its top was located 3 mm from the osseous crest on the buccal and lingual aspects of the tooth and 4 mm from the osseous crest interdentally (Fig 2-5).[5] This conclusion did not really modify dentists' therapeutic approach to tissue management, which has always been conditioned by the claim that maintenance of biological tissue health depends on supragingival margin placement of the restoration since it appeared that careless invasion of sulcus depth invariably generated permanent or punctual periodontal tissue damage. Indeed, studies have shown that the further subgingivally a restoration is placed the greater the chance of plaque accumulation, inflammation, and periodontal breakdown.[6–8] But for fear that an unpredictable passive eruption may occur after final cementation, thereby exposing margins, restorations are usually buried to attain an immediately pleasing esthetic result.[9]

Esthetic considerations drive the world and guide our hands, and despite the possibility of tissue damage, subgingival margin placement has become routine. To overcome its negative effects while still conserving tissue health, certain precise clinical approaches have been proposed.[10,11] They all directly depend on the skill of the dental team, particularly its mastery of four components:

- Atraumatic clinical procedures
- Proper margin placement of restorations
- Coordinated tooth preparation according to the requirements of the selected restorative material
- Precise fit and marginal design of the restoration.

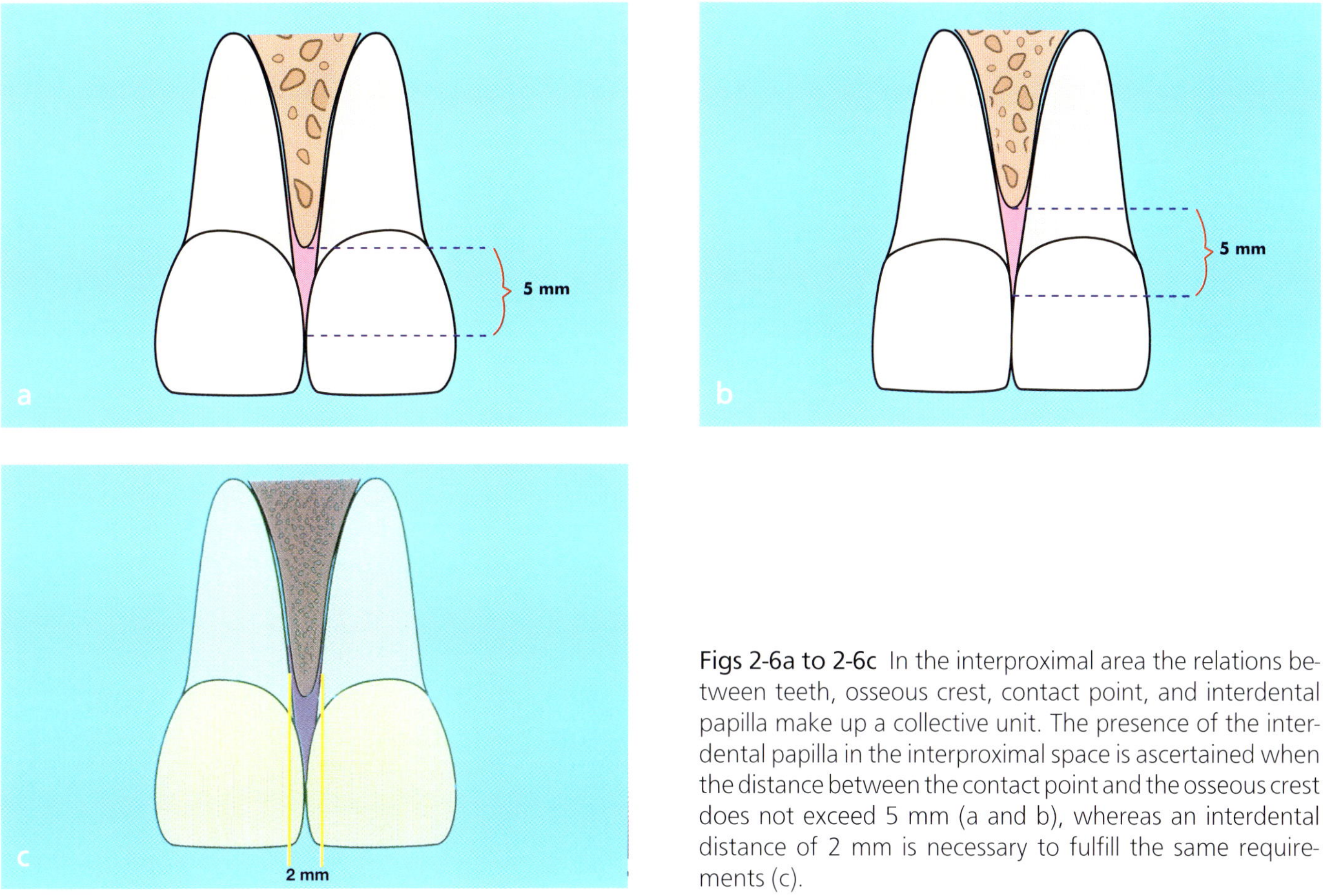

Figs 2-6a to 2-6c In the interproximal area the relations between teeth, osseous crest, contact point, and interdental papilla make up a collective unit. The presence of the interdental papilla in the interproximal space is ascertained when the distance between the contact point and the osseous crest does not exceed 5 mm (a and b), whereas an interdental distance of 2 mm is necessary to fulfill the same requirements (c).

In our eyes the notion of emergence profile, often advocated as an important factor in tissue maintenance, needs to be precisely defined before it can be included in the above list.

From a frontal point of view the maintenance of the interdental papilla, whose loss constitutes another hallmark of dental pathology and a regular complaint of esthetically inclined patients, is attained when the distance from the interdental contact point to the osseous crest level does not exceed 5 mm and the distance between the two adjacent teeth reaches at least 2 mm (Figs 2-6 to 2-8).

Sound knowledge of these elements is mandatory to achieve in the entity of the prosthesis-dentogingival unit the same good esthetic relations usually associated with healthy biological relations in the attachment of the gingiva to the tooth.

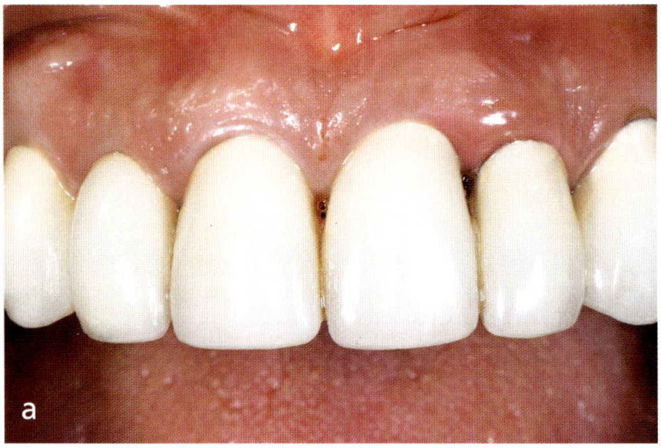

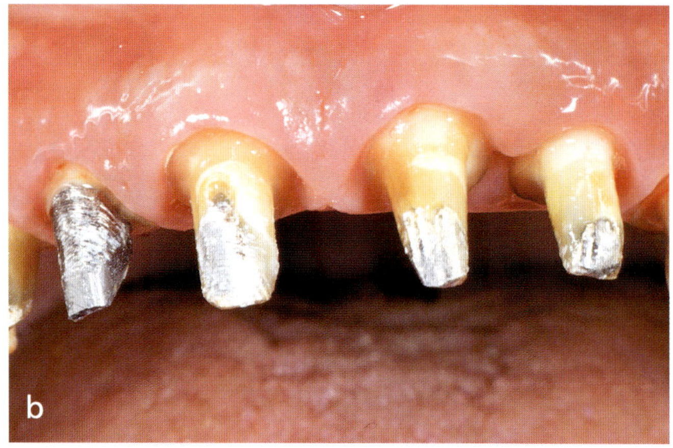

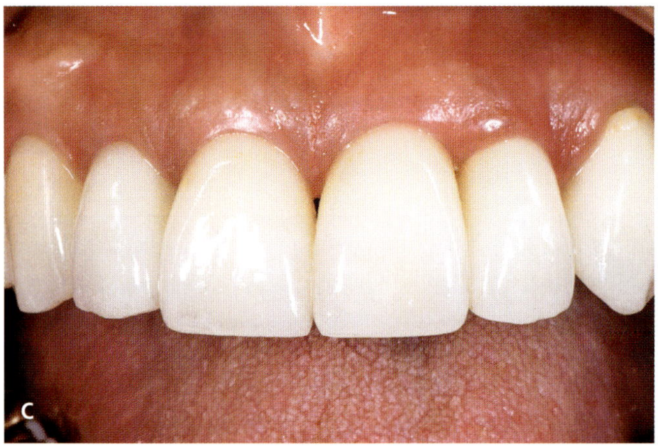

Figs 2-7a to 2-7c (a) Initial clinical situation with wide-open interproximal areas. (b) Odontotomy and soft tissue conditioning have just succeeded in creating a concave interproximal tissue adaptation between left central and lateral incisors, where interdental distance is reduced. (c) The restoration of a tooth design adapted to the marginal soft tissue design greatly improved esthetic appeal. However, 1 year postcementation, recurrent pathologic edematous manifestations can be seen in the area where the interdental distance does not reach 2 mm.

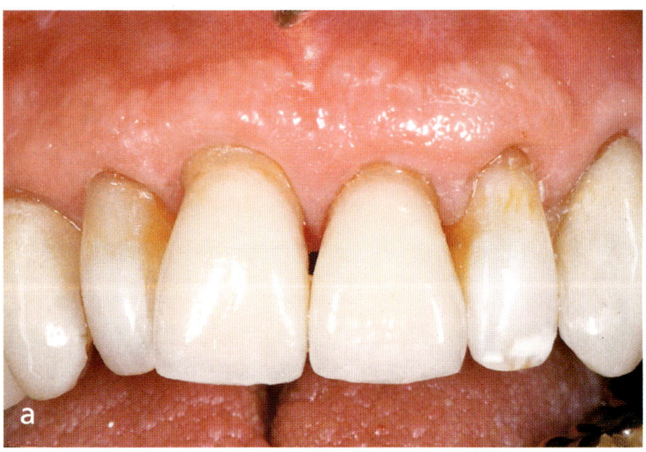

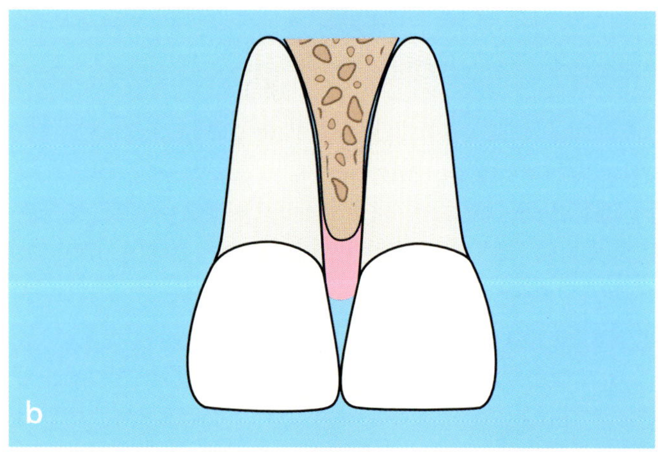

Figs 2-8a and 2-8b A simple clinical visual examination shows that an approximate determination of the location of the interproximal tooth contact will not lead to tissue stability and prevent the progressive opening of the interproximal area. A precise determination of the osseous level before crown insertion could have given the information relative to the location of the interocclusal contact necessary to achieve tissue stability.

Tissue Management

With respect to sulcus depth invasion in tooth preparation, biological width consistency suggests the application of the same precepts for every tooth whatever its location on the maxilla or the mandible. These precepts hold that soft tissue preparation should always precede hard tissue preparation and require proper access and visualization for the introduction of the retraction cord.[11] To ease interproximal accessibility, this process naturally involves the removal of interproximal contacts prior to any soft tissue manipulation; nonetheless, the previous recommendations remain in force.

Cord retraction and margin placement

Contrary to common belief, the atraumatic introduction of the retraction cord is illusory. Slight insults to the junctional epithelium attachment, and even to the supracrestal connective tissue, are normal. However, it has been shown that these injuries to the attachment apparatus are reversible, fulfilling our expectations for the stability of the gingival level over time (Fig 2-9).[12–14] The importance of the clinical impregnation of the cord is self-evident,[15,16] as it gives better "retraction" and achieves complete tissue recovery within 10 days.[17–19] This chemicomechanical retraction is more properly described, however, as a lateral deflection of the marginal tissue, which provides adequate space for an atraumatic placement of the mass of the rotary instrument up to the cord level. The tooth should be prepared up to this cord level and the particulars of the preparation adapted to the requirements of the preselected restorative material. According to this method, all margins will become automatically intracrevicular upon cord removal and tissue rebound.

Bleeding at cord removal must and can usually be avoided with careful moistening, as it indicates tissue laceration and probably rapid tissue recession. It tends to delay the final impression for 2 or 3 weeks.[20,21] Injuries from rotary instruments and the resulting bleeding also lead to delayed impression-taking for the same amount of time (Fig 2-10).

Provisionalization

Provisionalization should be considered as another factor in tissue maintenance and as a therapeutic measure for complete tissue healing following injuries caused by retraction and preparation maneuvers.[22–25] Provisionalization should also be seen as tooth protective. Esthetic considerations should also be considered but at this point remain secondary.

The expectation of proper soft tissue healing with interim restorations must be coordinated with sufficient hard tissue reduction to permit self-curing resin, the most commonly used material, to express its qualities while hiding its deficiencies.[26] The different types of preparations proposed to receive modern restorative materials completely fulfill these requirements (Fig 2-11) and allow for the best possible marginal adaptation of the provisional restoration.

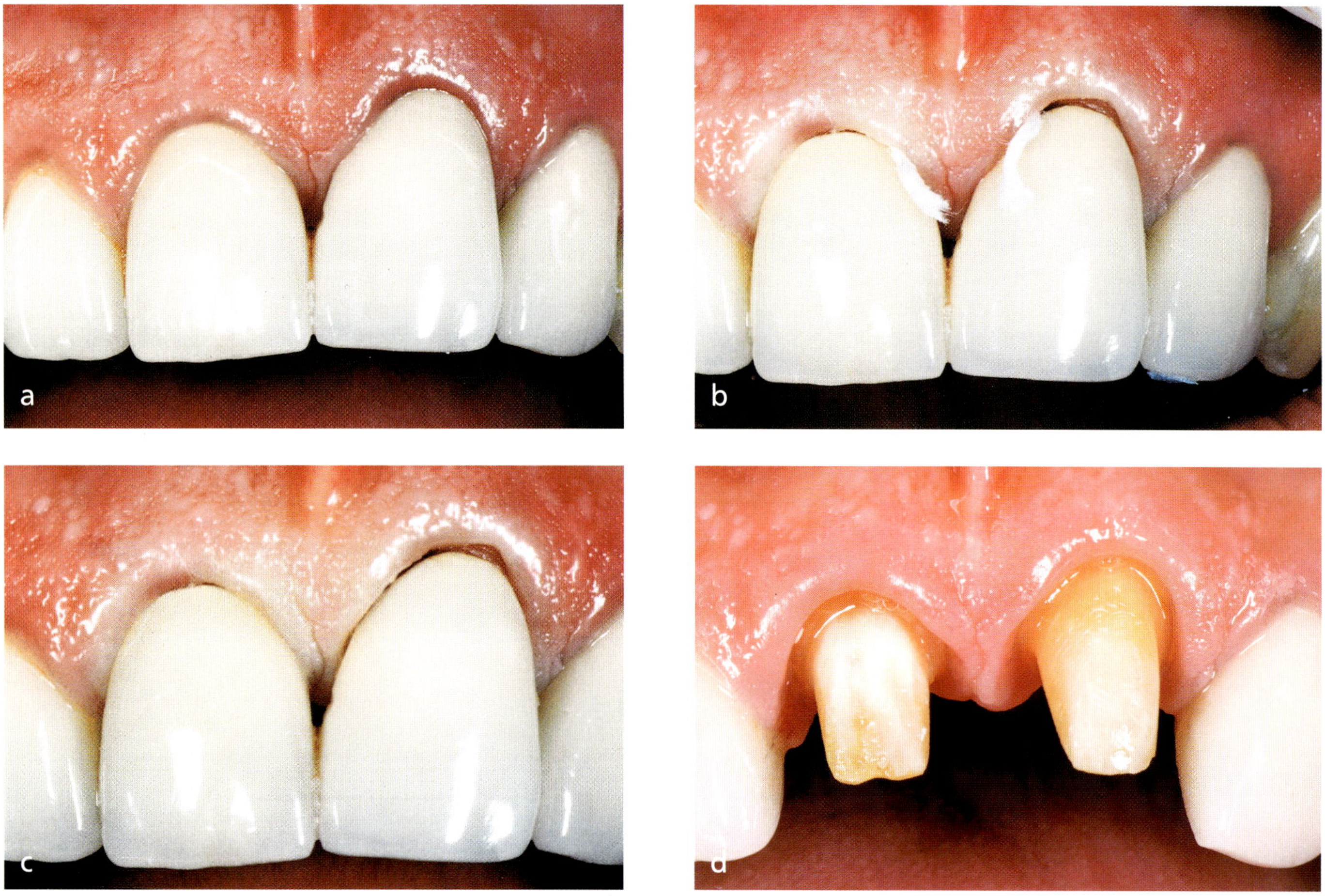

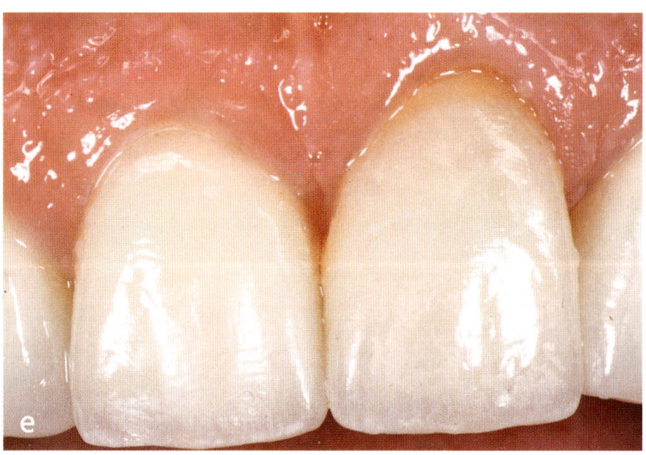

Figs 2-9a to 2-9e (a) Initial clinical situation. (b) Atraumatic introduction of the retraction cord. (c) Retraction and lateral deflection. (d) Tooth preparation. (e) Periodontal integration of ceramometallic crowns with ceramic margins.

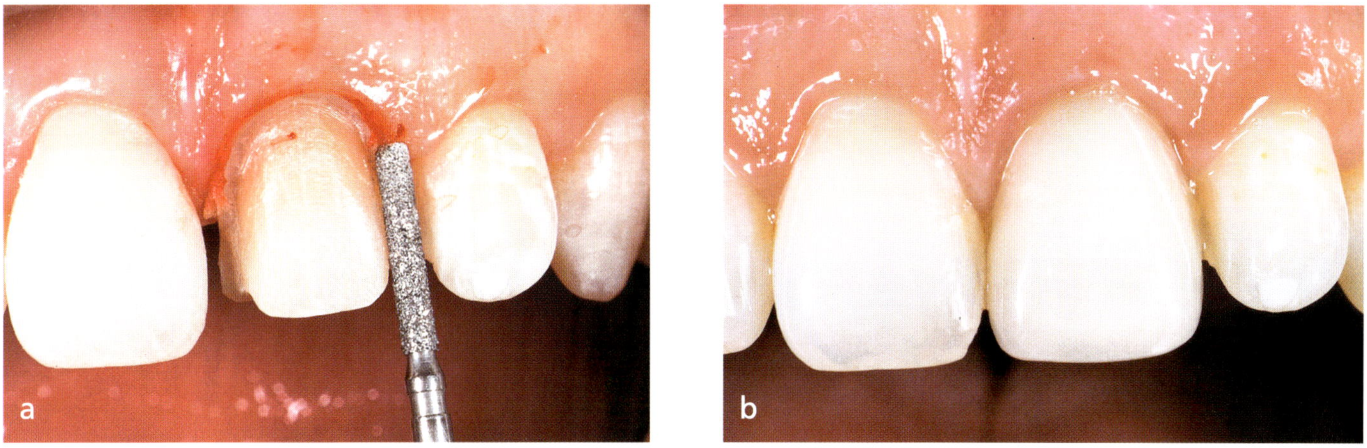

Figs 2-10a and 2-10b In logical sequential tissue management, hard tissue preparation follows the insertion and chemical impregnation of the cord. This allows for a lateral deflection of the marginal gingiva and a tooth preparation up to the cord level. However, unexpected and undesirable injuries and bleeding from rotary instruments (a) necessitate a delay in impression taking. (b) A premature insertion of the veneer has resulted in faulty biological integration over time.

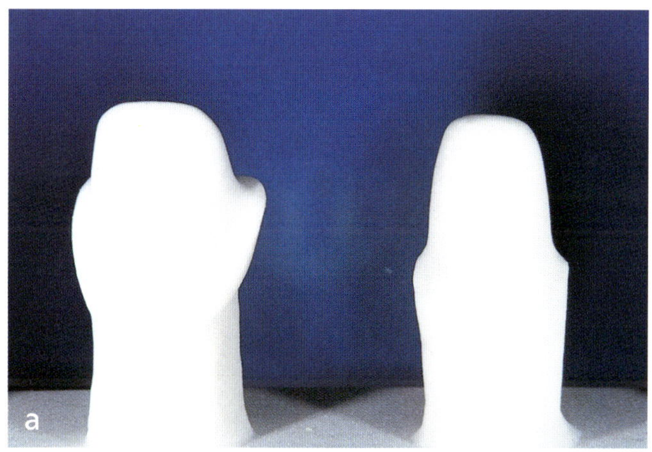

Figs 2-11a to 2-11c These types of preparation, proposed by Jeneric and foreseen for porcelain veneers, seem best suited to fulfilling the requirements of the usual conventional restorative materials.

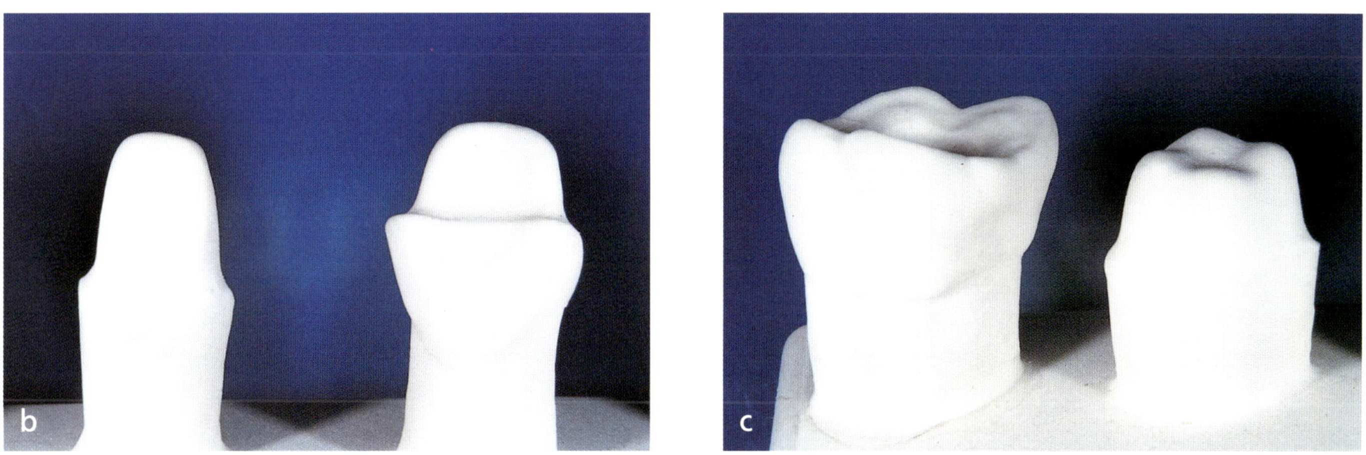

Implant-Mucosal Unit

Obviously, epithelial and connective tissue components are similar to the gingiva and the peri-implant mucosa.[27–30]

This fact has reinforced a conviction that the microenvironment of tooth and implant may be quite similar. Naturally, the necessity for a perimucosal seal of the soft tissue to the implant surface has been advocated as an important factor for long-term success.[31–35] It has even been reported that failure to achieve a perimucosal seal would allow for an apical migration of the epithelium into the implant osseous interface, which leads to the presumption of similarities with the mechanisms and pathogenesis at the origin of periodontal disease.

However, research has proved the importance of the distinction between the dentogingival unit and the implant-mucosal unit: the two differ anatomically, physiologically, and histologically.[36] The absence of a cementum layer on the implant surface creates fundamental differences between implant and tooth in regard to connective fiber arrangement and attachment.[37,38] Another histological dissimilarity is the absence of a periodontal ligament at the implant interface, which has brought up an interesting hypothesis: no ligament, no periodontal disease.[39]

This hypothesis has been reinforced by some significant observations:

1. The usual prosthodontic-periodontic soft tissue concerns relevant to prosthesis design and patient home care do not contribute to the process of implant loss. They have just been identified as "nuisances."
2. No correlation exists between the application of clinical parameters such as Plaque Index, Gingival Index, probing depth, and attached gingiva and the successful process of osseointegration.[40–43]

Yet it appears that the integrated implant is sealed from the adverse microenvironmental elements of the overlying soft tissue crevice by a mechanism different from the one around the tooth.

Histological examination of the supracrestal implant surface has revealed a discernible attachment of junctional epithelium and a repeated width of connective tissue approximating 2 mm, twice that of the gingival supracrestal connective tissue attachment, with collagen fibers originating from the osseous crest and running parallel to the implant surface.[44] More research is needed to determine whether the expansion of this zone results from a reaction between the connective tissue and titanium surface or should be regarded as a scar surface.

Comparative experimental breakdowns of the peri-implant mucosa and periodontal tissue demonstrate a more significant tissue destruction around implants than teeth, suggesting an impaired defense capability against exogenous irritation such as plaque accumulation.[45] Clinically, however, peri-implant breakdown of bacterial origin, referred to as peri-implantitis, is rather uncommon around functional osseointegrated implants.[46–50] This usually occurs in the postsurgical phase, mainly as the result of traumatic surgical techniques.[47]

Though supracrestal soft tissue thickness appears to bear no correlation to biological tissue health considerations, a sufficient amount of supracrestal soft tissue thickness greatly eases a surgical approach aimed at duplicating the morphological design of marginal periodontal tissue.

Peri-implant Tissue Management

Whereas the clinical approach to soft tissue management around natural teeth is aimed at an atraumatic intracrevicular placement of the prosthesis and at the preservation of the health integrity of the marginal papilla, peri-implant soft tissue management involves totally different objectives. We know that whatever the surgical approach and soft tissue thickness, peri-implant histological characteristics will be identical and variations in abutment length will have no influence on peri-implant tissue health. The objectives of peri-implant tissue management will then consist in the creation around the titanium abutment of a soft peri-implant tissue anatomy imitating marginal periodontal design.

Both a tissue punch technique and a full-thickness flap elevation at the surgical reopening or second-stage implant surgery have proved inadequate in fulfilling esthetically satisfying marginal and interdental papillalike formation.[51–56] Indeed, the multiplicity and unpredictability of complementary surgical procedures necessary for obtaining an adequate anatomic design in a third-stage surgery may discourage patients and clinicians.[57–59]

To overcome these problems, a surgical approach has been proposed which consists in moving the mucosa covering the crest from a lingual to a buccal direction during the second-stage surgery. The amount of tissue obtained in this flap elevation not only increases tissue volume and height in the buccal aspect of the titanium abutment but also allows for the use of its free marginal aspect in designing and carving an interdental papillalike pedicle that will be rotated, moved back, and sutured along the initial lingual incision (Fig 2-12).[60,61]

In the clinical practice of this surgical procedure to recreate a morphological design of the marginal papilla, therefore, supracrestal tissue thickness is crucial to good esthetic results. Thus, whenever soft tissue thickness is insufficient, one should proceed to soft tissue thickness augmentation during or before[62] the first-stage surgery (Fig 2-13). In areas where soft tissue thickness is reduced, the restoration of an original morphological tooth design becomes aleatory because of width differences between implants and natural teeth at cervix, and the chances of recreating a scalloped marginal soft tissue design vanish.

At this stage of the procedure some attention should be paid to the presence or absence of a sufficient amount of attached gingiva. The idea that the absence of attached gingiva may jeopardize soft tissue health around implants has never found scientific support, yet its presence remains an important factor in esthetics.

The importance of first-stage surgery cannot be overemphasized as its purpose is not only objective fixture placement but also the preparation of environmental conditions permitting a duplication of the original tooth-periodontal morphological design at second-stage surgery. From the schematic representation of ideal maxillary and mandibular arch forms, it clearly appears that most variations between the interdental distance at cervix and interfixture distance at head platform occur in the anterior area (Figs 2-14 and 2-15).

Clinical practice fully confirms these restrictive parameters which, with the problem of advanced osseous tissue resorption (Figs 2-16 to 2-18), represent an ever-renewed challenge confronting every sur-

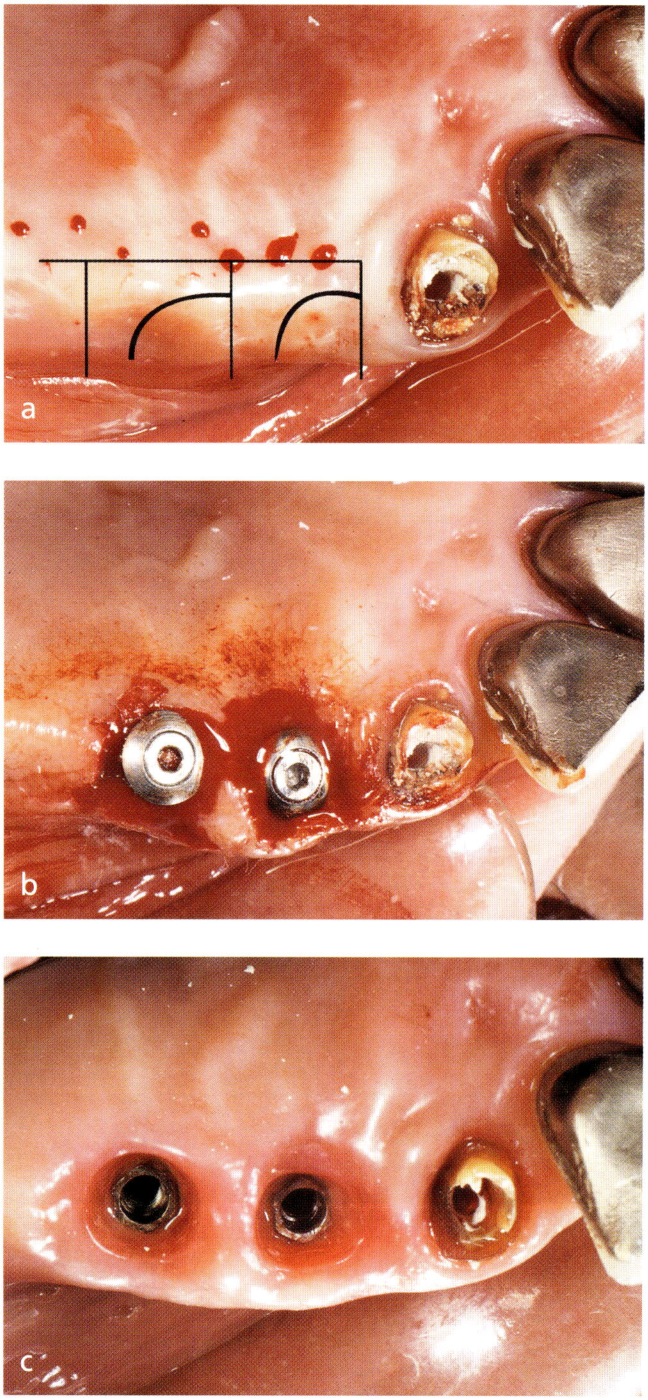

Figs 2-12a to 2-12c Second-stage surgery and peri-implant tissue preparation for the canine and first premolar. Incision along the crest, lingual to the lingual aspect of the implant's head, completed with three release incisions. (a,b) A pedicle is carved in the thickness of the tissue, rotated, and sutured back lingually. The excess of tissue is removed once the healing caps are positioned at a gingival level that attains a regular front-back progression. (c) Four weeks following surgery.

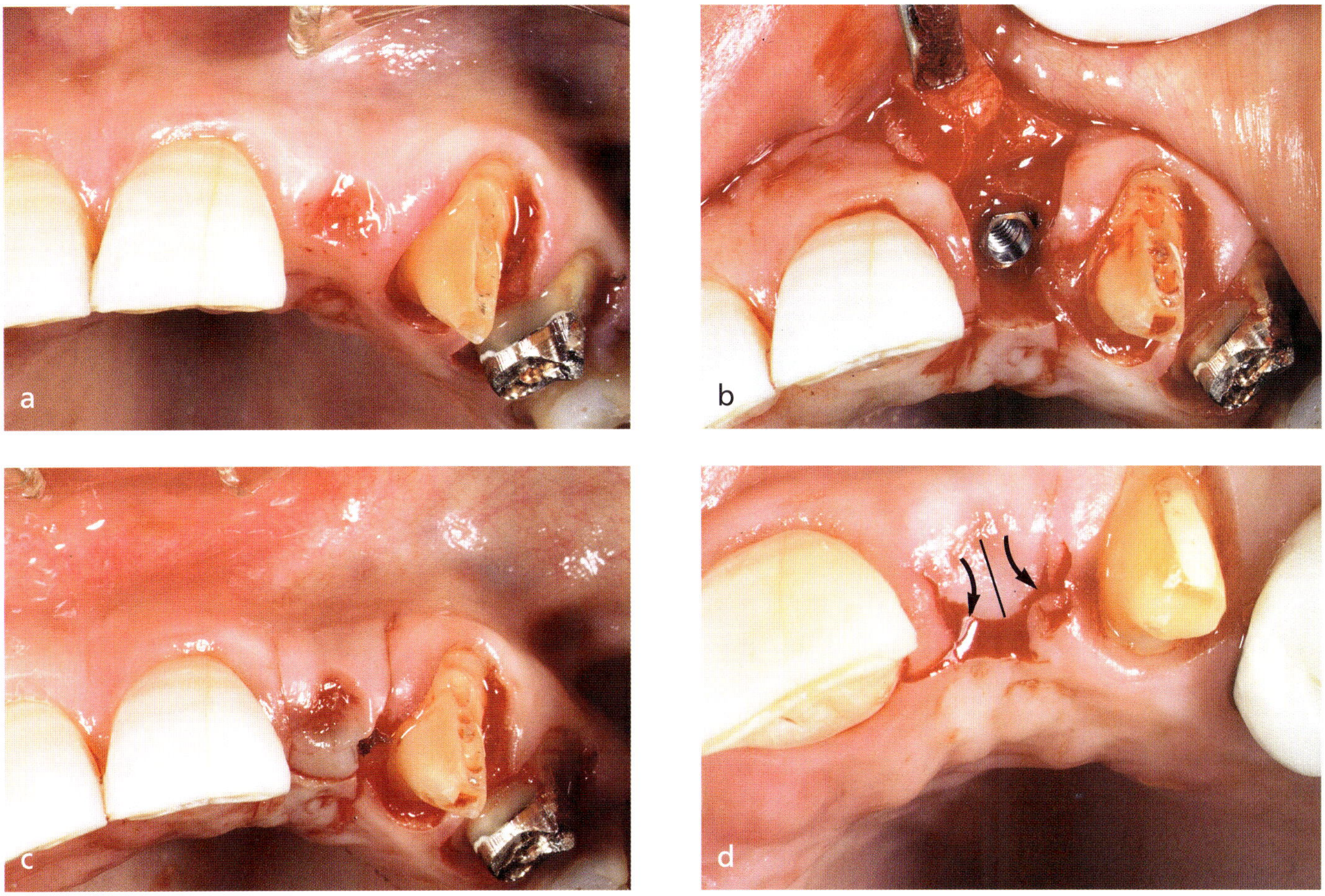

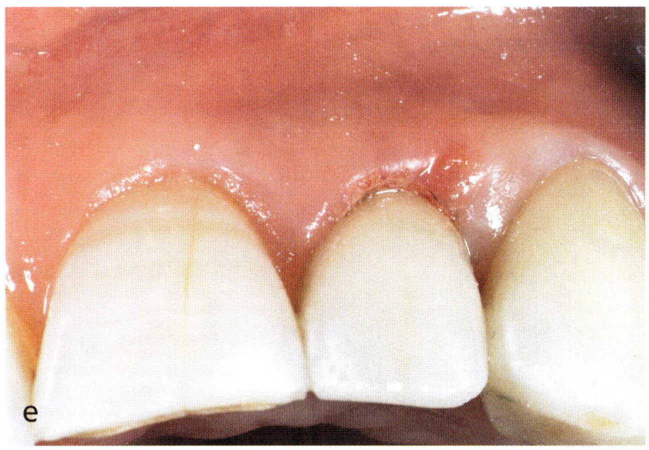

Figs 2-13a to 2-13e (a) To fulfill specific esthetic requirements in tissue height, tissue contour, and tooth placement, correct planning of fixture insertion includes an initial soft tissue preparation of the edentulous crest conditioned by the overlying pontic-gingival unit. (b) Its imprint will determine implant placement. (c) At wound closure, the area is ready to receive the same provisional pontic relation. (d) At reopening at second-stage surgery, a curved lingual incision designs the interdental papillae that will be sutured back lingually. (e) One week postsurgery with provisional abutment and prosthesis for tissue conditioning.

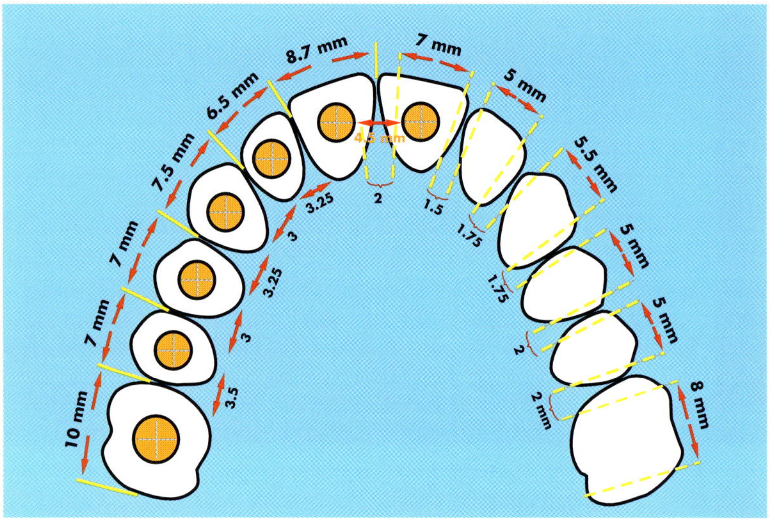

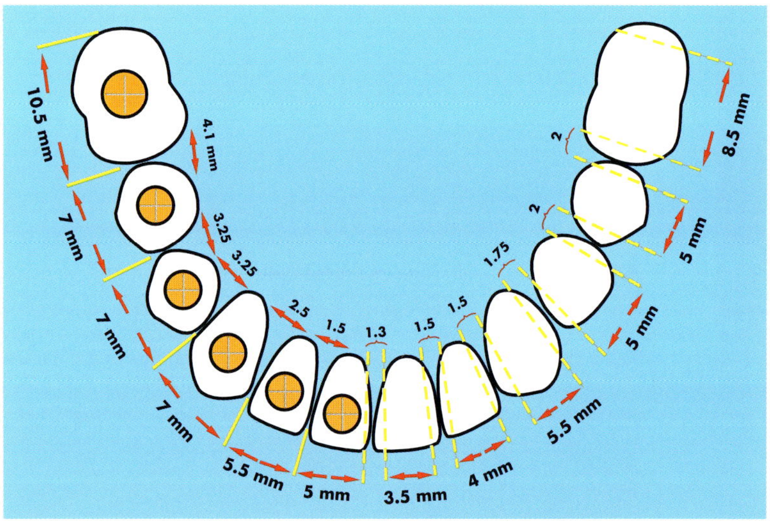

Figs 2-14 and 2-15 Sketch of maxillary (*top*) and mandibular (*bottom*) arches. The average incisal tooth width and average tooth width at cervix are inscribed on the buccal aspect of the arch. On the lingual aspect, the average interdental distance at cervix and the average interfixture distance when dealing with standard fixtures of 3.75 mm in diameter and of 5 mm for molars. The following conclusions can be drawn: most fixture head platforms and abutments should be systematically extended; standard fixtures are the most suitable with respect to the biological distance of 3 to 4 mm required between fixtures; fixture placement should also be considered with regard to its buccolingual location; complications and restrictions in proper fixture placement increase with the advancement of horizontal or vertical crest resorption which requires a fixture placement in the most buccal location of the crest. In edentulous maxillae the initial placement of a maxillary premolar implant using anatomical and facial landmarks should always precede additional implant placement. This is a condition for realizing an esthetic prosthetic outcome.

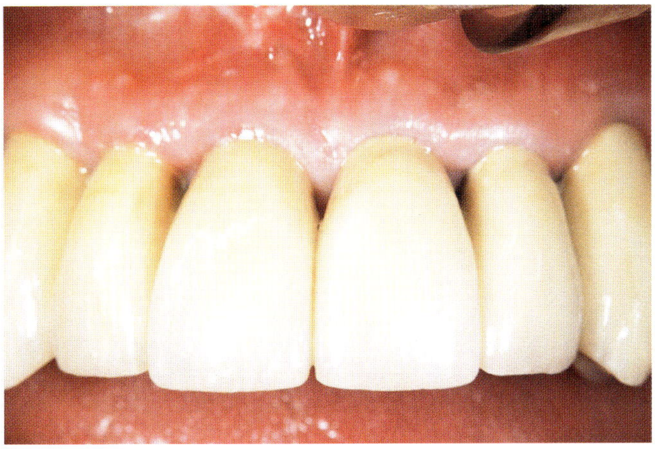

Fig 2-16 Mixed implant- and tooth-supported fixed denture prosthesis. Because of an important crest resorption, the inserted dental elements reach 18 mm in length for the central incisors and canines. This has been made possible thanks to a low lip-line level and the patient's reduced esthetic demand. Yet an evading anterior segment gives a strong feeling of instability.

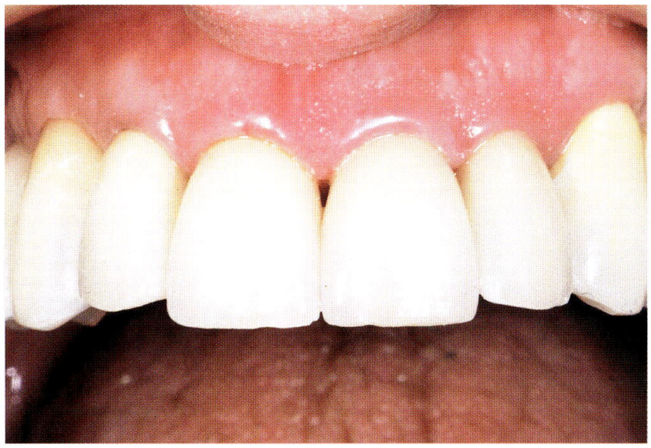

Fig 2-17 The feeling of instability generated by evading dental elements is common in fixed denture restorations supported by implants even if osseous crest resorption, vertical and horizontal, seems to be limited. Tooth-periodontal location and functional and interocclusal requirements have caused this situation.

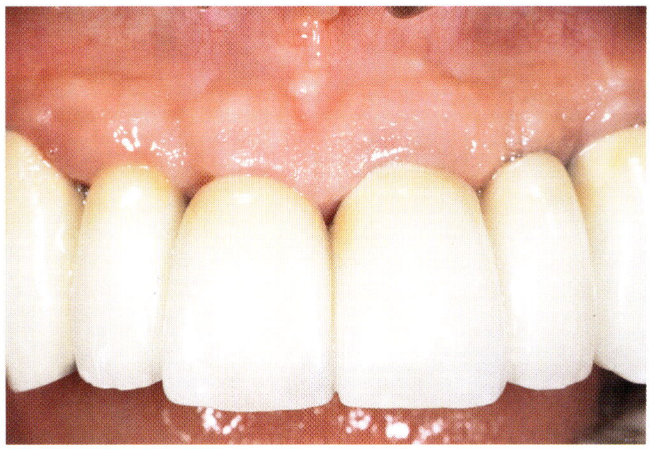

Fig 2-18 Full edentulous arch with severe vertical resorption corrected with multiple connective tissue grafts and HA allograft fillers. Eight fixtures support an11-unit fixed denture prosthesis. The maxillary central incisors (pontics) display a length of 14 mm, which is more compatible with mean tooth length, and the anterior flare, which usually characterizes tooth axial direction in similar cases, has been avoided. Yet this clinical picture, taken 2 years following insertion, shows that interdental papillae not benefiting from appropriate osseous support have vanished.

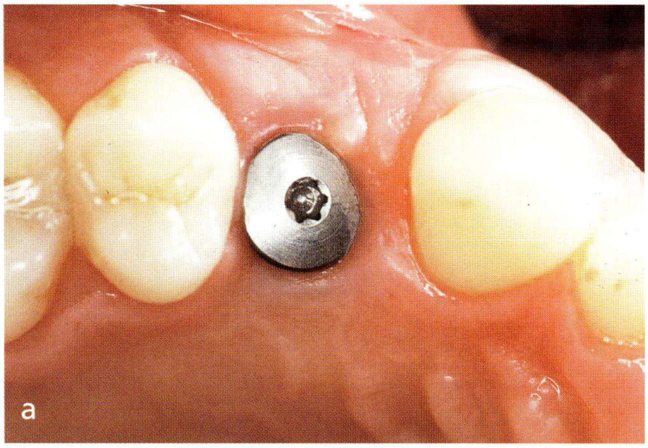
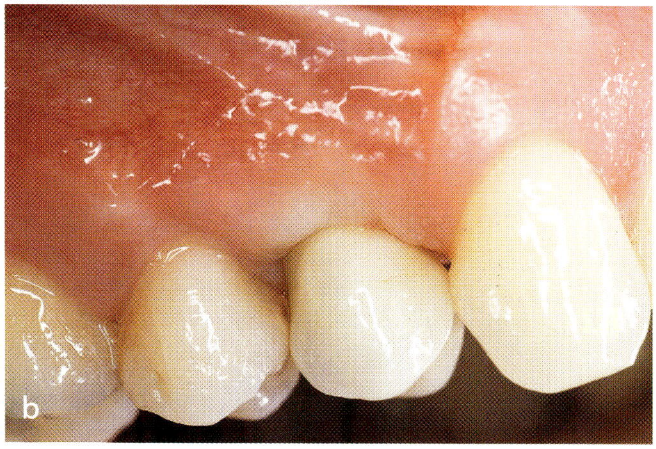

Figs 2-19a and 2-19b Clinical situation following extraction of the first premolar with preparation of the lingual root socket for immediate fixture placement. (a) At second-stage surgery with tissue healing cap. (b) Buccal view of the implant-mucosal unit that cannot hide its too-lingualized location.

geon in the selection of appropriate fixture sites and in the adequate preparation of surrounding soft tissue thickness. Clinical reality will sooner or later show that esthetic objectives will not only have to deal with the restrictive parameters of the mesiodistal width differences between teeth and implants but also with their respective buccolingual width.

The immediate fixture placement in fresh extraction sites, therefore, can only secure a good positioning of the prosthesis when sufficient soft tissue coverage can be achieved at first-stage surgery.[14–68] This tissue thickness will make it possible to provide correction of a spatial implant placement that will invariably be found in a too-lingualized position (Fig 2-19).

While the surgeon's participation in the collective visualization of the final esthetic result remains important, therapeutic efficiency is directly dependent on the capability of the restorative dentist to provide the surgeon with the guideline of a provisional prosthesis perfectly duplicating the final prosthesis in shape and spatial location. This will give the surgeon precise indications for implant placement and for provisional supra-implant soft tissue preparation at first-stage surgery. It should also be remembered that in a large edentulous area planned to receive a fixed denture prosthesis, the first-stage surgery should also be used to previsualize the reconstruction of the interdental papilla, which requires osseous support should it be foreseen for one, two, or multiple elements (Fig 2-18).

In today's dentistry we still have to acknowledge a decrease of esthetic quality in fixed restorations proportional to the increase of edentation and the associated loss of osseous support (Fig 2-19). This demonstrates that the width, shape, and size of the platform and related abutment designs of titanium fixtures, even if they are far from duplicating natural elements, have nothing to do with the esthetic outcome of dental rehabilitation.

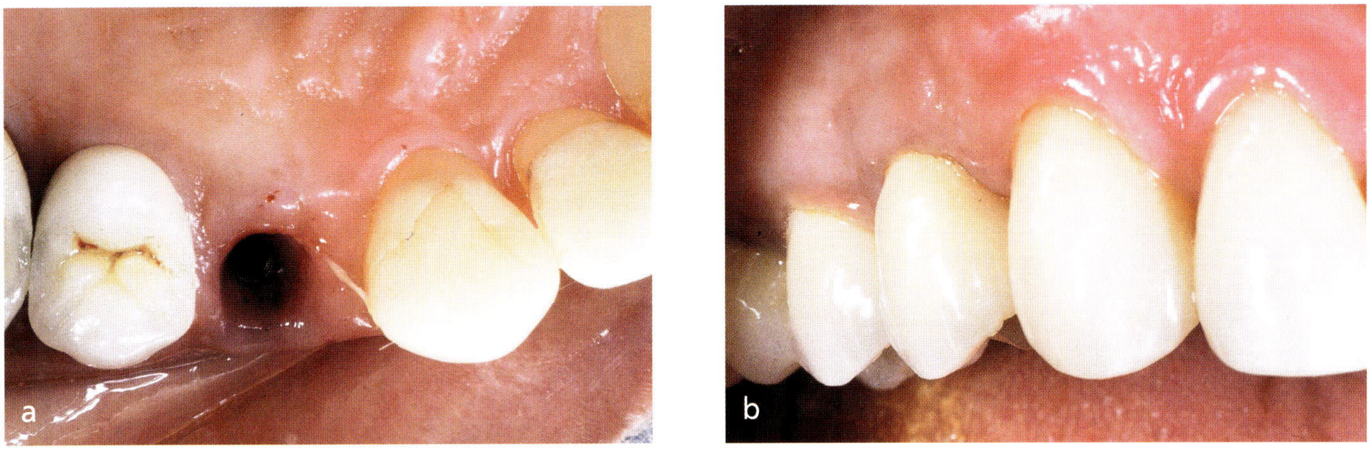

Figs 2-20a and 2-20b (a) A similar situation at second-stage surgery following immediate fixture placement in the buccal root of a first premolar. (b) Buccal view of the implant-mucosal unit respecting the alignment of the front-back progression. For improved esthetics, the ideal fixture placement should always be realized in the most buccal part of the buccolingual tooth width unless a fair amount of soft tissue thickness allows for adequate tissue conditioning, thus improving the emergence profile.

Pontic-Gingival Unit

The pontic-gingival unit may be one of the most ignored and mistreated relational entities in restorative dentistry. The loss of dental elements following trauma, carious lesions, or periodontal disease invariably modifies the shape of the supporting structures. A large variety of procedures, including root technique and pouch technique, aimed at preserving or restoring hard and soft tissue morphology, has been proposed to the restorative dentist. These procedures can be used should the restored crest serve as a recipient site for a pontic-gingival or implant-mucosal unit.

Yet if we assume that the edentulous ridge may retain or regain a shape identical to that existing prior to the extraction of teeth, soft tissue contour will nonetheless no longer display specific particularities such as root prominence or marginal and interdental papillae, and tissue structure will no longer exhibit its characteristic orange-peel appearance. The scalloped form of the gingiva that attained the biological and esthetic tooth-gingiva relationships no longer exists; therefore, specific clinical preparation of the pontic-gingival area is necessary to restore similar relationships.

The plastic quality of these relationships depends on the material or visual reproduction of two elements, the marginal and interdental papillae, conditioned and maintained by an appropriately designed pontic recipient site, and the pontic shape and its emergence profile. Assuming that the ovate pontic is the rule, the clinical approach to duplicating these elements will be dictated by an evaluation of the quality and quantity of soft tissue supporting the pontic. This evaluation will decide the depth of the pontic excavation, commonly and probably best achieved with electrosurgery followed by immediate and careful relining of the provisional's pontic base. Yet excavations are only excavations (Fig 2-20), whereas proper mor-

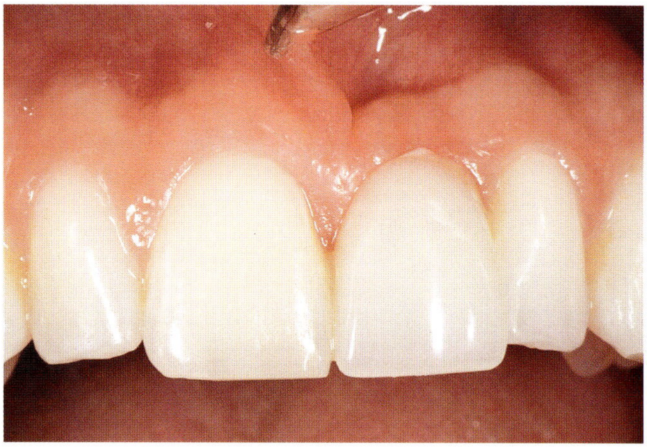

Fig 2-21 When adjacent interdental papillae do exist and when crest resorption is absent, duplication of original morphological conditions with implant-supported fixed restorations remains a realistic objective.

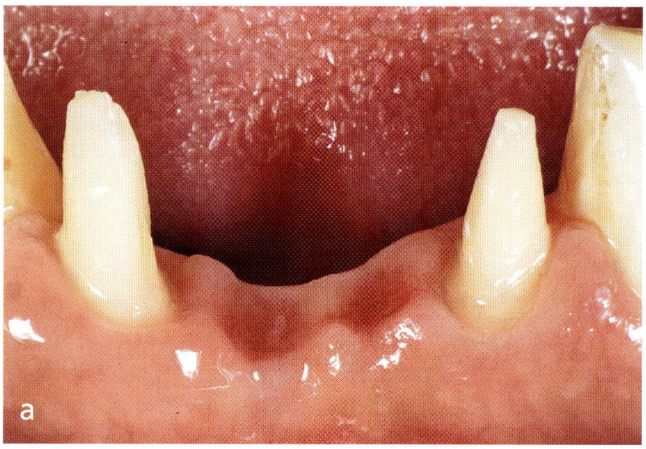

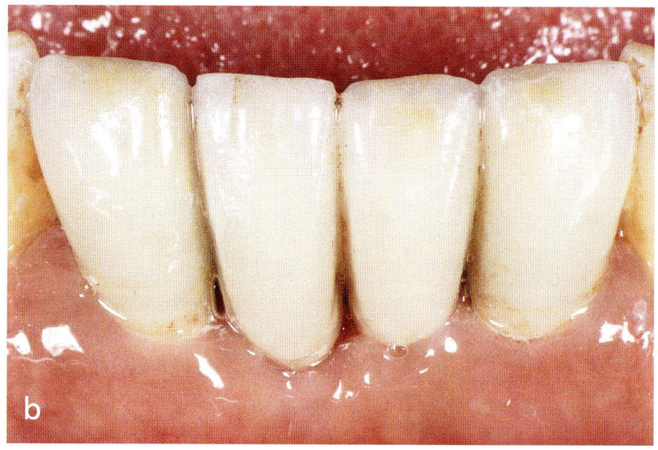

Figs 2-22a and 2-22b (a) In edentulous areas, prepared or unprepared soft tissue excavations are nothing but excavations. (b) A simulation of original tooth-periodontal relationships can only be illusory without proper tissue conditioning from well-designed provisional and final pontic restorations. This involves a perfect adaptation of pontic design to the soft tissue recipient site and a mild circumference "pressure" at prosthesis insertion.

phology demands root prominences, or marginal and interdental papillae. The duplication of these elements requires a sequential therapeutic approach. The preparation of the pontic sites' excavation width is dictated by overlying tooth width; the excavation depth remains limited by tissue thickness, and the simulation of the periodontal characteristics of the original dentogingival unit is linked to the excavation depth and the nature of the contacts exerted by the pontic (Figs 2-21 and 2-22).

In the phase of tissue conditioning that depends totally on a dentist's sensibility, it has been observed that where thin tissue permits only a shallow excavation, the lateral tissue pressure will create a lateral

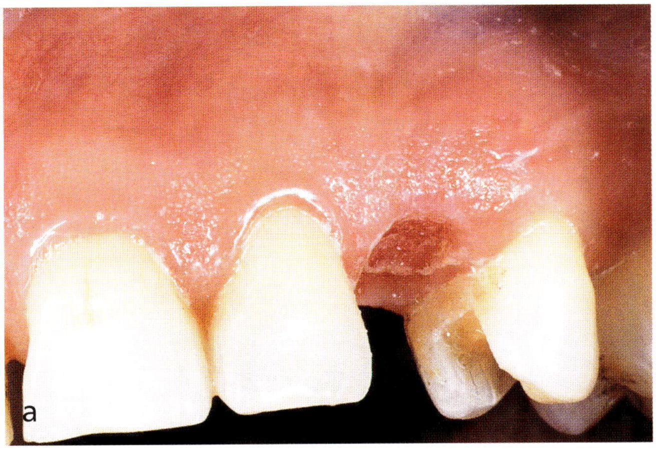

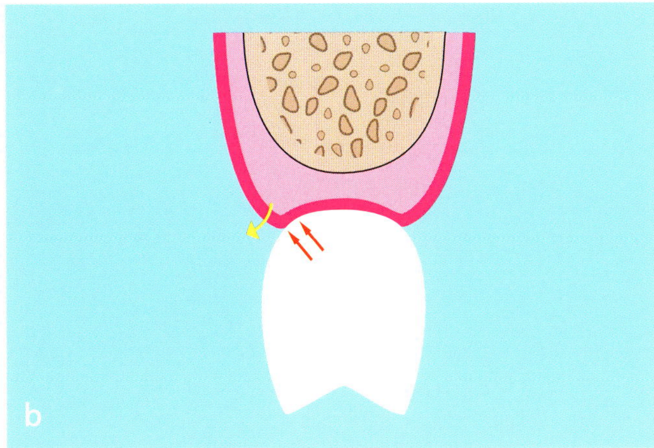

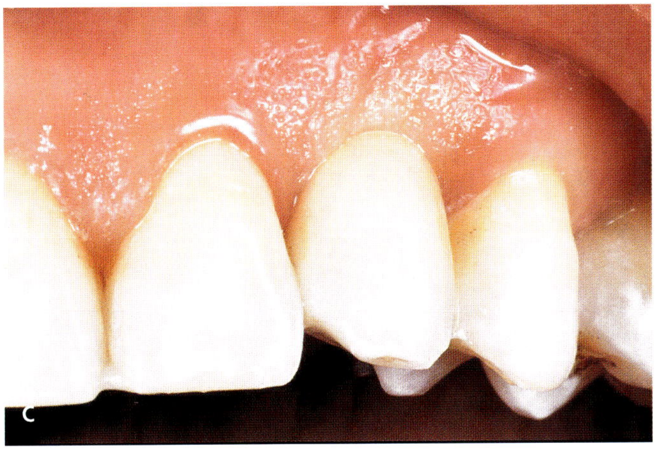

Figs 2-23a to 2-23c (a,b) In thin tissue thickness and limited excavation depth, one should exert at the insertion of the pontic base a lateral pressure that should take place 1 mm from tissue margin both on the buccal and proximal aspects of the excavation. (c) Tissue necrosis may occur if tissue blanching lasts more than 30 seconds, yet shallow excavations show minimal tissue rebound at tissue conditioning.

tissue rebound simulating marginal papillae, while thick tissue, permitting deeper excavation, may duplicate root prominence if lateral pressure is applied from pontic design (Figs 2-23 to 2-27). With sensitive management of soft tissue and pontic design, a satisfactory esthetic result duplicating the characteristics of the tooth-gingival unit can be expected in the pontic-gingival unit thanks to the qualities of the gingiva for natural tissue rebound.

The conception of the dentogingival unit, implant-mucosal unit, and pontic-gingival unit can succeed only when it takes into account biological and esthetic relational characteristics. These characteristics arise from the structural particularities of forms subjected

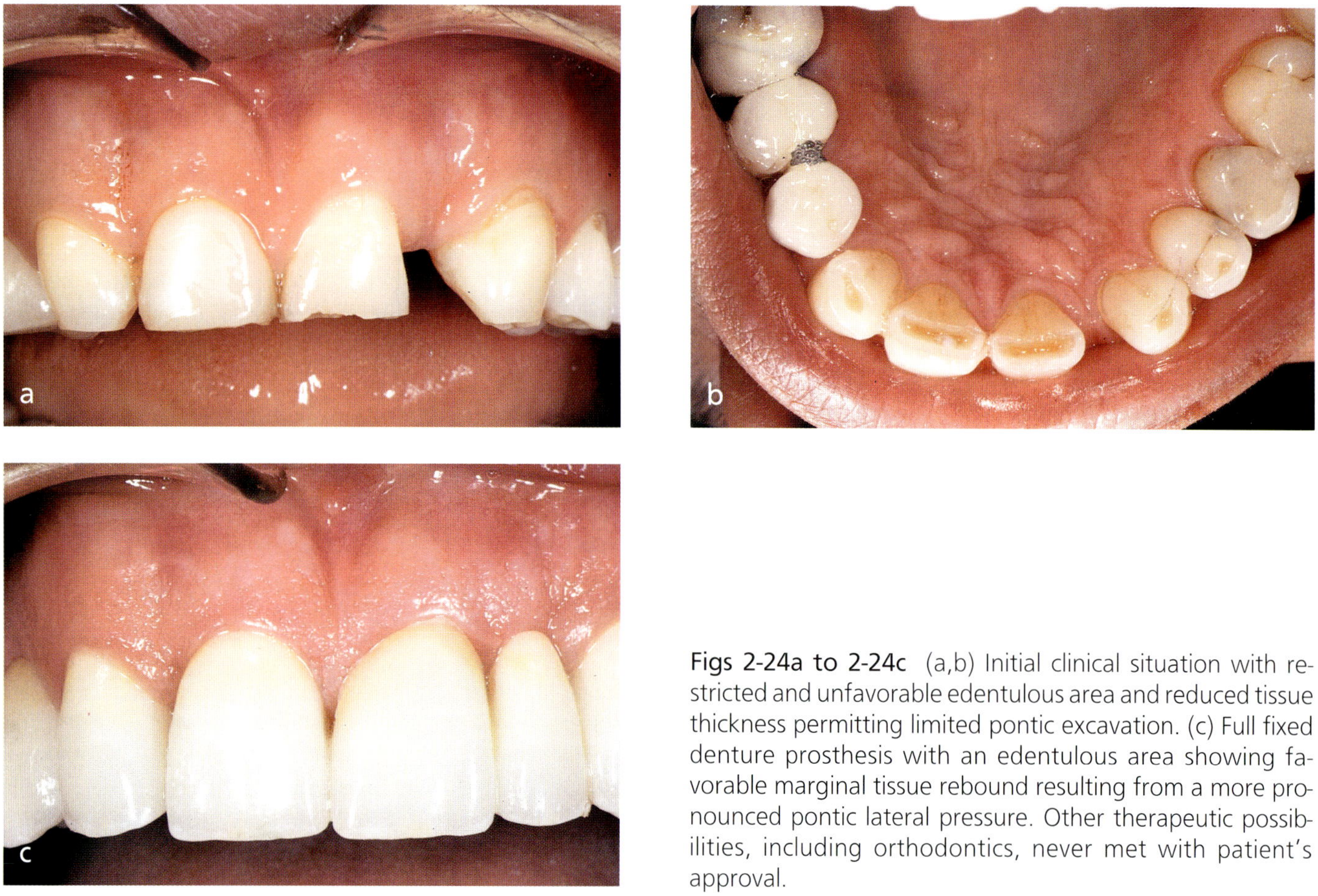

Figs 2-24a to 2-24c (a,b) Initial clinical situation with restricted and unfavorable edentulous area and reduced tissue thickness permitting limited pontic excavation. (c) Full fixed denture prosthesis with an edentulous area showing favorable marginal tissue rebound resulting from a more pronounced pontic lateral pressure. Other therapeutic possibilities, including orthodontics, never met with patient's approval.

to the demands of function (Fig 2-26). In the duality of forms and relationships no one element takes precedence. Biological, functional, and esthetic considerations are not in conflict. They complete each other, support each other, and must be understood and visualized as a whole.

The objectives of oral rehabilitation are at the same time both functional and esthetic. They involve a realistic morphological duplication of the original elements of the dentofacial composition and the institution of harmonious relationships between each of these elements in relation to each other and to the whole.

The imitation of reality, an important goal of esthetic creation, implies in the restorative process the harmonious association of restored elements

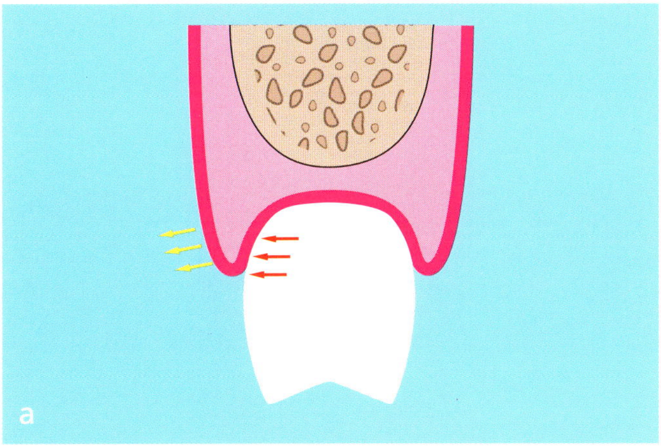

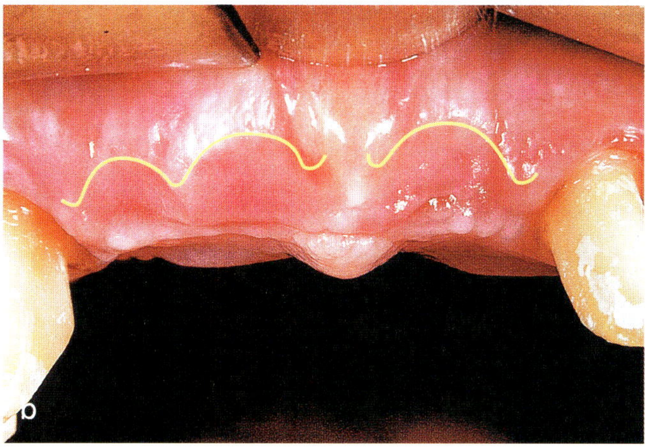

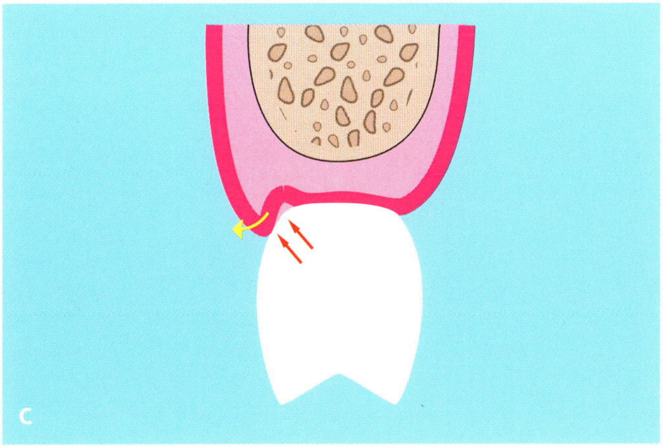

Figs 2-25a to 2-25c (a) In edentulous areas with important tissue thickness, it is extremely easy to carve appropriate pontic recipient sites to simulate normal tooth-gingival relationships, with root prominence and interdental papillalike tissue design. When tissue thickness is reduced a simulation of the marginal papilla remains possible. It requires (b,c) a 2-mm-deep incision with an upward inclination designed in the lateral and buccal aspect of tissue excavation. The flap is then reflected and maintained in a buccal position during pontic insertion.

with existing structures. To acquire the taste and judgment necessary to achieve this, to banish habitual norms and deal instead with individual components, to appreciate the nature of the necessary elements, progressive esthetic training and esthetic knowledge remain indispensable.

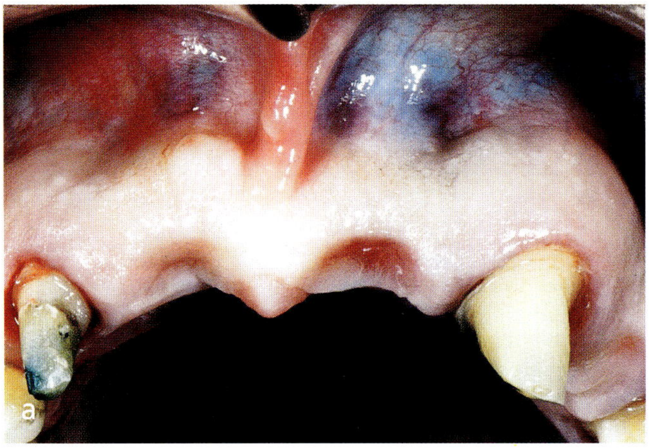

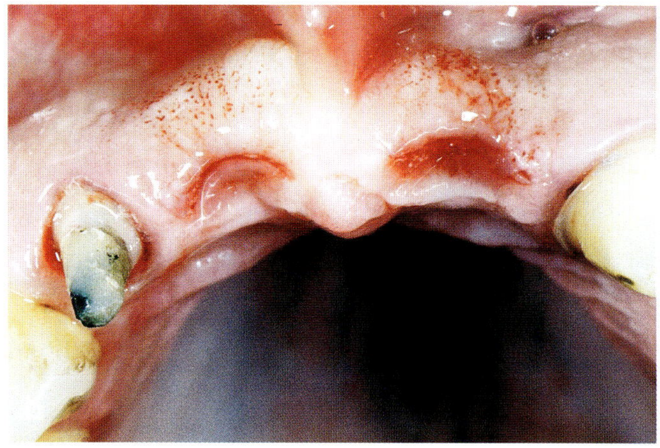

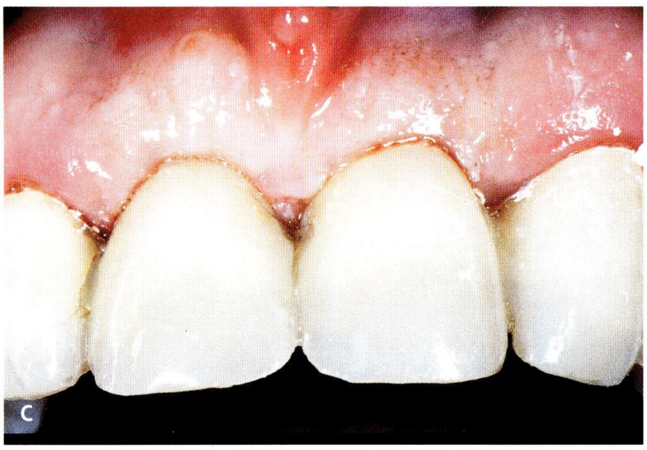

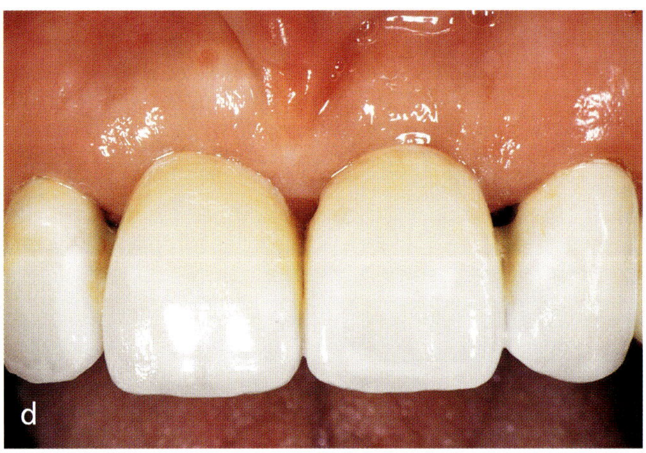

Figs 2-26a to 2-26d (a) Initial clinical situation. (b) Preparation of a 2-mm-deep curved incision. (c) Following completion of a release incision, the pontic design, of which the marginal width has been increased, is introduced into the prepared site. (d) Final fixed restoration of an area originally provided with a large diastema. Marginal papillae are well designed and in continuity with tooth prominences.

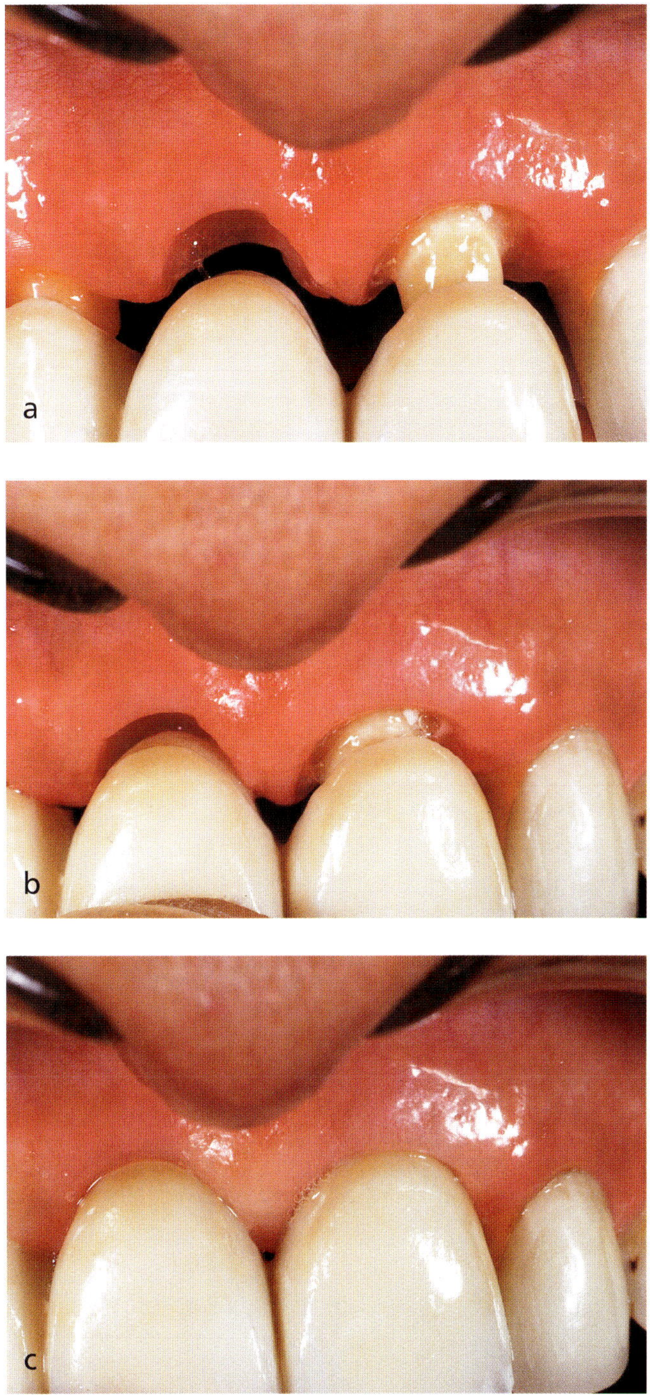

Figs 2-27a to 2-27c In the creation of tooth-gingival units, pontic-gingival units, and implant-mucosal units, biological conditions should be considered with the objective of simulating original tooth-gingival morphological design.

References

1. Garguilo AW, Wentz FM, Orban B. Dimension and relations of the dento-gingival junction in humans. J Periodontol 1961;32:261–267.
2. Sicher H. Changing concepts on the supporting dental structures. Oral Surg 1959;12:31–35.
3. Schroeder HE, Listgarten RA. Fine structure of the developing epithelial attachment in human teeth. Monographs in Developmental Biology. Basel: S. Karger, 1971:2–134.
4. Ingber JS, Rose LF, Coslet JG. The "biologic width"—A concept in periodontics and restorative dentistry. Alpha Omegan 1977;70:62–65.
5. Maynard JG, Wilson RD. Physiologic dimensions of the periodontium significant to the restorative dentist. J Periodontol 1979;50:170–174.
6. Waerhaug J. Presence or absence of plaque on subgingival restorations. Scand J Dent Res 1975;83:193–201.
7. Waerhaug J. Histologic considerations which govern where the margins of restorations should be located in relation to gingiva. Dent Clin North Am 1960;5:161–176.
8. Marcurm JS. The effect of crown marginal depth upon gingival tissue. J Prosthet Dent 1967;17:479–487.
9. Dello Russo NM. Placement of crown margins in patients with altered passive eruption. Int J Periodont Rest Dent 1984;4:58–65.
10. Becker CM, Kaldahl WB. Current theories of crown contour, margin placement and pontic design. J Prosthet Dent 1981;45:268–277.
11. Shavell HM. Mastering the art of tissue management during provisionalization and biologic final impressions. Int J Periodont Rest Dent 1988;8:24–43.
12. Kay HB. Criteria for restorative contours in the altered periodontal environment. Int J Periodont Rest Dent 1985;5:42–63.
13. Tarnow DP, Magner AW, Fletcher P. The effect of the distance from the contact point to the crest of bone on presence or absence of the interproximal dental papilla. J Periodontol 1992;63:995–996.
14. Löe H. Reactions to marginal periodontal tissues to restorative procedures. Int Dent J 1968;18:759–778.
15. Nevins M, Skurow HM. The intracrevicular restorative margin, the biologic width, and the maintenance of the gingival margin. Int J Periodont Rest Dent 1984;4:30–39.
16. Shavell HM. Mastering the art of tissue management during provisionalization and biologic final impression. Int J Periodont Rest Dent 1988;8:25.
17. Woycheshin FF. An evaluation of the drugs used for gingival retraction. J Prosthet Dent 1964;14:769–776.
18. Anneroth G, Nordenram A. Reaction of the gingiva to the application of threads in the gingival pocket for taking impressions with elastic materials. Odontol Revy 1969;20:301–310.
19. Harrison JD. Effect of retraction materials on the gingival sulcus epithelium. J Prosthet Dent 1961;11:514–521.
20. Löe H, Silness J. Tissue reactions to string packs used in fixed restoration. J Prosthet Dent 1963;13:318–323.
21. de Gennaro GG, Landesman HM, Calhoun JE, Martinoff JT. A comparison of gingival inflammation related to retraction cords. J Prosthet Dent 1982;47:384–386.
22. Wilson RD, Maynard G. Intracrevicular restorative dentistry. Int J Periodont Rest Dent 1981;1(4):34–49.
23. Duncan JD. Reaction of marginal gingiva to crown and bridge procedures. Part I. Miss Dent Assoc J 1979;35(2):26–28.
24. Dragoo MR, Williams GB. Periodontal tissue reactions to restorative procedures. Part II. Int J Periodont Rest Dent 1982;2(2):34–45.
25. Löe H. Reactions to marginal periodontal tissues to restorative procedures. Int Dent J 1968;18:759–778.
26. Barghi N, Simmons EW. The marginal integrity of the temporary acrylic resin crown. J Prosthet Dent 1976;36:274–277.

27. Adell R, Lekholm U, Rockler B, Brånemark P-I, Lindhe J, et al. Marginal tissue reactions at osseointegrated titanium fixtures (1). A 3-year longitudinal prospective study. Int J Oral Maxillofac Surg 1986;15:39–52.

28. Akaawa Y, Takata T, Matsumoto T, Nikai H, Tsuru H. Correlation between clinical and histological evaluations of the peri-implant gingiva around single-crystal sapphire endosseous implant. J Oral Rehabil 1989;16:581–587.

29. Jansen JA, de Wijn JR, Wolters-Lutgerhorst JML, van Mullem J. Ultrastructural study of epithelial cell attachment to implant material. J Dent Res 1985;64:891–896.

30. Lekholm U, Ericsson I, Adell R, Slots J. The condition of the soft tissues at tooth and fixture abutments supporting fixed bridges: A microbiological and histological study. J Clin Periodontol 1986;13:558–562.

31. Gould TRL, Brunette DM, Westbury L. The attachment mechanism of epithelial cells to titanium in vitro. J Periodont Res 1981;16:611–616.

32. Brånemark P-I. Introduction to osseointegration. In: Brånemark P-I, Zarb GA, Albrektsson T (eds). Tissue-Integrated Prostheses: Osseointegration in Clinical Dentistry. Chicago: Quintessence, 1985:11–76.

33. Ten Cate AR. (1985). The gingival junction. In: Brånemark P-I, Zarb GA, Albrektsson T (eds). Tissue-Integrated Prostheses: Osseointegration in Clinical Dentistry. Chicago: Quintessence, 1985:145–153.

34. McKinney RV, Steflik DE, Koth DL. The epithelium-dental implant interface. J Oral Implantol 1988;13:622–641.

35. Meffert RM. The soft tissue interface in dental implantology. J Dent Educ 1988;52:810–811.

36. Carmichael RP, Apse P, Zarb GA, McCulloch CAG. Biological, micro-biological and clinical Aspects of the periimplant mucosa. In: Albrektsson T, Zarb GA (eds). The Brånemark Osseointegrated Implant. Chicago: Quintessence, 1989:39–78.

37. McCulloch CAG, Melcher AH. The periodontium. In: Smith DC, Williams DF (eds). Biocompatibility of Dental Materials. Vol 1. Boca Raton: CRC Press, 1982.

38. Buser D, Stich H, Kreker G, Schroeder A. Faserstrukturen der periimplantären Mukosa bei Titanimplantaten. Eine experimentelle Studie am Beagle-Hund. Zeitschrift für Zahnärzt Implantologie 1989;5:15–23.

39. Zarb G. Osseointegration: A requiem for the periodontal ligament. Guest editoral. Int J Periodont Rest Dent 1991;11(2):28–91.

40. Adell R, Lekholm U, Rockler B, Brånemark P-I. A 15-year study of osseointegrated implants in the treatment of the edentulous jaw. Int J Oral Surg 1981;10:387–416.

41. Lekholm U, Adell R, Lindhe J, et al. Marginal tissue reaction of osseointegrated titanium implants II. A cross-sectional retrospective study. Int J Oral Surg 1986;15:53–61.

42. Bower RC, Radney NR, Wall CD, Henry PJ. Clinical and microscopic findings in edentulous patients 3 years after incorporation of osseointegrated implant-supported bridgework. J Clin Periodontol 1989;16:580–587.

43. Apse P, Zarb GA, Schmitt A, Lewis DW. The longitudinal effectiveness of osseointegrated dental implants. The Toronto Study: Peri-implant mucosal response. Int J Periodont Rest Dent 1991;11:94–111.

44. Berglundh T, Lindhe J, Ericsson I, Marinello CP, Liljenberg B, Thomsen P. The soft tissue barrier at implants and teeth. Clin Oral Implants Res 1991;2:81–90.

45. Ericsson I, Berglundh T, Marinello CP, Liljenberg B, Lindhe J. Long-standing plaque and gingivitis at implants and teeth in the dog. Clin Oral Implants Res 1992;3:99–103.

46. Adell R, Lekholm U, Roskler BJ, et al. A 15-year study of osseointegrated implant in the treatment of the edentulous jaw. Int J Surg 1981;10:387–416.

47. Albrektsson T, Zarb GA, Worthington P, Eriksson AR. The long-term efficacy of currently used dental implants: A review and proposed criteria of success. Int J Oral Maxillofac Implants 1986;1:11–25.

48. Zarb GA, Schmitt A. Osseointegration and the edentulous predicament. The 10-year-old Toronto study. Br Dent J 1991;170:439–444.

49. Lindquist LW, Carlsson GE, Glantz PO. Rehabilitation of the edentulous mandible with a tissue-integrated fixed prosthesis: A six-year longitudinal study. Quintessence Int 1987;18:89–96.

50. Smith DE. A review of endosseous implants for partially edentulous patients. Int J Prosthodont 1990;3:12–19.

51. Adell R, Lekholm U, Brånemark P-I. Surgical procedures. In: Brånemark PI, Zarb GA, Albrektsson T (eds). Tissue-Integrated Prostheses: Osseointegration in Clinical Dentistry. Chicago: Quintessence, 1989:221–232.

52. Moy PK, Weinlaender M, Tenney EB. Soft tissue modifications of surgical techniques for placement and uncovering of osseointegrated implants. Dent Clin North Am 1989;33:665–681.

53. Hertel RC, Blijdorp PA, Kalk W, Baker DL. Stage 2 surgical techniques in endosseous implantation. Int J Oral Maxillofac Implants 1994;9:273–278.

54. Israelson H, Plemons JM. Dental implants, regenerative techniques, and periodontal plastic surgery to restore maxillary anterior esthetics. Int J Oral Maxillofac Implants 1993;8:555–562.

55. Sullivan D, Kay H, Schwarz M, Gelb D. Esthetic problems in the anterior maxilla. Int J Oral Maxillofac Implants 1984;(Suppl 9):64–74.

56. Ibbot CG, Kovach RJ, Carlson-Mann LD. Surgical correction for esthetic problems associated with dental implants. J Can Dent Assoc 1992;58:561–562.

57. Silverstein LH, Lefkove MD. The use of the subepithelial connective tissue graft to enhance both the aesthetics and periodontal contours surrounding dental implants. J Oral Implantol 1994;20:135–138.

58. Palacci P. Amenagement des tissus peri-implantaires intérêt de la régénération des papilles. Réalités Cliniques 1992;3:381–387.

59. Palacci P. Optimal Implant Positioning & Soft Tissue Management for the Brånemark System. Chicago: Quintessence, 1995:59.

60. Wennström JL, Bengazi F, Lekholm U. The influence of the masticatory mucosa on the peri-implant soft tissue condition. Clin Oral Implants Res 1994;5:1–8.

61. Strub JR, Garlerthël TW, Grunder U. The role of the attached gingva in the health of peri-implant tissue in dogs. Part I. Clinical findings. Int J Periodont Rest Dent 1991;11:317–333.

62. Parel SM, Triplett RG. Immediate fixture placement: A treatment planning alternative. Int J Oral Maxillofac Implants 1990;5:337–345.

63. Garber DA, Rosenberg ES. The edentulous ridge in fixed prosthodontics. Compend Continue Educ Dent 1981;2:212–223.

64. Seibert JS, Cohen DW. Periodontal considerations in preparation for fixed and removable prosthodontics. Dent Clin North Am 1987;31:529–555.

65. Lazzara RJ. Immediate implant placement into extraction sites: Surgical and restorative advantages. Int J Periodont Rest Dent 1989;9:333–343.

66. Gelb DA. Immediate implant surgery: 3-year retrospective evaluation of 50 consecutive cases. Int J Oral Maxillofac Implants 1993;8:388–399.

67. Rosenquist BA. A comparison of various methods of soft tissue management following the immediate placement of implants into extraction sockets. Int J Oral Maxillofac Implants 1997;12:43–51.

68. Landsbert CJ. Socket seal surgery combined with immediate implant placement. A novel approach for single-tooth replacement. Int J Periodont Rest Dent 1997;17:141–149.

CHAPTER 3

Esthetic Integration

Esthetic taste, though universal, is based upon one highly subjective element: the feeling that arises when human beings encounter shapes and colors. Through the centuries philosophers have tried and failed to understand this feeling and, since its sources are indefinable, have attributed it to irrational and individual causes. As a result, Cartesian spirits feel uncomfortable in the esthetic world; they consign beauty to intuition and to lyric effusions, whatever the degree of emotion generated.

Yet esthetic knowledge, consisting of an accumulation of intuitions, feelings, and sensations, may be acquired through patient and repetitive interrogations and a constant effort of perception. Esthetic knowledge can be reduced to no other because absolute criteria do not exist. Therefore, we need to be trained to bring to the level of consciousness the common factors in the variety of entities that generate beauty. This chapter will focus on the description of these esthetic factors.

Logic, based on human constants, is both an instrument of control and, for the inventive, a route to discovery. Logic guides the march of intuition. However, logic without the complementary support of intuition will merely remain a sterile device.

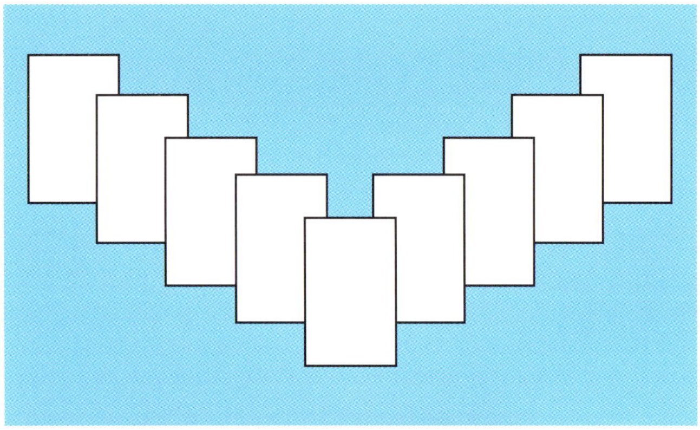

Fig 3-1 Western estheticism is based on strictly mathematical considerations. A perfect schema of repeated or similar elements generates in the human mind a uniquely intense sense of esthetic delight. A perfect dental alignment, enhanced with similitudes of shape and color and an architectural design based on the addition of similar elements, illustrates this concept of esthetics.

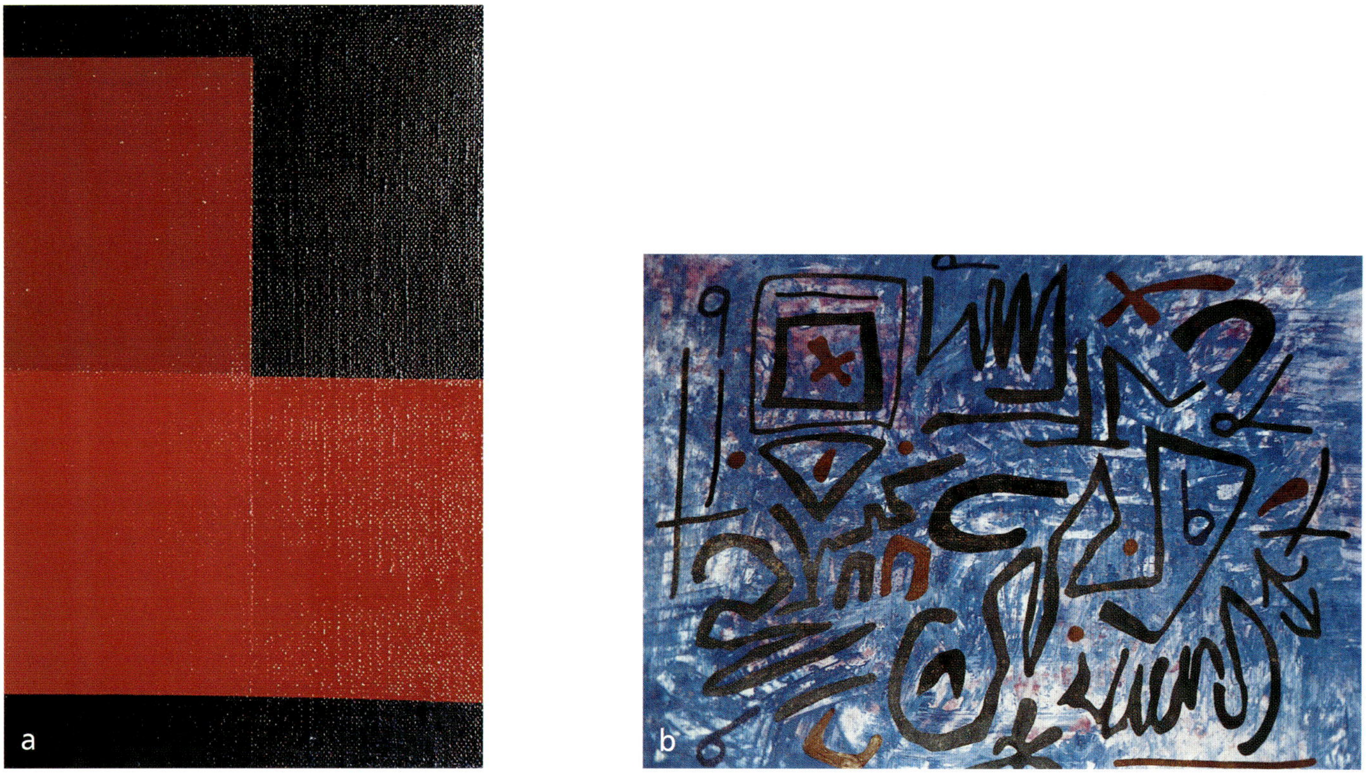

Figs 3-2a and 3-2b Beauty can be analyzed with regard to its own form or with regard to human perception. Yet the nature of the alchemy that takes place between these different entities and human sensibility defies explanation. These figures show that the beauty of a composition does not proceed from an identity of forms or relations but from the specific position of its constitutive elements in response to the requirements of sensibility. (a) When perception of a composition promotes collective sensations of the primary order, like the perception of squares in a rectangular support for example, the specific location of these squares and their differences in coloring introduce elements of tension, generating sensations of the secondary order (A. Nemours, private collection). (b) This art composition, on the contrary, mainly creating sensations of the secondary order, may only satisfy those in complete resonance with the creator (O. Nebel, private collection).

Order of Sensation

Esthetic sensations are not all of the same degree of intensity and quality. They may be arranged according to some type of hierarchy. One of the highest delights of the human mind is to perceive the order of nature and of its own participation in the scheme of things. This gives us the feeling that the world obeys the laws man has assigned it. A law is nothing other than the verification of an order expressed "mathematically."

We have been raised in the clear perception of a mathematical order because the Western estheticism born from the Mediterranean estheticism is based on strictly mathematical considerations. And even if shapes and colors seem to have to address the senses more directly, pure mathematics, which acts on the symbolic level, appears to trigger in the mind reactions of a superior order that occupy the highest level in the hierarchy of sensations (Fig 3-1). As a result, for us the release of feelings generated by shapes and colors can hardly predispose the mind to subjective reactions without the addition of a mathematical order.

We can define two distinct orders of sensation: primary and secondary. The primary order of sensations is determined in all human beings by the simple play of colors and forms. For example, a sphere will create in each individual an identical reaction because of its spherical form, even if that form is only partially seen. This sensation is a constant. It constitutes the basic element or the fixed vocabulary of the esthetic language.

A sphere will always be a sphere and a square a square, and each of these shapes causes specific perceptual and esthetic reactions. What is true for the sphere is just as true for the cube, the cylinder, the cone, and the pyramid, as well as for the constituent elements of these entities: the triangle, the square, and the circle. This statement can be extended to straight and broken lines; right, acute, or obtuse angles; and all elements eliciting in all individuals identical reactions.

Sensations of the secondary order graft themselves on these sensations of the primary order but include the intervention of the subject's hereditary or cultural composition. In the case of the sphere, for example, a Brazilian will associate it with a football, a Papounasian with the idea of divinity, and an astronaut with the planet earth, the central point of his or her vision and preoccupations.

To a certain extent one could make the statement that a piece of art, using exclusively the primary order of sensations, would be reduced to an ornament without human resonance. Reciprocally, a piece of art based only upon the secondary order of sensations would be devoid of any esthetic quality and might only satisfy those intimate with the creator (Fig 3-2).

Unlike the primary sensations, the secondary sensations are unlimited in number so that the universality of the esthetic language, formal and explicit, remains theoretical and will always determine subjective reactions of an individual origin. Superior sensations of a mathematical order can only be born of primary sensations combined with secondary ones.

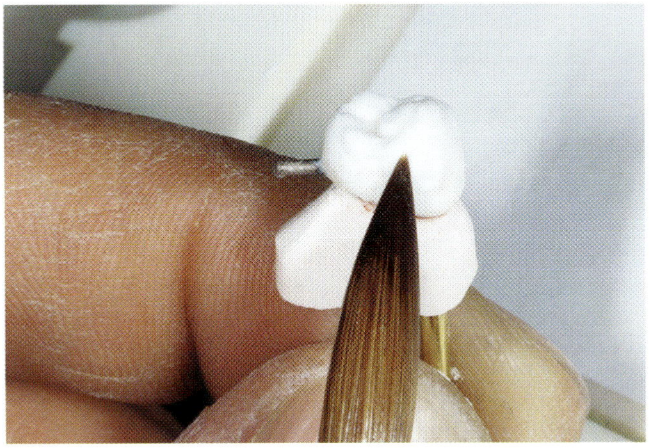

Fig 3-3 The conception of an artistic creation is an operation of the mind that foreshadows the finished work, which is realized by means of specific ingredients such as powders, water, brushes, and refractory stones.

Conception and Composition

An esthetic creation uses a variety of means for specific results. To conceive such a thing one must first know what one wishes to do. Should one try to satisfy the senses, to please the eye, or to satisfy at the same time the sense and the mind? Conception is, in fact, an operation of the mind that foreshadows the general appearance of a piece of art. For that, one must bring to bear the associations of natural and artificial forms to create a symphony of sensations in the spectator (Fig 3-3).

At the laboratory level, prosthetic dentistry presents perfect conditions for such creation. An abundant variety of natural or artificial shapes, colors, and materials provide all the ingredients for a dental symphony. The dental team are privileged participants with unusual opportunities for accomplishment or deception. The dental team is organized to produce carefully selected forms and arrangements to fulfill functional needs (Figs 3-4 and 3-5). The conception

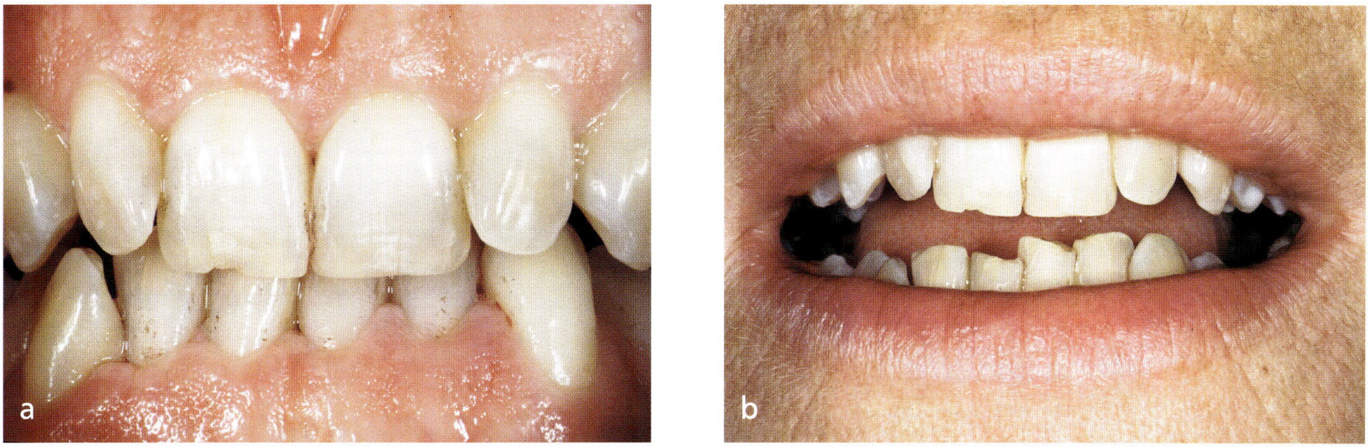

Figs 3-4a and 3-4b The term *composition* refers to the inner organization of a work of art. The organization of a dental composition is based on the perception of constant and variable elements. Two central incisors surrounded by two lateral incisors and canines represent the constant, while tooth shape, tooth position, the specific characteristics of the dental arrangement, and the surrounding facial structures represent the variables. But which criteria can be used to determine these variables within the conception of a dental arrangement in harmony with its environment? (a) Poor dental arrangement according to Western concepts, (b) yet needing little correction to be in full harmony with its environment.

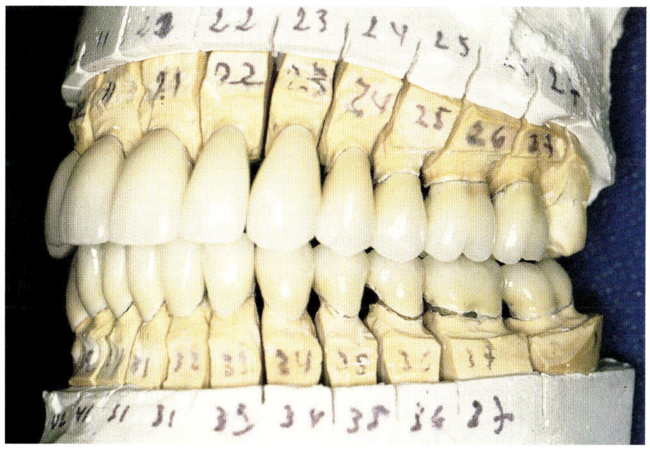

Fig 3-5 Can we really expect a favorable esthetic result from a dental composition born from the imagination of the dental technician confronted with surrounding structures? Knowing that esthetic qualification is based on the privileged relationships between different elements, a dental arrangement restricted to the architectural frame of the articulator can only be considered erroneous. It is illusory to believe that all the elements of the dentofacial puzzle will automatically find esthetic concordance when the related facial parameters have been ignored during the conceptual phase.

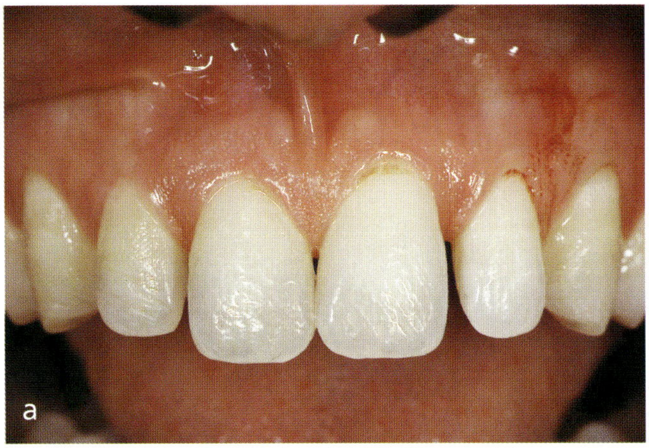

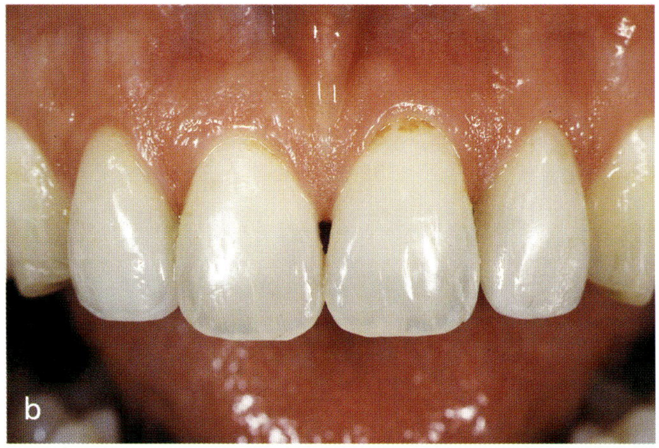

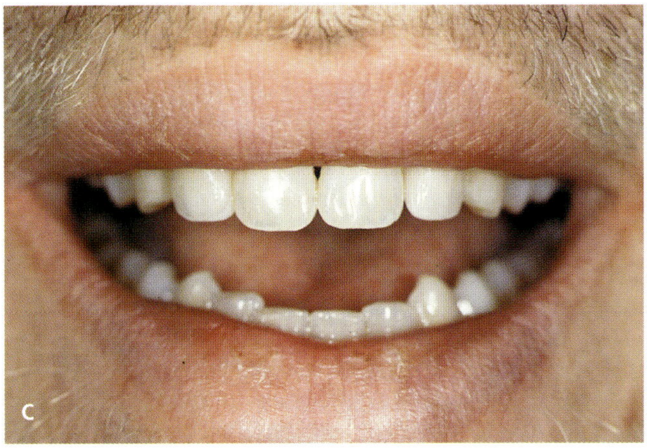

Figs 3-6a to 3-6c (a) The esthetic effect of the dental composition is impaired by the presence of multiple diastema. (b) Treatment planning has consisted of restoring normal tooth shape with porcelain veneers for the lateral incisors and slightly increasing, using composite bonding, the distal contour of the central incisors, which apparently improves the esthetics of the dental composition. (c) Yet in relation to its surrounding structures, the dental composition, displaying a monotonous horizontal symmetry, is an esthetic failure. This arrangement even increases the feeling of characterial laxness generated by upper and lower lip design and structure.

of these elements, made up of constants and variables, takes place at the laboratory level, where the field of vision is restricted to a fragment of an architectural space that in reality extends to the whole facial structure.

The difficulty of taking in this space, and of transferring and reproducing highly volatile facial elements at the laboratory level, explains the preponderance given to function in prosthetic dentistry and the commonness of a misconceived esthetic approach (Figs 3-6 and 3-7).

An organization of shapes and colors dedicated to transmitting an emotion requires an architectural space for materialization. This materialization is best perceived when it appears in the eye's normal field of vision. The eye should be confronted with a space that gives the impression of a whole. This explains why for years many painters use traditional formats.

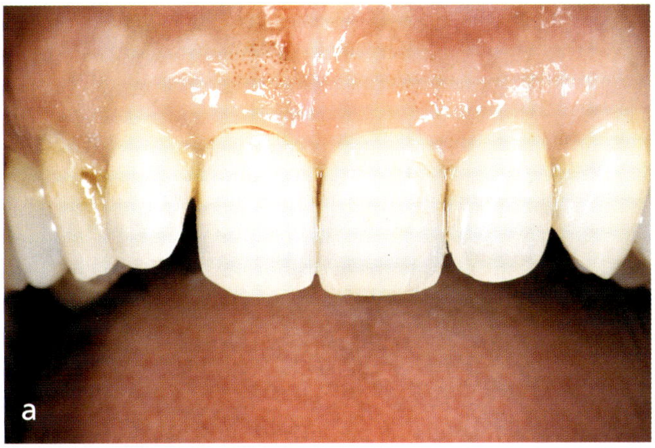

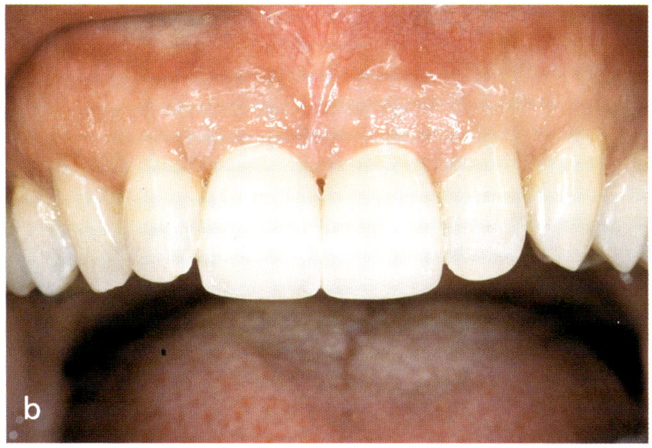

Figs 3-7a to 3-7c (a) The esthetic quality of the dental composition suffers from the location of the right lateral incisor, which emerges from the curve of the arch. (b) Yet the specific design of the lip, suggesting the maintenance of knots of attention, calls for a vestibularization of the two central incisors. (c) A correct evaluation of relational elements allows us to improve the harmony of the dentofacial composition.

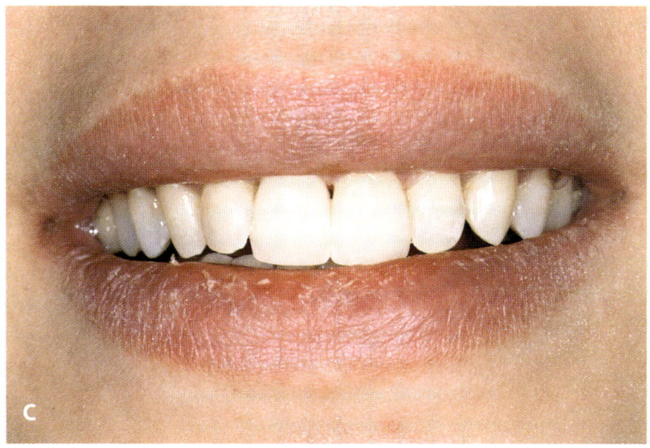

These formats satisfied personal visual needs and could be grasped in a single glance.

Observed through a large window or a bull's-eye, a landscape will always contain the same details. But modifications of the distance of focus will subject the architectural space to apparent variation and lead to new compositions emphasizing various specific elements. A composition can be defined as a realistic or imaginary space perfectly delimited by its geometric dimensions and characterized by the elements that it contains.

The nature of the elements of the facial structure, in their shape, position, and dimension, is already fixed. As a consequence, the conceptual capabilities of the dental team are restricted to the harmonious integration of the dental elements into this predetermined structure. Unfortunately, no material or practical framework governing the esthetic relations

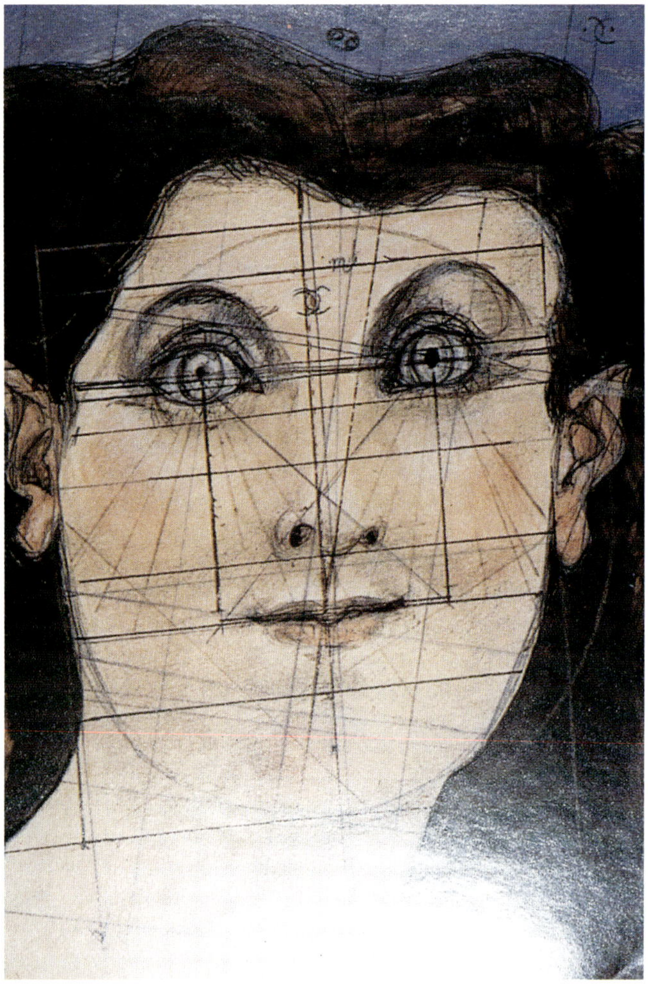

Fig 3-8 From Greek antiquity to the Italian Renaissance the theory of the proportionate body has served as a constant reference point for the secular understanding of universal harmony. Modern sensibility has been influenced primarily by Rafael and Leonardo da Vinci, and this head of a woman by John Graham (1954, private collection), incorporating parts of the facial composition into a mechanical system of lines, rectangles, and squares, illustrates this influence and suggests the way to apprehend dentofacial esthetics.

between the elements of the dentofacial composition has yet been proposed, and the objectives of esthetic integration therefore seem governed by the laws of chance. Such frameworks incorporating ideals of human beauty as have been proposed have seldom served a practical use and never incorporated elements of dentofacial esthetics (Fig 3-8).

Therefore, in the absence of ready-made recipes for beauty, one must develop a basic esthetic knowledge, a sensitive approach to the relation of things. This will make possible a methodology of esthetic analysis and a clinical setup that will allow the harmonious integration of dental elements into environmental structures.

The dentofacial parameters necessary to this integration will naturally need to be appraised from a frontal point of view, a unique point of view that will lead to a variety of consequences: the conditions of perception of a surface in its shape and dimension should be ideal; the location of points of perception, close to or far from the spectator, should exist along a single line; the elements that belong to these different points of perception will be subject to minor deformations; other points of view can be briefly considered when a more global spatial perception becomes necessary.

Esthetic dentistry will have to visualize the frontal composition from three or four basic, different distances (Fig 3-9) associated with different dynamic relations between the lips and other dental elements (Fig 3-10). The frontal composition should be viewed from distances that reveal the dental composition constituted by upper and lower teeth with supporting structures; the dentofacial composition constituted by teeth and lips in various possible oral movements; the facial composition in its vestibular

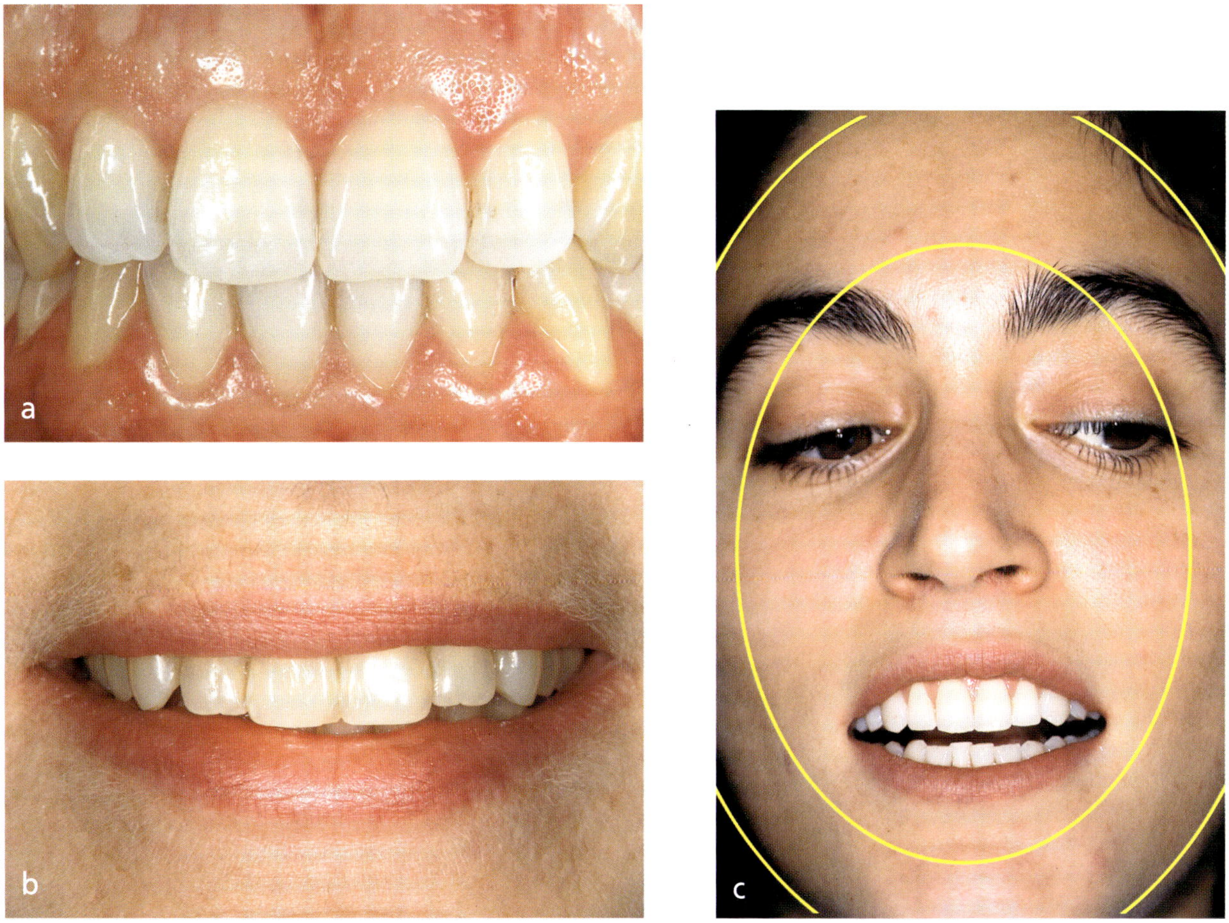

Figs 3-9a to 3-9c To become familiar with dentofacial esthetic analysis and the dentofacial conceptual setup, it is important that we approach the dental composition from four different basic distances of focus: (a) the dental composition; (b) the dentofacial composition; and (c) the facial composition in its vestibular frame surrounding ocular, nasal, and oral receptors, and in its totality.

limitation, containing mouth, nose, and eyes; and the facial composition in its general morphological design.

Constant confrontations with these various planes and dynamic dentofacial situations are mandatory in the restoration of dental elements. The production of dental elements apart from or without reference to their future surroundings will lead to failure even if functional requirements are perfectly fulfilled.

The esthetic perfection of a composition does not rest on the perfection of the entities that it contains. The history of esthetics has demonstrated that all the artists who over the centuries attempted to build up an ideal body composition by assembling ideal small-

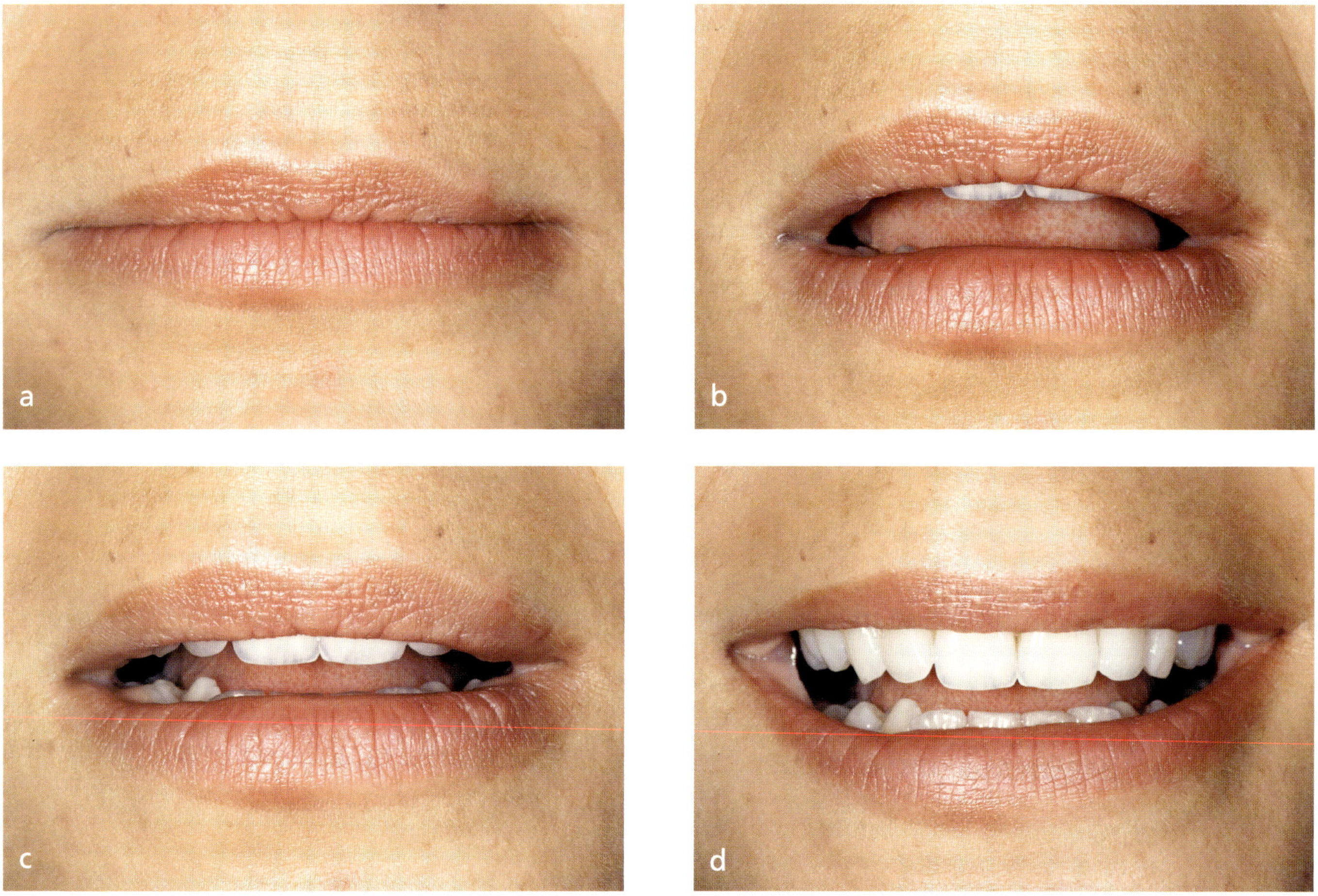

Figs 3-10a to 3-10d These basic frontal compositions, selected during the dynamic of oral movements, will permit us to determine the nature of relational elements, which create shapes: (a) closed mouth, (b) rest position, (c) quarter of a smile, and (d) full smile.

er entities such as nose, arms, legs, or eyes experienced, like Dürer, esthetic failure. We face identical restrictions. Ideal dental elements introduced into an ideal lip-frame design do not attain an ideal dentofacial esthetic. Facial harmony cannot be achieved by assembling ideal individual elements into a whole. Rather, such harmony can be achieved only when elements showing no identity of shape, color, and position can be visualized in a common relationship. The nature of these relationships constitutes the rationale of esthetics even if this rationale hides a preponderance of the irrational.

Nothing less than repetitive visual training will allow us to grasp the irrational aspect of the esthetic science, to bring it to the level of consciousness, and to discover the way to use it methodically in order to integrate dental elements esthetically in their environment.

In choosing to refer to various frontal facial compositions, all characterized by the presence of dental elements, we react to the human habit of confronting one another face to face, eye to eye. But this field of vision cannot avoid the irrational, manifested in optical illusions and the effects of perspective.

Perspective Effects

The Cartesian philosophy at the base of our medical education does not accept any type of phenomenon, simple or complicated, that cannot be verified. However, analysis of the simplest elements suggests that the really simple does not predominate. Each element hides a complicated phenomenon.

Every object can be subject to apparent deformation in geometric shape whenever observed from certain positions. These deformations result from two types of phenomena: (*1*) the effect of perspective and (*2*) the effect of optical illusion. Though they seem to show specific properties, one esthetic, the other scientific, a precise distinction between these two phenomena is difficult to establish. Our interest will be limited to the description of these phenomena and to the evaluation of their characteristics and impact on a composition. At the same time we will neglect no opportunity of suggesting clinical application so as to help clinicians correct these deformations in their dentofacial compositions.

Perspective is the science and art of representing three-dimensional objects on a flat surface according to optical and mathematical principles. It has been observed that objects seem to diminish in size as they recede further from the eye and that, in general, the appearance of objects differs from the reality. The two basic rules upon which the whole science of perspective rests can be formulated as follows: (*1*) when a line is parallel to the picture plane, its perspective will be parallel to the line itself (Fig 3-11); (*2*) when a line is inclined to the picture plane, its vanishing point may be found by drawing from the eye a visual ray parallel to this line and noting where this ray pierces the picture plane (Fig 3-12).

These two rules indicate that the adoption of a unique point of view displaying selected frontal compositions at different distances already involves elements of deformation, affecting especially its most lateral elements (Fig 3-13).

As a matter of fact, the facial, dentofacial, and dental compositions that seem linear respond or correspond in reality to a spatial organization. This suggests that a shape is never perceived in its real physical properties. "Normal perception is an anomaly" (Helmholz). Illusion and deformation are the rule, leaving our intellect the task of restoring the physical reality.

A cube, for example, is a solid constituted of six equal square faces. However, no point of view is able to embrace the whole reality. Since the capabilities of visual registration are opticophysiological by nature, the characteristics of any shape are always reconstituted by reasoning. The angle of registration of a shape is of primary importance as, depending on the multiplicity of the points of view, a shape may appear more or less identical to that disclosed by the material reality. Whatever the nature of the deformation, on no occasion will more than an appearance by registered.

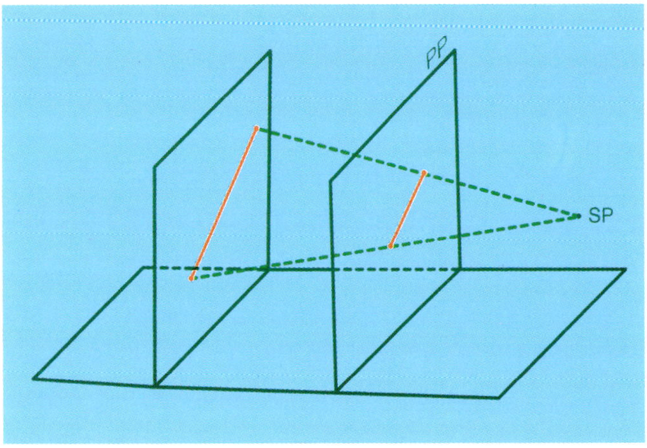

Fig 3-11 When a line is parallel to the picture plane, its perspective will be parallel to the line itself. PP = picture plane, SP = station point.

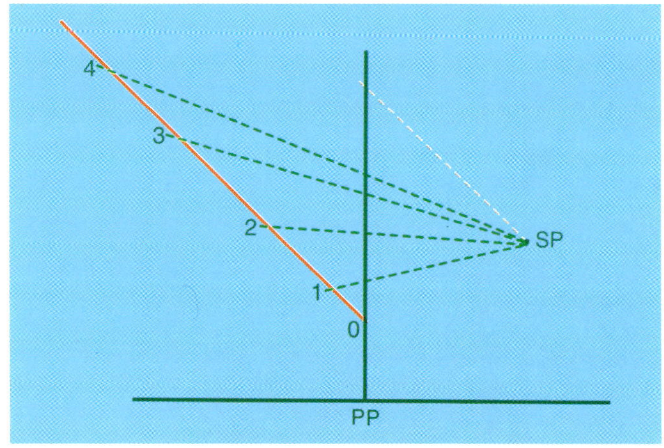

Fig 3-12 When a line is inclined to the picture plane, its vanishing point may be found by drawing from the eye a visual ray parallel to this line and noting where this ray pierces the picture plane. PP = picture plane, SP = station point.

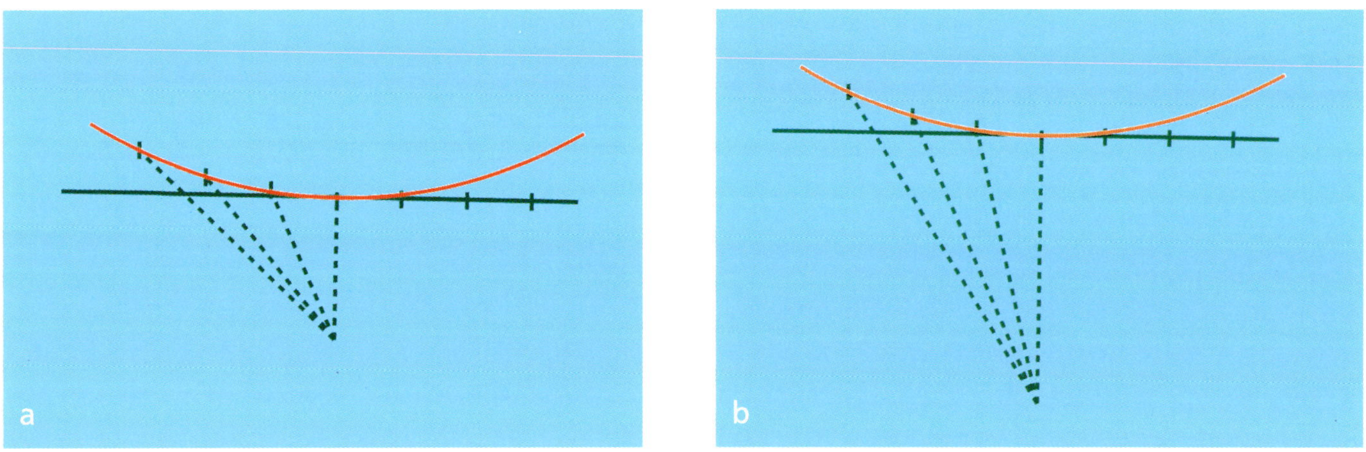

Figs 3-13a and 3-13b The perception of a frontal composition at different distances of focus already involves elements of deformation mainly affecting its most lateral elements. This also includes the perception of the anterior dental segment at different focal distances.

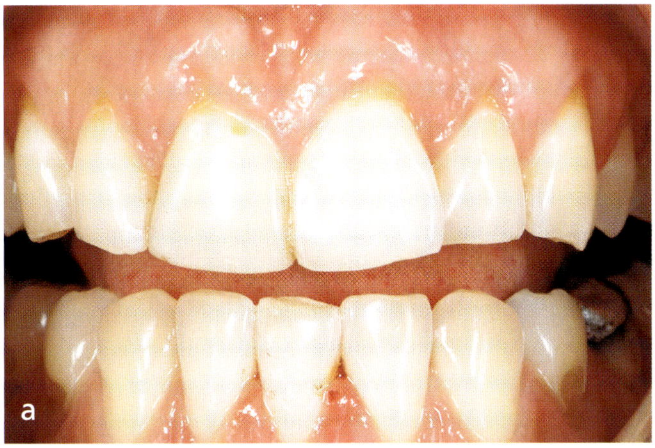

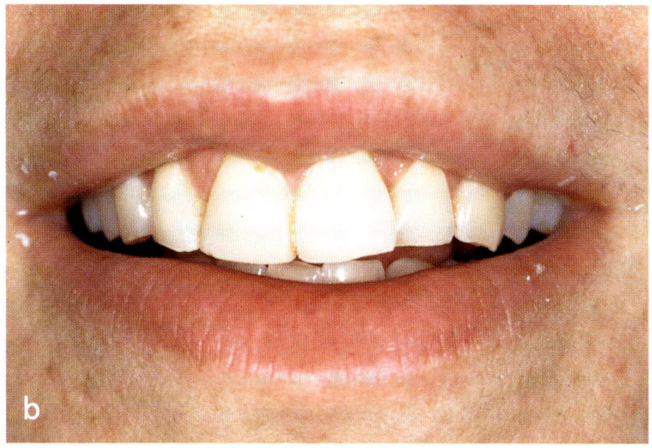

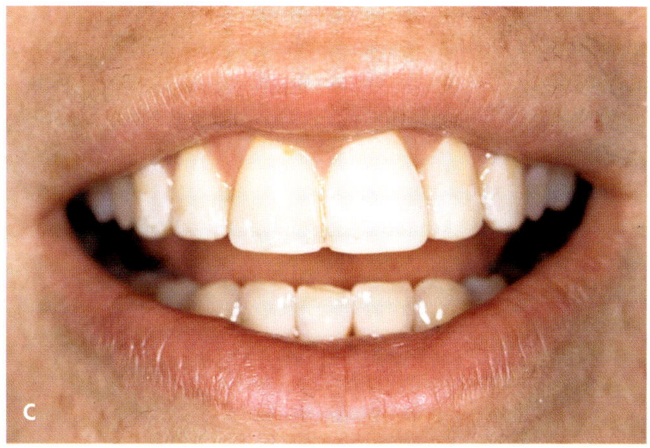

Figs 3-14a to 3-14c From a frontal point of view, the canine displays an appearance that is far from its geometric reality. It has been proposed that half the width of the canine should be in golden relation to the width of the lateral incisor, in turn in golden relation to the width of the central incisor. (a) If this proportional relation can be applied more or less successfully to the right canine, it seems more difficult to apply it to the left canine without introducing an element of visual disturbance into the dental composition. (b) At an increased distance of focus, the absence of proportional relationships affecting the left canine is clearly apparent. It seems that this tooth, presenting morphological manifestations of wear with a distalization of the incisal tip and an effacement of the mesial incline, has gained in width. (c) The effect of perspective is immediately eliminated with a diagnostic tooth reshaping using temporary composite bonding.

The appearance of the canine as registered in a frontal picture plane is far from its geometric reality, but it contributes to the perception of the rhythmic properties of the anterior segment. Objective criteria have established a golden relationship between the width of the central incisor and that of the lateral incisor and in turn between the width of this incisor and half the width of the canine. It can be stated that any incorrect shaping of the canine affects the quality of this relationship. For example, an increase of the axial curvature, an increase of the mesiodistal curvature, a distalization of the incisal tip, and an effacement of the mesial incline are the most common deformities introduced into the morphological design of the canine by accidental aging or during the restorative process through a simple lack of knowledge or a too-close working distance to the object that misses whole perception and therefore fails to detect deformities (Figs 3-14 and 3-15).

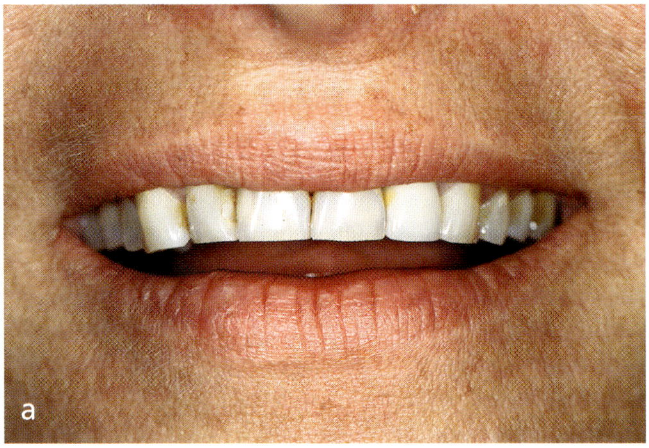

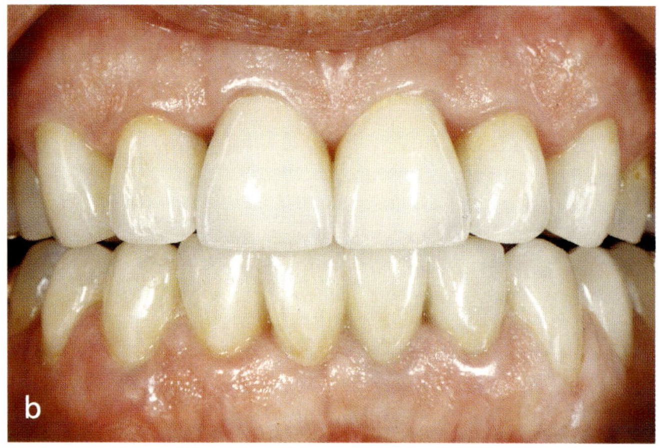

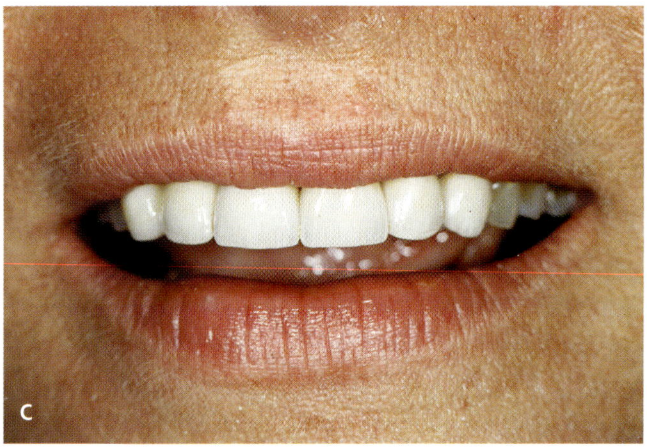

Figs 3-15a to 3-15c (a) At this distance of focus the anterior segment does not present ideal proportional relationships, mainly because of the excess of width affecting the maxillary left lateral incisor. It reflects the nature of a horizontal symmetry, the poor esthetic qualities of which are not enhanced by the reversed curvature of the incisal line. (b) A close view of this restored composition does not reveal any specific morphological distortion either in the upper or lower segments. (c) At this distance of focus the design of both canines, with an excess of incisocervical curvature, increases the canines' apparent width and affects the proportions that should rule the relationships between the elements of the anterior segment.

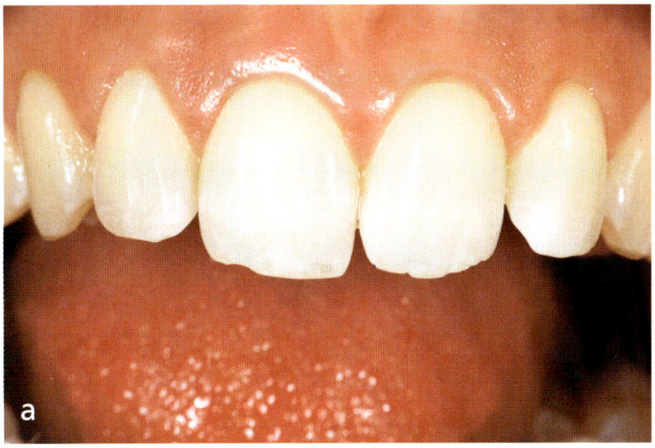

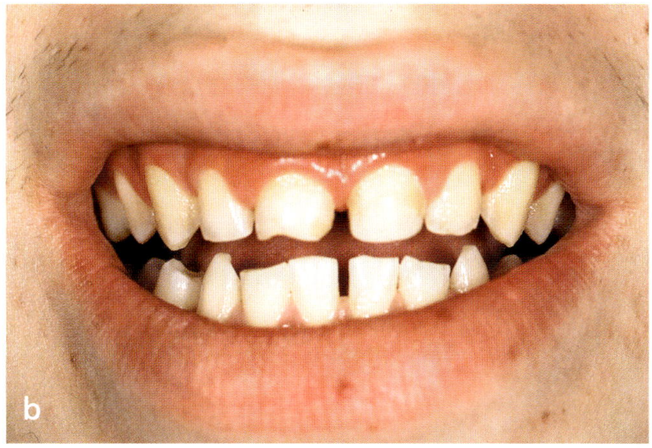

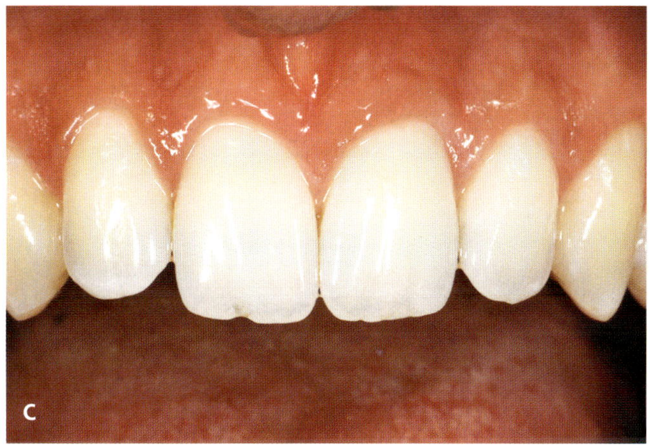

Figs 3-16a to 3-16c The canine often presents a more or less pronounced curvature in its incisal third (a, c) that seems to have been introduced by nature to decrease and so correct in optical appearance the amount of mesial axial inclination of the front-back progression, perceptible at another distance of focus (b).

A frontal view, even if it results in deformations of lateral elements, requires for these elements consideration of their physical design. Observation suggests that adjustments by which architects correct for optical illusions have been already introduced by nature in the anterior dental segment. The morphological design of the canine very often presents in its incisal third a slight concavity (Fig 3-16). It is surprising to note that this morphological particularity most often takes place in a composition characterized by a pronounced mesial inclination of the front-back progression.

Similarly, the Greek architect Vitruvius, noting an apparent enlargement of a square or rectangular architectural surface in its upper portion (Fig 3-17), so that columns perfectly positioned in the vertical plane give a definite feeling of upward divergence, gives precise instructions for correcting these deformities

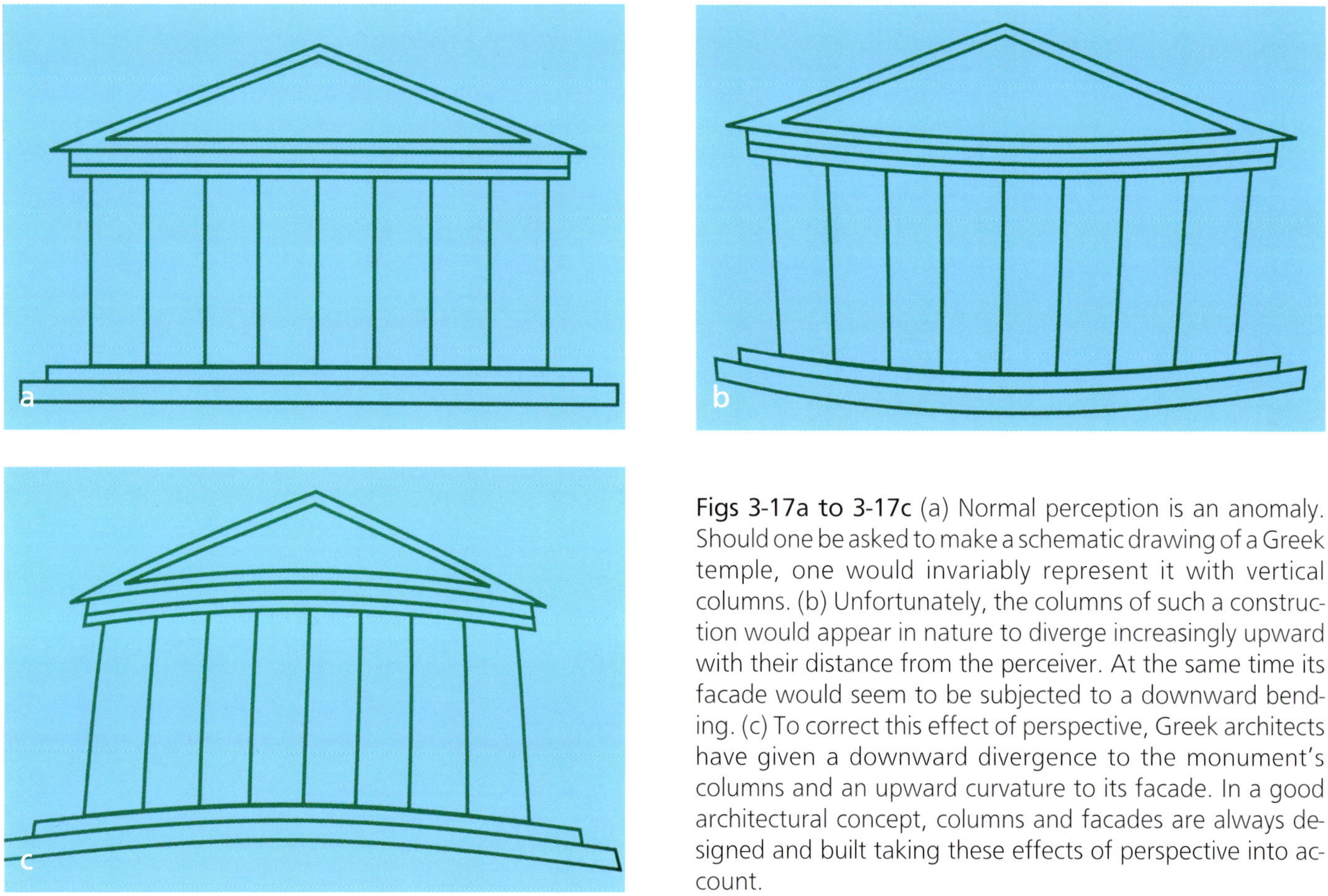

Figs 3-17a to 3-17c (a) Normal perception is an anomaly. Should one be asked to make a schematic drawing of a Greek temple, one would invariably represent it with vertical columns. (b) Unfortunately, the columns of such a construction would appear in nature to diverge increasingly upward with their distance from the perceiver. At the same time its facade would seem to be subjected to a downward bending. (c) To correct this effect of perspective, Greek architects have given a downward divergence to the monument's columns and an upward curvature to its facade. In a good architectural concept, columns and facades are always designed and built taking these effects of perspective into account.

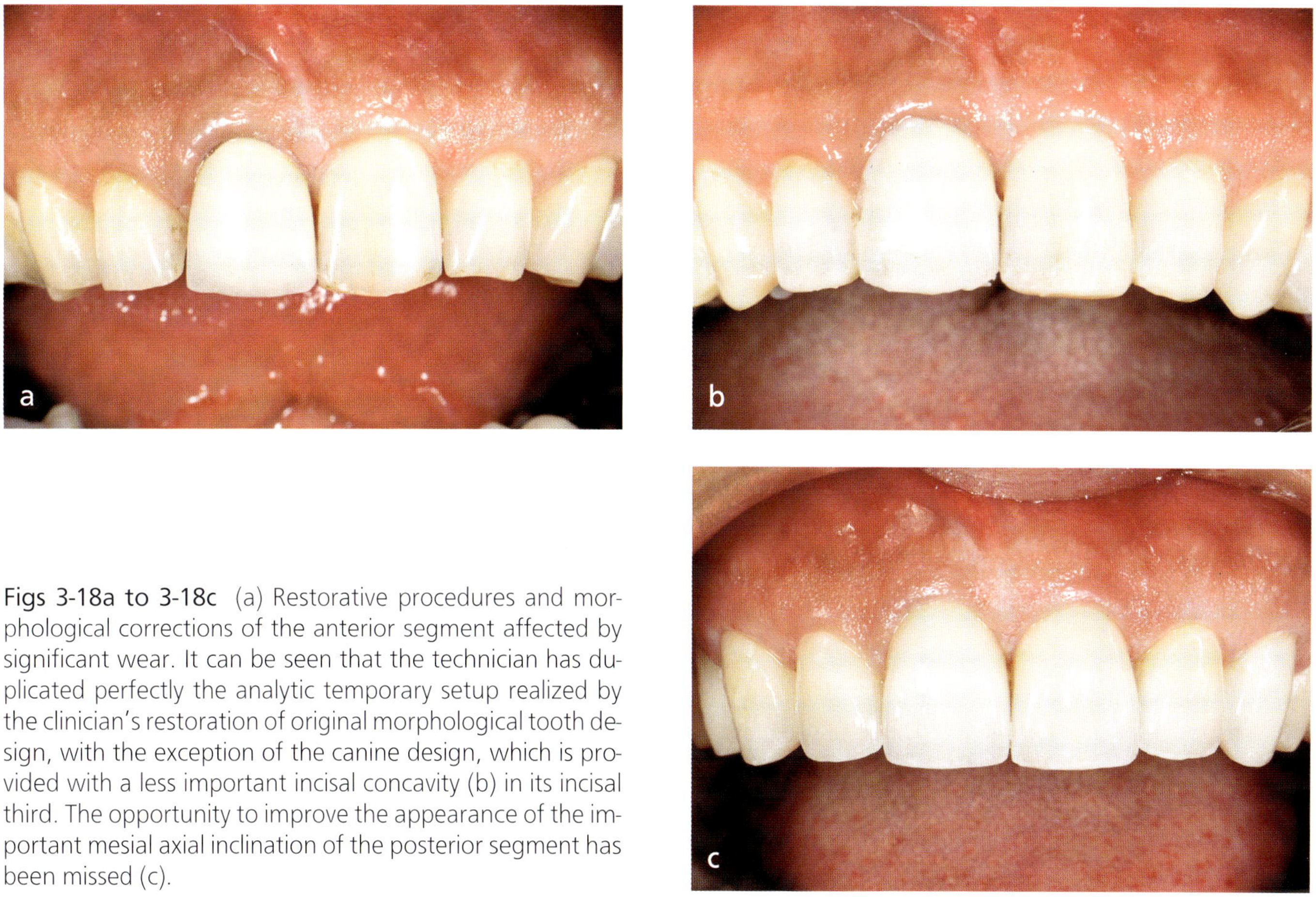

Figs 3-18a to 3-18c (a) Restorative procedures and morphological corrections of the anterior segment affected by significant wear. It can be seen that the technician has duplicated perfectly the analytic temporary setup realized by the clinician's restoration of original morphological tooth design, with the exception of the canine design, which is provided with a less important incisal concavity (b) in its incisal third. The opportunity to improve the appearance of the important mesial axial inclination of the posterior segment has been missed (c).

by placing the base of the columns slightly further apart in the lower portion, leaving to the optical properties of the eye the task of restoring their verticality.

These considerations suggest that a minor modification in the design of the buccal cusp of canines and premolars may reduce the effects of an overpronounced mesial inclination of the posterior segments and break the feeling of a small mouth affecting a number of dentofacial compositions, in particular Class II, division 2 dental arrangements (Figs 3-18 and 3-19).

Such problems as vertical bone loss leading to increased tooth length, divergent tooth axial direction, and overbulked canine curvature to meet with occlusal requirements require familiarity with the particulars of optical effects in the clinician, who may then compensate for the resulting morphological deficiencies. Yet it must be stressed that perspective deformation only explains a limited number of modifications of forms.

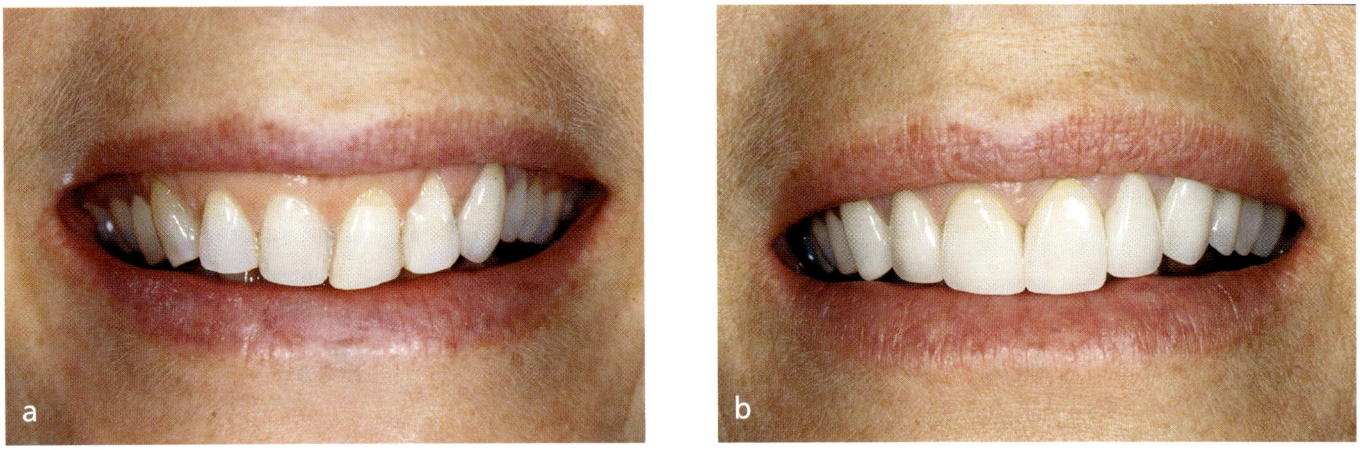

Figs 3-19a and 3-19b (a) An attractive smile composition despite a high lip-line level and anterior malpositions. A too-bulky restored maxillary left canine and a left posterior segment in passive eruption break the continuity of the front-back progression. (b) Restoration of the anterior segment with a slight tooth lengthening to reduce gingival display. The maxillary left canine and premolar are designed with an incisal concavity to optically correct the posterior inward axial inclination of the restored front-back progression.

Optical Illusions

When rules of perspective cannot be applied and deformation results from specific conditions, defying logical explanation, the terminology *optical illusion* is usually applied. For example, perfectly square shapes are formed by two horizontal lines and two vertical lines. In one of them, we take out the two vertical lines and fill the square exclusively with horizontal lines. In the other, we take out the two horizontal lines and fill the square exclusively with vertical lines. Without the introduction of any type of dimensional change, the square with horizontal lines will seem longer, the square with vertical lines will seem wider (Fig 3-20). This is an optical illusion.

This phenomenon is irrational, as is another involving the appearance of identical square shapes of different colors. A dark red square, for example, will appear larger, a blue one smaller (Fig 3-21). White and yellow objects will appear larger than identically shaped dark ones.

Further, a vertical line looks longer than a horizontal of the same length. This appearance, however, can be explained by the physiological capacities of the muscles of the eye, which execute a horizontal movement more easily than a vertical one (Fig 3-22).

The multiple vertical and horizontal linear tracings that distort the appearance of squares have no such effect on other shapes (Fig 3-23). One must keep in mind the particular impact of light reflection on curved or flat surfaces (Fig 3-24) and remain aware

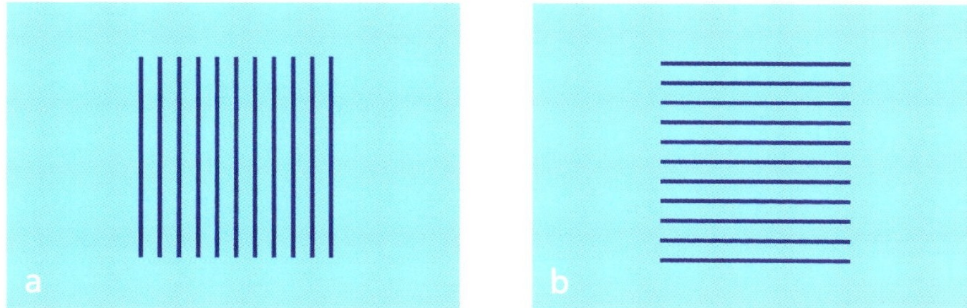

Figs 3-20a and 3-20b A square is constituted by two vertical and two horizontal lines. (a) If provided with vertical lines the square will seem wider; (b) if provided with horizontal lines, it will seem longer.

Figs 3-21a to 3-21c Colors also generate optical phenomena. (a) The red expands while (c) the blue reduces the same square shape. This principle of surface expansion is currently used in tooth bleaching and in the application of lipstick.

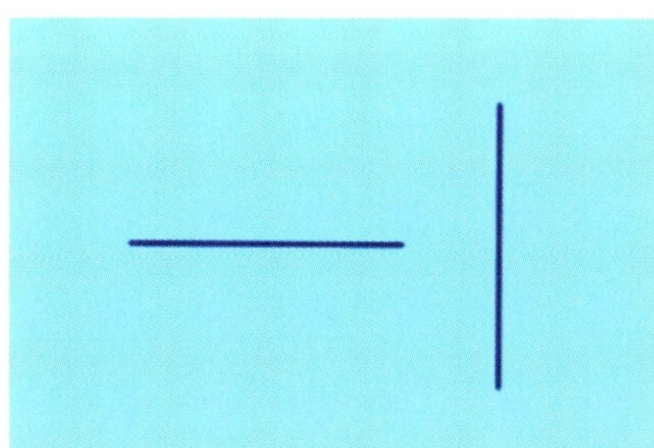

Fig 3-22 Because of the eye's ability to move more easily on a horizontal than on a vertical plane, a vertical line seems longer than a horizontal line of the same length.

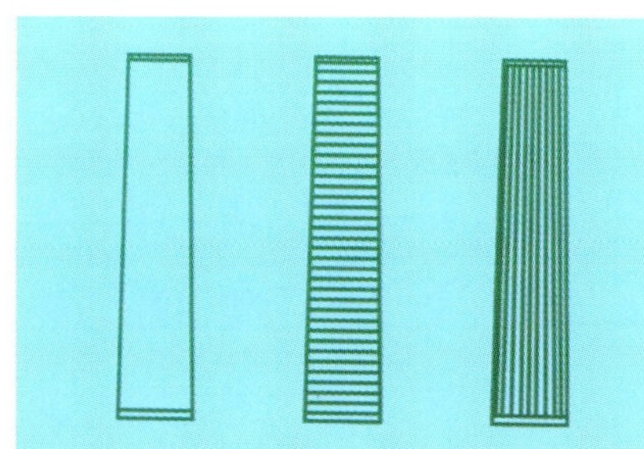

Fig 3-23 The accumulation of lines on a rectangle no longer creates the optical effects produced by such lines on a square. On an elongated tube, column, or tooth, it creates an opposite effect; horizontal lines shorten and vertical lines lengthen the appearance of the structure.

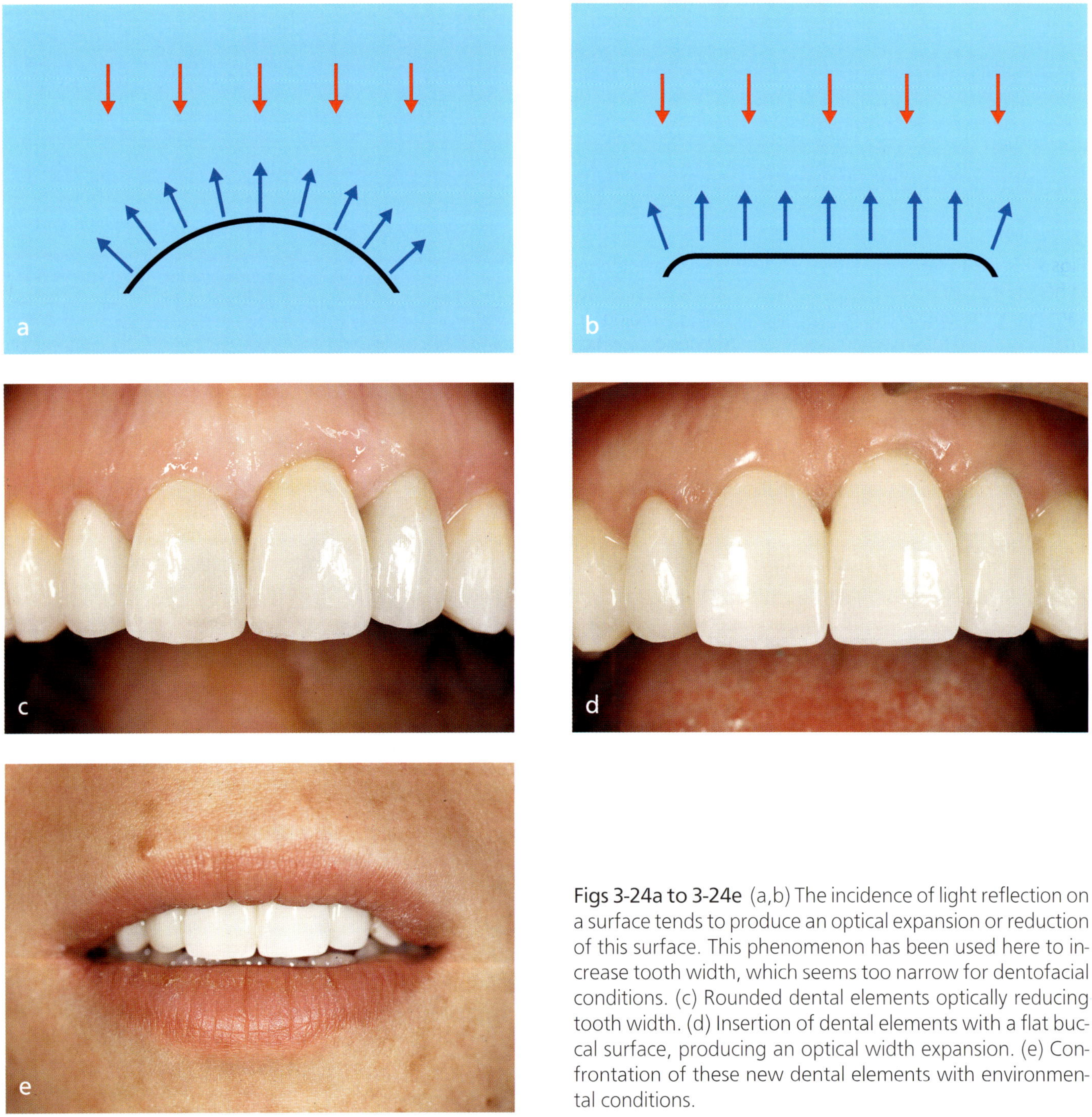

Figs 3-24a to 3-24e (a,b) The incidence of light reflection on a surface tends to produce an optical expansion or reduction of this surface. This phenomenon has been used here to increase tooth width, which seems too narrow for dentofacial conditions. (c) Rounded dental elements optically reducing tooth width. (d) Insertion of dental elements with a flat buccal surface, producing an optical width expansion. (e) Confrontation of these new dental elements with environmental conditions.

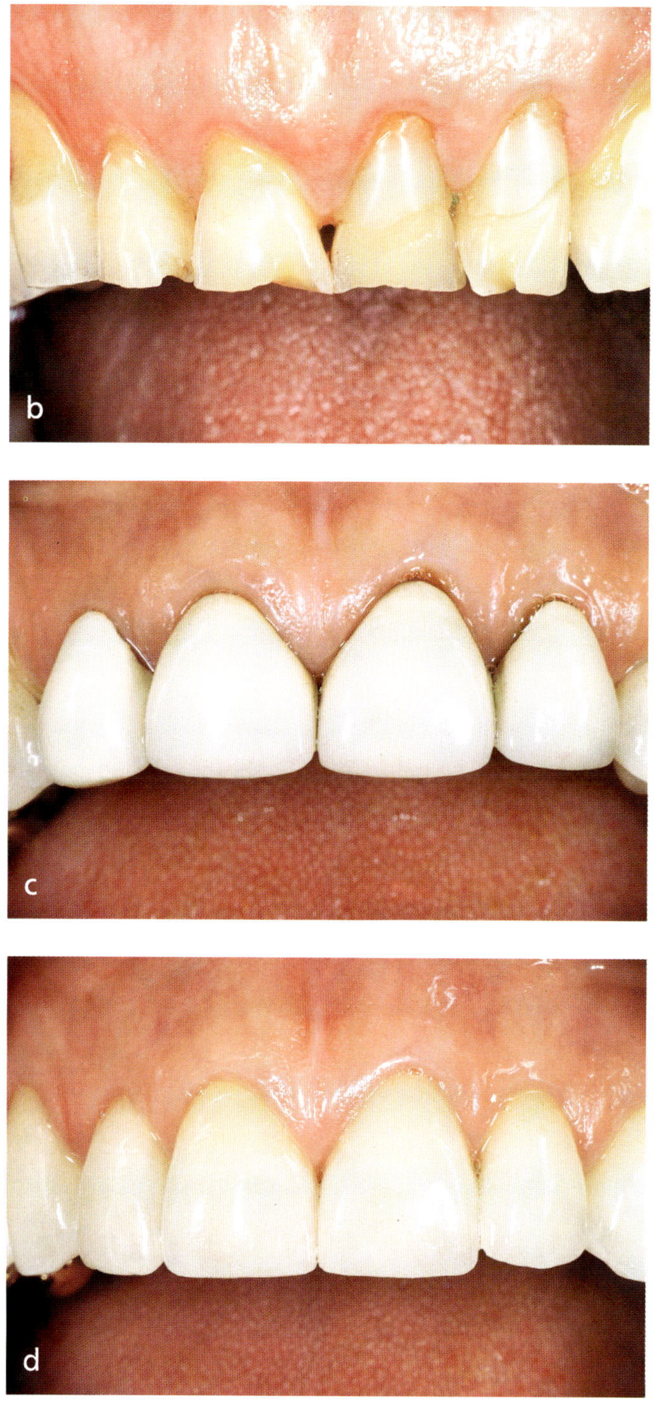

Figs 3-25a to 3-25d (a) An equilateral triangle appears longer in height than in width. (b) Nature seems to have taken advantage of this optical illusion by systematically providing victims of aging dental elements with tapered designs, which optically elongate reduced tooth length. (c) Contrary to what has been claimed, tapered tooth design is unusual in young individuals and results either from faulty restorative procedures or from pathological periodontal tissue conditions. (d) A better laboratory approach could have totally corrected this triangular tooth design.

of other illusions created by the physiological capabilities of the eye.

An equilateral triangle, for example, will always appear longer in height than in width. This means that a tapered tooth design will make a tooth seem longer than it is and so should always be avoided when an important resorption has affected the dental crest, imposing an elongated tooth design, whether a pontic or tooth implant unit. A tapered tooth shape should only be used with short dental elements, where apparent elongation is desirable, just as nature models compensatory tapered tooth designs when parafunctional habits (Fig 3-25) have progressively shortened tooth morphology.

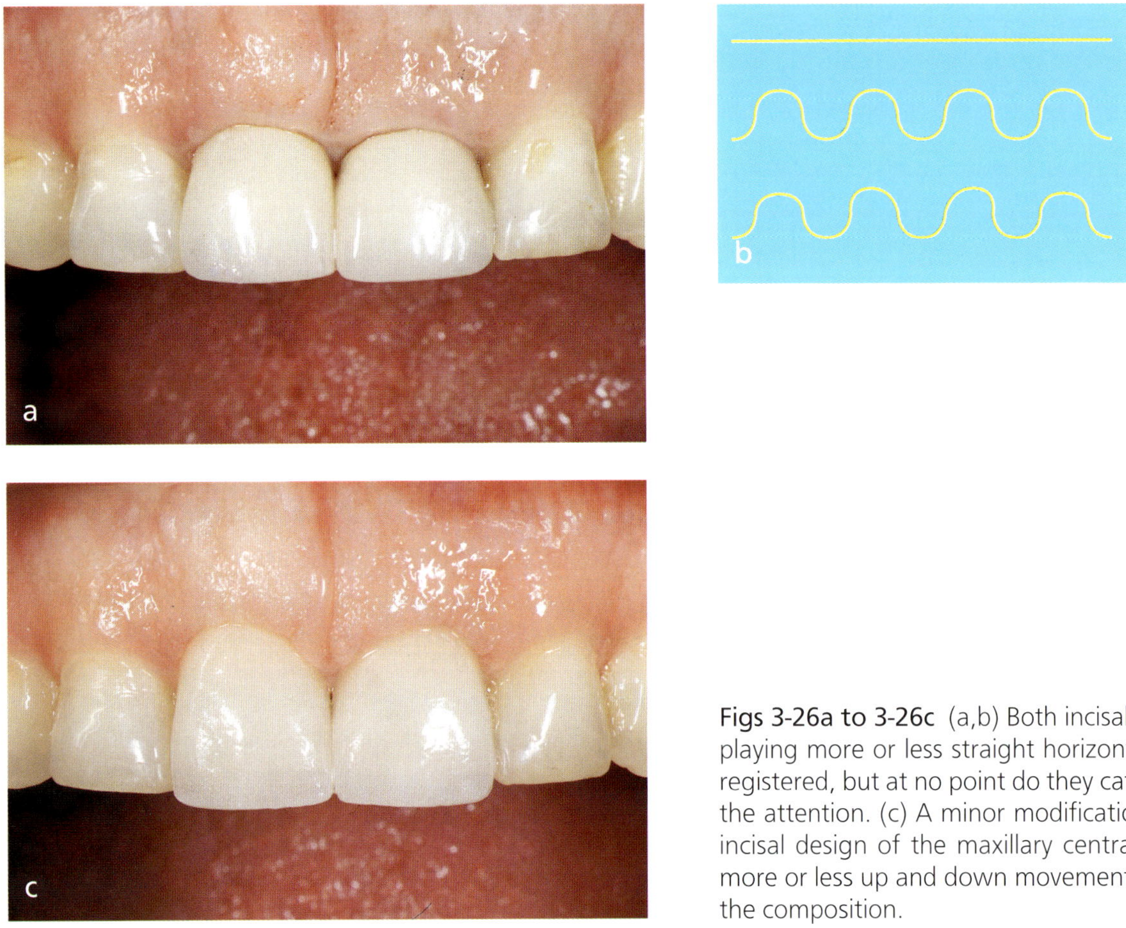

Figs 3-26a to 3-26c (a,b) Both incisal and gingival lines displaying more or less straight horizontal designs are rapidly registered, but at no point do they catch the eyes and focus the attention. (c) A minor modification of the gingival and incisal design of the maxillary central incisors, requiring a more or less up and down movement of the eye, enhances the composition.

Whereas the registration of a horizontal line requires a simple movement of the eye, the registration of an undulating line requires an up and down ocular movement, which may leave time for the appreciation of its characteristics and generate esthetic appeal. The field of optical illusion is replete with linear elements able to arouse our esthetic sensibility (Fig 3-26). It has been observed, for example, that a dotted line generates less directional strength than a full line of the same length and is usually registered as shorter (Fig 3-27).

An alignment of dental elements provided with well-marked incisal spaces, simulating—at a proper distance of focus—a dotted line, promotes an apparent reduction of the anterior segment, whereas the absence of interdental spaces in an incisal alignment, such as occurs in completely worn dentitions, simulates a straight line and so results in the apparent enlargement of the anterior segment (Fig 3-28). This phenomenon concerns every practitioner who deals with the restoration of the anterior segment.

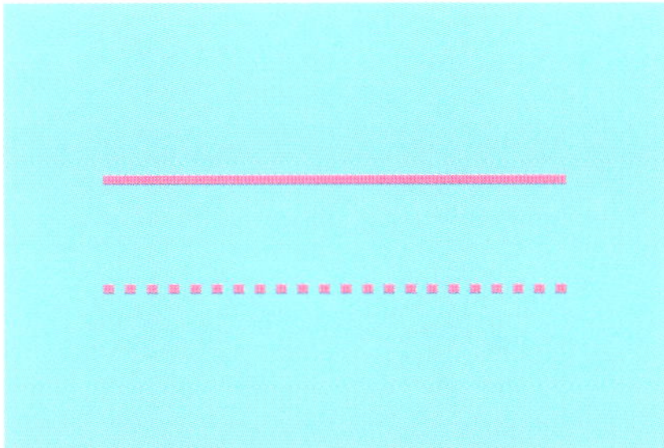

Fig 3-27 A dotted line suggests less directional strength than a straight line of the same length.

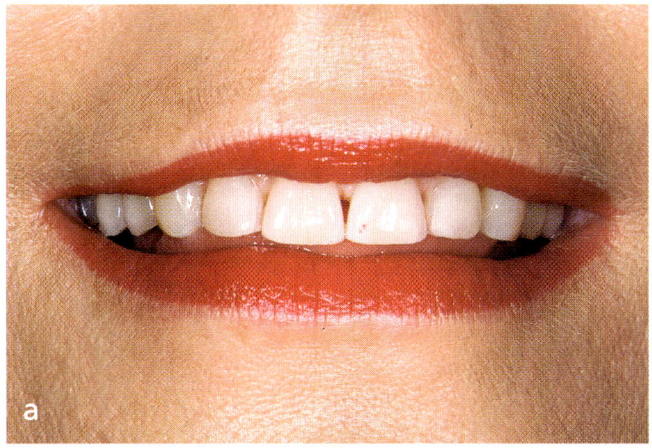

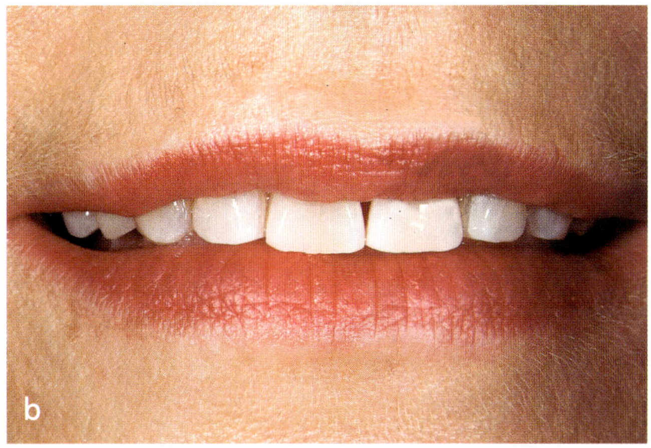

Figs 3-28a and 3-28b (a) The apparently straight incisal line with worn dental elements seems to extend the width of the dental segment. (b) A modification of maxillary incisor tooth length, where interincisal spaces simulate a dotted line, optically shortens the width of the dental segment.

How many times do practitioners limit therapeutic modalities to the restoration of four to six anterior teeth when the whole dentition reflects the impact of abrasion, unaware that the patient will complain of reduced "mouth width"? Marked interincisal spaces breaking the incisal line and a tooth length that slightly exceeds that of the previous elements simulate a dotted line, and the resulting apparent loss of directional strength will deeply affect the patient's satisfaction. It must be kept in mind that patients are influenced by magazine photos of smiling people with large, straight, white incisal lines, whatever the variations affecting the spatial position of the teeth.

The feeling of reduced mouth width, however unjustified, leads to deep patient resentment and yet is extremely difficult for the practitioner to identify at close range, since it results from an optical phenomenon arising from ruptures in the continuity of the linear reading of the dental composition.

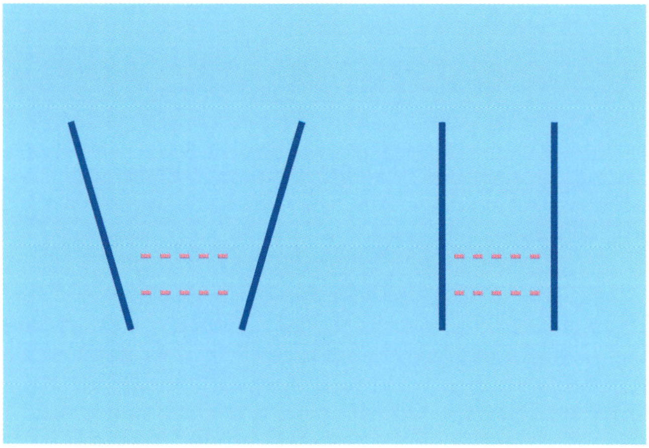

Fig 3-29 In the confrontation of a full line and a dotted line, the full line is experienced first. In the confrontation of two dotted lines, the rapidity of registration of one or the other line will depend on the nature of the surrounding structures. Embedded between a full linear angle design, the dotted line close to the angle will be registered first and as longer than the second one, which is affected by the preceding registration.

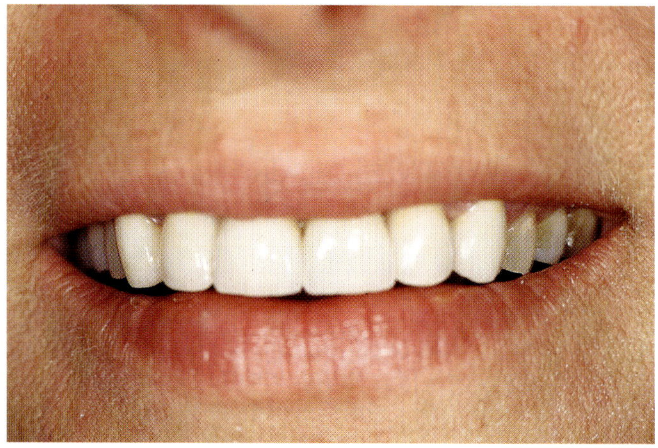

Fig 3-30 When shadow, darkness, or malposition reduce the visibility of the posterior segments, only the anterior segment embedded between mouth corners, simulating a dotted line, is registered. The rhythm of successive readings that usually takes place when coordination between anterior and posterior planes does exist is broken, and the whole dental segment appears reduced in width.

When these two types of lines, dotted and full, are present, the eye is first attracted by the registration of the full line and in a second stage by the dotted line, which generates less visual attraction or, as it has been called, directional strength. If we take, for example, two dotted lines parallel to each other, equal in length and embedded in an acute angle, the line closer to this angle will appear longer than the other. They will appear of equal length again as the angle is opened (Fig 3-29).

This phenomenon has opticophysiological causes. Only after the easily individualized full line is registered does the eye perceive the dotted line, which, because it maintains very close contact with the angular full line, will resist identification and consequently require more time to be individualized. This will make it appear to have a more important linear length than the second dotted line, which not only benefits from the previous identification but also generates less interest by reason of its retruded position (Fig 3-30).

This means that in the frontal evaluation of the dentofacial composition, the anterior segment is first registered as a dotted line surrounded by the full line of mouth corner and negative space. Only then will the posterior area be registered in a progressive rhythmic reading when presenting elements of visual attraction like well-designed canine tips invading the negative space.

As to disturbances affecting the development of the posterior front-back progression and resulting from malposed dental elements, unfavorable tooth axial directions, or differences in gingival margin levels, illusion and reality can generate identical percep-

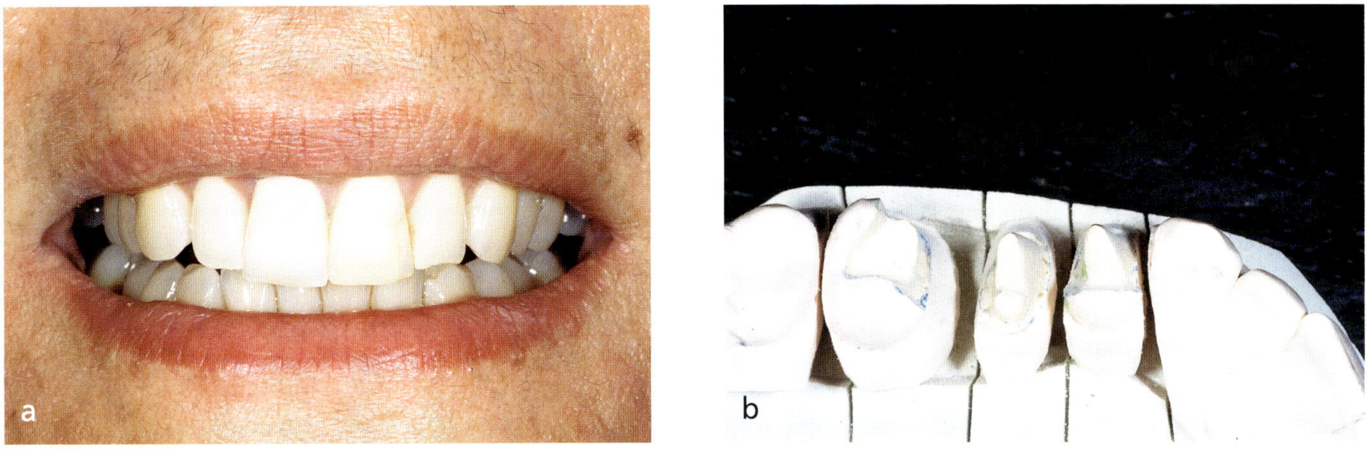

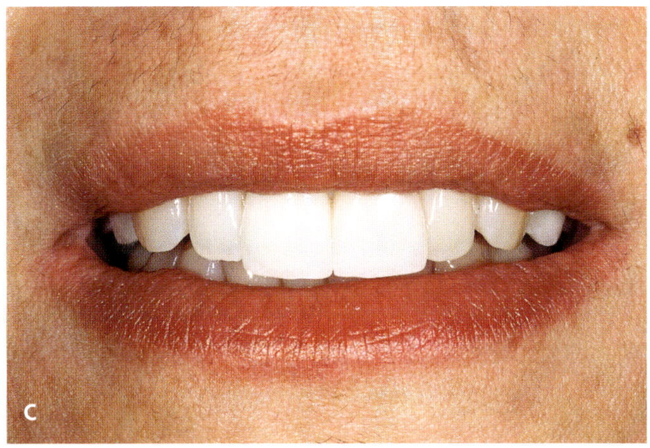

Figs 3-31a to 3-31c (a) Malposed posterior dental segments produce a feeling of reduced mouth width. (b, c) A material expansion of the posterior segment using bonded porcelain veneers provided with sharp incisal tips invading the negative space attracts visual attention and progressive optical registration, producing the expansion of the dental composition with respect to the front-back linearity.

tions. But there is no difference in treatment modalities that require a lateral extension of the restorative process involving first and second premolars and sometimes first molars to remove the illusion or reality of a linear rupture (Fig 3-31). In practice, bonded additive veneers applied to the buccal and occlusal surfaces of well-prepared dental elements will restore the continuity of the front-back progression and increase the perceptive registration of the posterior segment during the development of the smile.

All these observations confirm the complexity of a comprehensive esthetic setup that will provide the composition with elementary optical corrections. They also confirm the importance of understanding the nature of the optical phenomenon involved. However, understanding remains useless where perceptive capabilities fail. Both knowledge and esthetic perceptive capabilities require constant effort and repetitive training. Creativity and visual perception represent the two extremes of esthetic communication, which can communicate only when a common language has been developed.

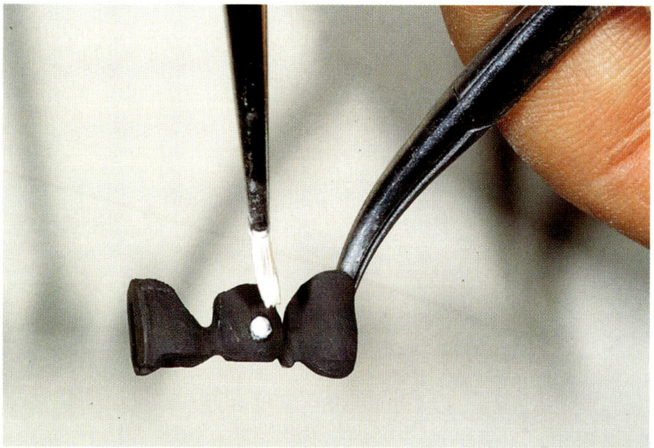

Fig 3-32 The material event of creativity involves no more than the meeting between tool and esthetic support. The result of this meeting is the point.

Esthetic Means

Esthetic language

The phenomenon of creativity in all fields is felt as an answer that suddenly overwhelms the questions, as the accomplishment of the laborious search with which one has identified one's existence. It expresses the buried tendencies of the subconscious. It involves at the same time emotion and sensory spirit. It unifies the moment of invention and realization, the knowing and the making. It involves a definite though temporary rupture with negative cultural experiences and social structures. However, though isolated in their own world, creators can never fully escape environmental influences and structures; they must return to them when creation has been achieved, if only for the purpose of communication.

In art, the material elements of creation have varied little during the last centuries: brushes, paints, charcoals, stones, wood, canvas, paper. The material act of creation involves no more than the meeting between the tool and the support, the result of which is a point, the primary element of esthetic language (Fig 3-32).

The point

In geometry, the point is a totally abstract element, invisible and immaterial. Finding materialization in the written language, the geometric point becomes a sign, a useful element with a practical application, but at the same time a habit that has lost expressivity through this restrictive use. In written language, it has taken on the symbolic signification of the interruption of connection between two elements, a signification with both negative and positive connotations. This has contributed to concealing its multiple properties.

If, however, it is isolated from this field of action its inner characteristics, which have been strangled, will appear. The geometric point, from being invisi-

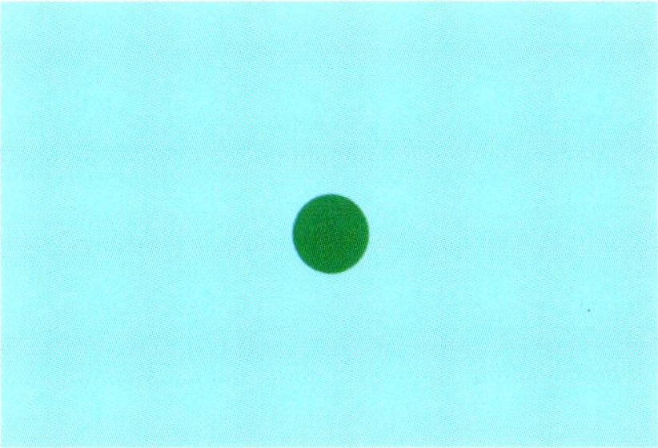

Fig 3-33 From a geometric point of view, the point is invisible, immaterial, abstract. In its esthetic realization it can be defined as the smallest basic shape but may grow and occupy a certain surface. In abstract thought, it cannot be other than ideally round, ideally small. It is static, isolated, turned toward itself, completely introverted. These qualities, at the same time both geometric and psychological, constitute the basic elements of esthetic language.

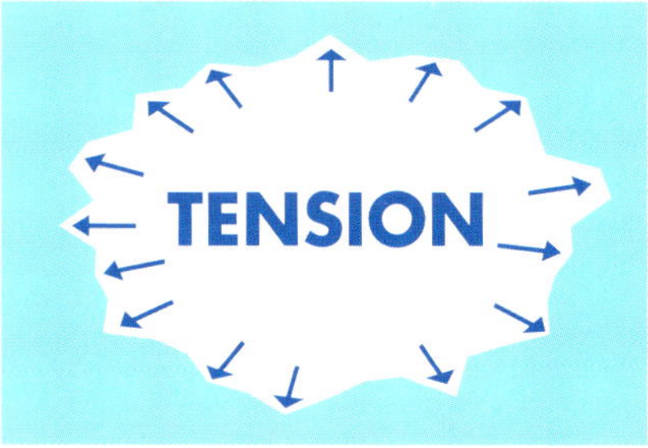

Fig 3-34 Each shape is the result of its inner significance expressed by tension. No shape says nothing.

ble, suddenly becomes perceivable, reaches a certain dimension, occupies a certain surface, possesses contours and limits (Fig 3-33). In its material form, of which the shape and dimension may vary, the point can be defined as the smallest basic shape. But the notion of the smallest basic shape defies definition. The point may grow, and in the absence of any possibility of precise measurement one must accept the idea that only intuition can evaluate its extreme limits. This evaluation of the exterior limit of the point will define its exterior form.

In abstract thought, the point cannot be anything other than ideally round, ideally small. In its interior significance, it constitutes a notion subconsciously linked to a great restraint. It is a world by itself, isolated from surrounding structures and manifesting no inclination to integrate. It firmly maintains its position, shows no tendency to any movement—horizontal, vertical, forward, or backward. It is totally static. It represents absolute conciseness. It is an introvert. It never loses these characteristics, whatever the irregularities developed by its exterior design. Its basic tension remains concentric, even when eccentric tendencies interfere.

The exterior limits of a material shape are only the expression of intrinsic constraints at work within that shape. Indeed, the point's contours, like its dimensions, can take on multiple appearances. From its circular shape it can assume other geometric shapes with unlimited variation: dentated, pointed, triangular, or square. These characteristics define the exterior limits of its material shape.

The physical materialization of the point that constitutes the basic esthetic element arises not from chance but from the living tensions that form it. "Each shape is the result of the inner constraints contained in the element, expressed by tension. Each shape is the expression of its significance" (Kandinski) (Fig 3-34).These considerations distinguish the point as the primary element of esthetic language. Its qualities, at the same time both geometric and psychological, are never dissociated. In fact, no shape exists which says nothing.

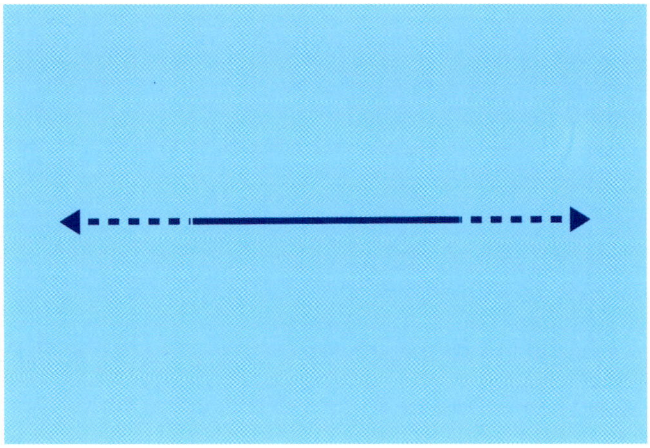

Fig 3-35 The line—invisible, immaterial—arises from an impulse given to the geometric point in one direction or another. This direction gives the line its significance.

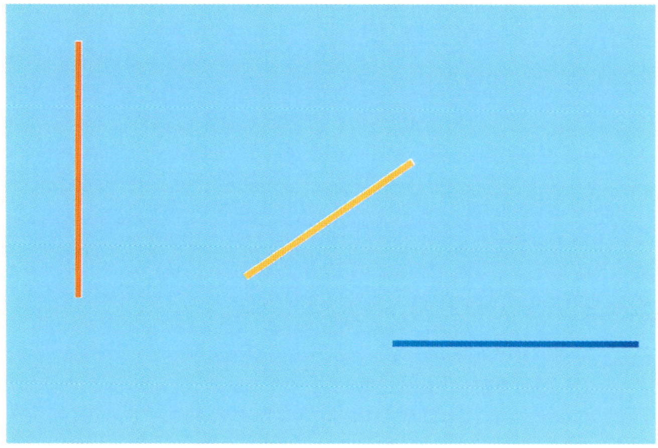

Fig 3-36 The horizontal line corresponds to the surface on which we live, walk, and die. It has cold associations. The vertical line, on the contrary, is associated with warmth, with activity and physical vitality and with psychic and physical excitement. The diagonal line represents the infinite possibilities of cold-warm movements. It introduces a dynamic arising from unresolved tension between cold and warm.

The perception of the tensional strength displayed by a variety of shapes is a characteristic of human sensibility. This results from the suggestive action of direct or allegoric symbols. Abstraction in no way dilutes the subconscious effect of symbols; in fact, it has long been demonstrated that "abstract" shapes seem to have more expressive strength than natural ones. Every element conceived as an entity will invariably generate a chain of reaction:

- inner tension
- shape materialization
- perception
- receptivity

This chain of events will subconsciously determine the specific significance of this element.

The line

The line is born of the destruction of the immobility of the point and introduces an element of dynamism. The geometric line—invisible, immaterial—results from an impulse given to the geometric point. When an exterior force induces the movement of a point in a determined direction with a tendency to continue toward infinity, we have a straight line (Fig 3-35). The straight line represents the most concise form of the infinite possibilities of movement.

The tension that represents the live forces of an element constitutes only one part of the movement. The other part is the direction. These are the two characteristics that mark the difference between point and line and permit us to differentiate a horizontal from a vertical or diagonal line (Fig 3-36). This differ-

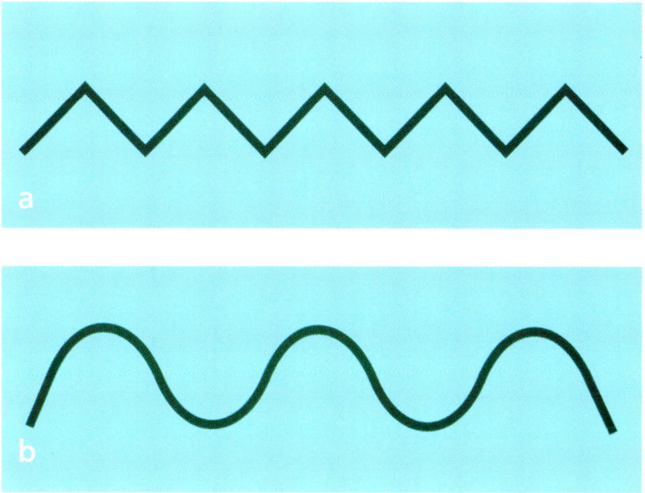

Figs 3-37a and 3-37b (a) Contrary to the straight line, which expresses a unique significance, broken lines reflect a conflict and the alternate application of other forces. (b) Curved lines are nothing other than straight lines subjected along their course to a constant tension. They express the qualities associated with the most open angles: psychological and physical stability and maturity.

entiation is important because of the specific significance associated with each line direction. The horizontal line suggests the surface on which we move, live, and die. It has a "cold" significance and can be considered the most concise form of the infinite possibilities of cold movement (Fig 3-36). Opposed to this line, and at a right angle to it, the vertical line (Fig 3-36) develops in height and represents the most concise form of the infinite possibilities of warm movement. Vertical movement is "warm" because it expresses a primordial significance: the desire of humanity to free itself from the forces of gravity or to elevate itself spiritually and socially.

These denominations of cold and warm that define the inner properties of the lines represent phenomena universally accepted by psychologists, physicists, and artists. It has been demonstrated that these physio-psychological phenomena are associated with others: cold with calm, passivity, and depression; warm with activity, excitement, and intensity. The meeting of these two lines represents the symbol in human experience of absolute equilibrium, of vertical tension on a horizontal plane.

The diagonal line (Fig 3-36), presenting the same inclination toward horizontal and vertical, is the most concise form of the infinite possibilities of cold-warm movement, since the diagonal possesses both qualities. Diagonal lines introduce strong directional impulses, a dynamic arising from unresolved tendencies toward the vertical or the horizontal. All other lines represent only variant forms of these three lines.

Straight lines express a single significance; broken or curved lines express conflict. Curved lines and broken lines originate from two forces either simultaneously or alternately applied (Fig 3-37). The significance of such a line is linked to that of its constitutive elements and to the nature of its angles: straight, acute, or obtuse (Fig 3-38).

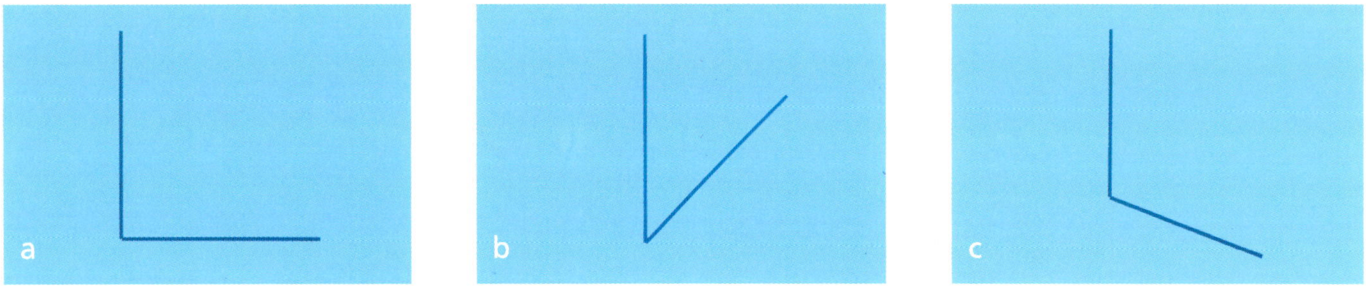

Fig 3-38a to 3-38c Human sensibility attributes to straight, acute, or obtuse angles qualities of color, rhythm, temperature, or action. Lines, colors, and shapes possess their own forms of expression independent of any association with the external aspects of the world. Their actions are self-conditioned phenomena, rooted in human nature.

	Straight angle (a)	Acute angle (b)	Obtuse angle (c)
Temperature	Cold-warm	Warm	Cold
Action / Dynamic	Deliberate	Spontaneous	Mental static
Rhythm	Moderato	Presto	Adagio
Color	Red	Yellow	Blue
Musical sound	Calm	Acute	Deep

The right angle can be described as the most objective, expressing self-control, reflection, and maturity, though variations in the length of its segments can modify its significance. The acute angle stresses activity, capabilities of action and execution, dynamism and aggressiveness—characteristics linked to the capabilities of the young. The obtuse angle suggests passivity and weakness, and the progressive opening of this angle that results from a proportionate diminution of tension can be interpreted as an increase of these qualities.

The curved line is nothing other than a straight line subjected, along its course, to a constant tension (Fig 3-37). The growth of stability and reliable maturity, in the sense of physical and psychological development, characterizes the curved line. The difference between a straight and a curved line lies in the number and the nature of the tensions that are applied to them. Whenever the straight line is subjected to two primary tensions, these tensions are overpowered in the curved line by a third tension working with constant pressure in opposition to the others.

The harmony of the curved line can be directly opposed to that of the straight line, and the broken line suggests a transition between these. The geometric qualities of broken and curved lines are linked to the nature of their angles. They are not mere abstract elements but manifest specific qualities of significance rooted in human sensibility.

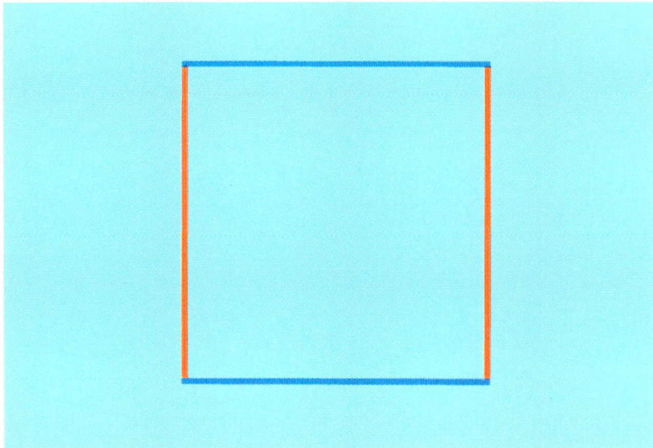

Fig 3-39 Two elements of warm opposed to two elements of cold determine the calm serenity of the square plane.

The plane

The line possesses the ability to generate a plane when exterior forces superimpose their action on that of its primary tension. At the same time, the material point, in reaching a certain dimension, may also become a plane but will lose its pure significance in this transformation. However, the geometric boundaries between these two entities, point and plane, are imperceptible.

But whatever its origins, any form or shape can indifferently take part in or support a composition. The distinction between a shape, a form, and a plane is purely academic. A schematic design facilitates the qualification as artistic support and takes the denomination of plane. In its most fundamental manifestation, the plane can be schematically reduced to a space limited by two horizontal and two vertical lines. We know the significance of a horizontal and a vertical line: two elements of warm calm and two elements of cold calm whose combination defines the resonance or the calm serenity of the square plane (Fig 3-39). The predominance of one tendency over the other or the predominance of length or width that takes place, for example, in a rectangle according to its position promotes the prevalence of an objective sonority of cold or warm. As a result, identical elements placed in a plane reflecting a cold or a warm resonance, whatever the positioning, can hardly completely dissipate the quality of this atmosphere (Fig 3-40). But a multiplication of upward active tensions, for example, in a cold plane will create by opposition a dramatic, though purely psychological, tension (Fig 3-41). We may thus conclude that the plane is a deliberate visual limitation of a portion of space in which a composition will take place.

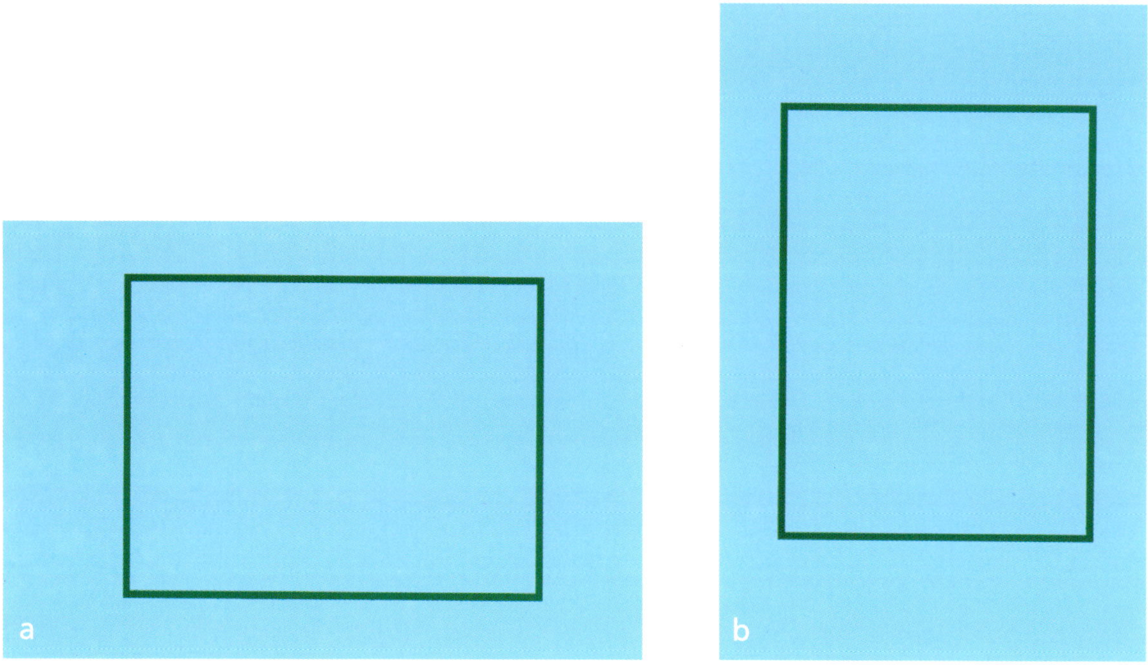

Figs 3-40a and 3-40b The predominance of one tendency over the other—the predominance of length or width in the rectangular plane, for example—promotes for the plane an objective sonority of warm (a) or cold (b).

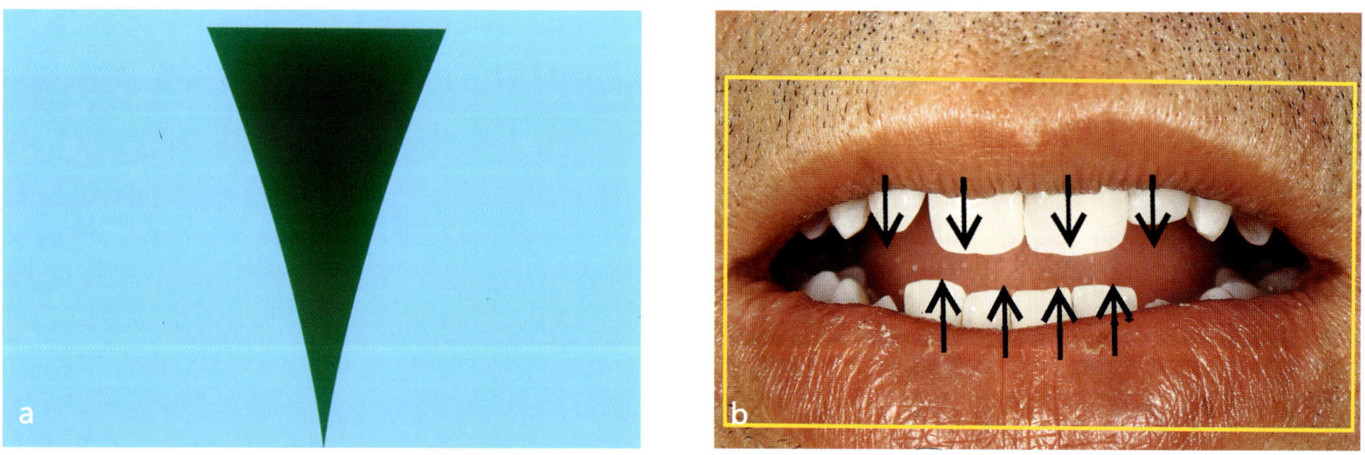

Figs 3-41a and 3-41b (a) The multiplication of upward or downward active tensions located in a cold plane, for example, will generate a dramatization of these tensions by simple opposition. Yet when too strongly opposed, the confrontation of these tensions may become unbearable. This play of tensions is dictated by the geometric shape of the basic plane. (b) In this particular case, individualized dental elements generate upward and downward tensions in strong opposition to the position and design of the supporting plane.

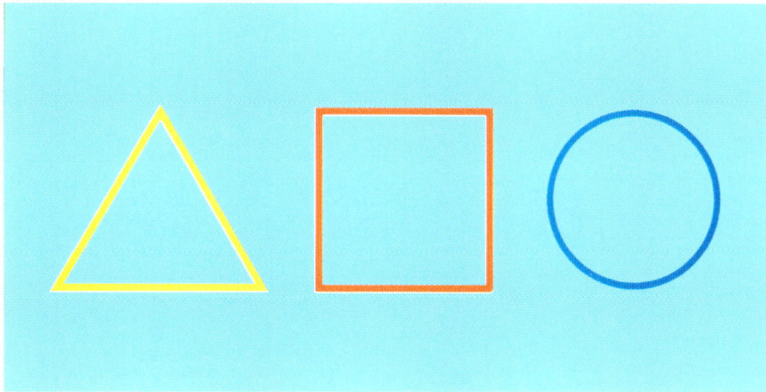

Fig 3-42 Shapes stand as limitations of space or surface. Each shape has its inner substance with its own resonance. The perception of this resonance is not objective but linked to the receptivity of the observer. Natural or abstract, no shape says nothing. The perception of its significance is innate in human sensibility. Three acute tensions for the triangle, four calm tensions for the square, and a constant concentric tension for the circle determine the significance and properties of the three basic shapes.These three basic shapes are associated with certain qualities of rhythm, color, activity, temperature, and musical sound (Fig 3-38). A combination of identical shapes and color—a yellow triangle, for example—increases the effect of each property while a confrontation of opposed shapes and colors—a blue triangle, for example—greatly reduces the effect of each property.

Triangle	Square	Circle
Three starting points	Four starting points	No identifiable starting point
Rapid rhythmic properties	Reduced eccentric tensions	Concentric tension
Expressivity	Complementary concentric tension	Absence of rhythm interiority
Acute resonance	Moderate rhythmic properties	Deep resonance
	Medium resonance	

The form

By definition, a composition is a precise and logical organization of a variety of elements; its shape reflects the tensions expressed by the live forces contained in these elements. It has a meaning. We defined the point as the most concise shape, introvert and concentric, stressing the geometric and psychological duality of its significance. Similarly, every form has its inner significance, which originates from its own form. The perception of this significance is not objective; rather, it depends on the receptivity of the observer. The objective consideration of shapes as normal or natural only emerges from habit.

Forms are abstract limitations of space or surface. In a narrow sense they are nothing but the separating line between surfaces. This is their outer meaning, which results from the tensions expressed by their inner constraints. Every form has its inner substance. No form says nothing. The esthetic evaluation of a form is based upon the perception of its universal geometric and sensory qualities.

Every shape can be reduced to one of three basic shapes: the circle, the square, and the triangle (Fig 3-42). The curved line, arising from the pull of two constant forces applied to the point, carries in itself the promise of a plane, since sooner or later in the development of its movement it will rejoin its starting point, converge into it, and vanish. The circle, so generated, is a solid but at the same time transitory form. A straight line also has the potential to produce a shape, even if this potential is hidden. But achieving this goal will require no less than the application of three successive forces, so that start and end remain indefinitely pointed at three different places for the constitution of the triangle.

These two shapes, triangle and circle, oppose one another and present the greatest contrast. The square, though one of the basic shapes, can be considered transitional between the triangle and the circle. All three shapes express specific qualities susceptible to soliciting our esthetic sensibility.

Points, lines, and shapes represent the basic words of a language accessible to all human beings and make up the key elements of esthetic communication. But esthetic knowledge can be reduced to no other. Its accessibility does not result from learning but from constant visual interrogation and repetitive training, by which alone one may develop esthetic sensitivity and receptivity.

The character and significance of forms

Points, lines, and shapes that have been defined by the active tensions inherent in every formal element express at the same time their interior significance. Necessity creates shapes.

The character of a form is closely linked to its physical and geometric constitution and so remains constant and displays the same properties in all circumstances. A circular form will never display the same character as an elongated one, whatever its perceiver does or feels. Round is always round; square is always square. Geometry predominates. But the geometric characteristics of a form are always associated with psychological connotations that determine its significance.

The significance of a form depends not only on its specific properties but also on the human perceiver's sensibility, feelings, and impressions. In generating the significance of a form, all those factors work simultaneously. Points, lines, and shapes which have been defined by the active tensions inherent in every esthetic element manifest at the same time specific qualities expressing their interior significance.

Whenever a straight line suggests continuity, its development in the horizontal or vertical plane generates a feeling of either inertia or dynamism. Yet most lines lack this relative simplicity of character. And each new presentation of a line, or any form, will invariably generate different feelings in direct relation to its design and position. For example, the character of a broken line will depend not only on its regularity or irregularity but also on the variations of its development in the horizontal or vertical plane.

A regular and symmetrical undulating line drawn in a horizontal plane will have a static character enhanced by the dynamism reflected in the succession of upward and downward movements. This predominance of the static may be affected by irregularities in the undulations (Fig 3-43). A vertical spatial position of the same line will inevitably have a predominately dynamic character.

These characteristics are confirmed in the significance expressed by the three original planes, triangle, square, and circle: three acute tensions for the triangle; four calm tensions for the square, at the same time eccentric and concentric; and a concentric

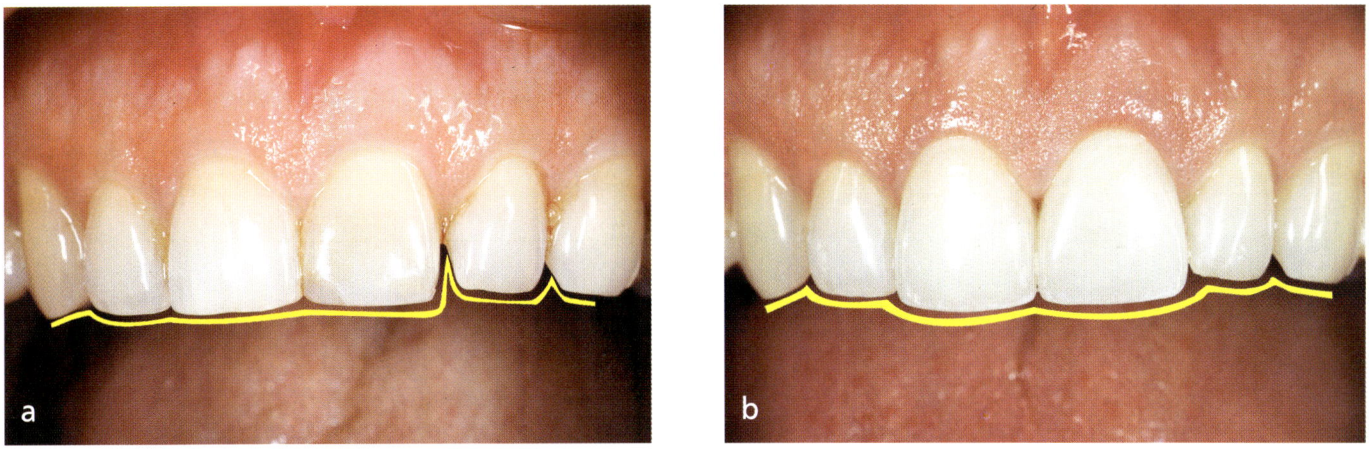

Figs 3-43a and 3-43b (a) A static and monotonous development of the incisal line in the horizontal plane disturbed by an abrupt interruption generates a loss of control of ocular movements, which does not enhance the composition's appearance. (b) A more pronounced, regular, up and down movement of the eye introduces a dynamic and appealing element in the static appearance of the incisal line, which stands in a horizontal plane.

tension closed on itself for the circle (Fig 3-42). These three basic shapes find themselves naturally represented in tooth design with unlimited variation.

We are dealing here with simple graphic means, suggesting in turn or at the same time dynamism, strength, inertia, and a variety of characterizing particulars (Fig 3-38). They constitute elements of reference to be introduced in any determined tooth design in an attempt to modify or accentuate the main resonance of the facial composition. The importance of the dental elements relative to the whole facial composition should keep us from any excess of pretension, but the necessity to characterize the elements of the anterior segment should nonetheless not be neglected.

Made up of broken and curved lines and of angles of various degrees, dental elements remain less significant than the predominant characteristics displayed by individual morphopsychology (Fig 3-44). But it is the privilege of human creativity to modify for expressive purposes the character of a form that is linked to its structure. To understand a form's significance one must accept those of its properties that generate on the spectator repetitive and identical impressions. This is in no way an objective statement since no shape is objective. Objectivity is merely appearance.

An arch form, for example, that introduces a notion of weight, distribution of force, and resistance generates as such an impression of stability (Fig 3-45). A parallel clinical situation that somehow mimics this design may be found in the undulating movement of the gingival design and the feeling of stability that it displays (Fig 3-45).

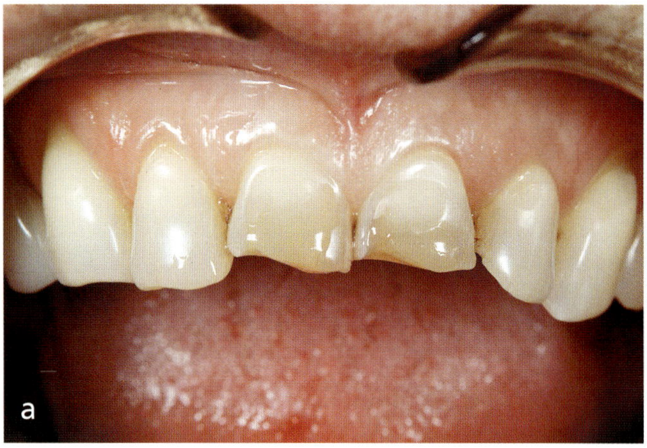
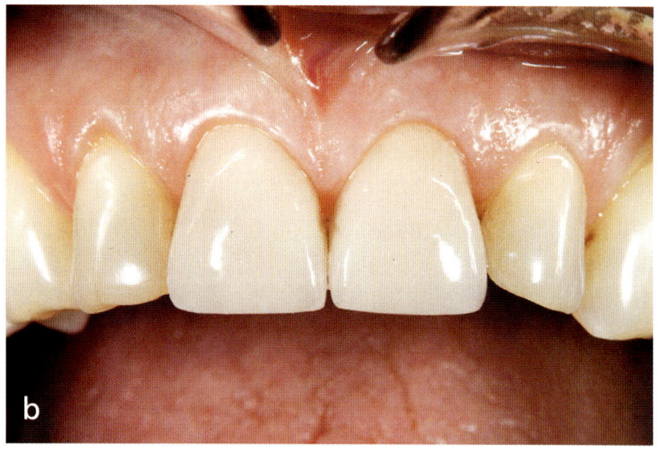

Figs 3-44a and 3-44b The characteristics of a tooth form, square, round, or tapered, correlate perfectly with the basic geometric forms. These geometric characteristics are related to specific character traits, a concept corroborated by the basic axiom of the esthetic language: "Each shape is the result of its inner significance." However, in the aging process these characteristics may (a) fade away, and therefore (b) the introduction into this dental composition of a slightly tapered tooth design loaded with a dynamic significance modifies the impact of the aging process.

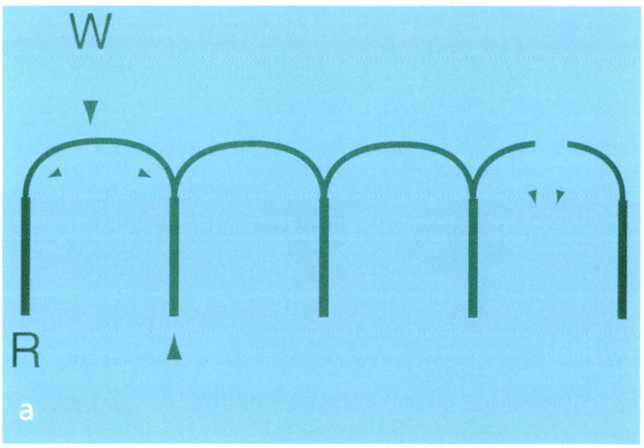

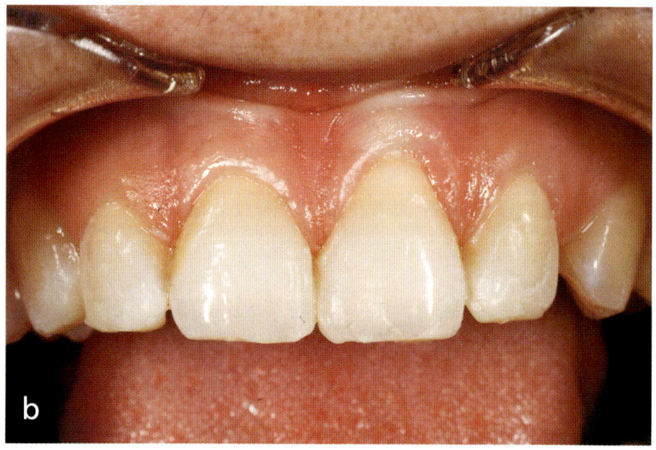

Figs 3-45a and 3-45b The acceptance of the significance of a form is dependent upon specific properties generating in the spectator repetitive and identical sensations. (a) An arch form introduces a notion of distribution of forces (W) and resistance (R). But when the original design displays elements of rupture (arrowhead), this feeling disappears. (b) Expectation of tissue resistance vanishes and a feeling of overload predominates when elements of rupture take place in the gingival undulating design.

The action of forces that take place in each of these systems is different and the adverse forces that can be applied to these constructions will produce different and selective impacts.

Forms only manifest the character that originates from their structure. Introduced into a context that contains other forms, these characteristics will be reinforced or reduced in response to the esthetic qualities of surrounding structures. This language of shapes and colors is not restricted to simple geometric shapes, lines, or angles or to suggestive elementary designs; it involves more complicated geometric shapes.

Morphopsychological theory has long held that the variety of facial morphological developments may signify specific character traits. "The shape of the face is modeled by the forces of life contained in each individual" (Corman). This basic axiom of the morphopsychological concept perfectly coincides with the statement of the German Bauhaus developed extensively in the preceding pages.

The statement, "The shape of an element is the result of the constraints contained in this element, expressed by tensions," stresses the direct dependence existing between simple or complex geometric forms and their psychological or characterizing expression on the psychological tendencies of the perceiver.

Moreover, the close relationships that can be established between these two movements of thinking throw a new light on the nature of human esthetics based on the subjectivity of individual sensibility and receptivity. Nothing other than individual sensibility allows accessibility to the specific character of shapes and colors.

Esthetic Factors

The definition of the basic esthetic elements and of specific elements of the facial composition will help improve esthetic knowledge and develop esthetic sensibility. The calm of the point or the active tension born from a movement at the origin of the line generates a language inaccessible to words but necessary to esthetic expression. Yet the perception of the significance of a form, the perception of the morphopsychological significance of human facial characteristics, cannot alone lead to esthetic judgments without the operation of subjective taste.

The fact that a form is closely linked to its historical development does not determine its esthetic quality. "Beauty is fitness expressed" (Walter Armstrong) suggests that the beauty of a form, organic or inorganic, emerges from successful efforts of adaptation to both environmental conditions and functional requirements and that this accomplishment is the result of a mathematical logic that will generate unanimous appreciation. This dictum reflects the often subconscious esthetic pleasure arising from the contemplation of an object that seems perfectly fitted to its function and environment. This fitness maintains its importance even in the mere image or projection of the object possessing it.

But to restrict esthetic explanation merely to the perspective apprehension of the language of forms is a facile oversimplification. Esthetic explanation must be extended to the analysis and understanding of the privileged and organized relationships between forms. The perception of the privileged relationships that take place in a composition, appealing to various aspects of our sensibilities, is crucial to esthetic analysis.

It is not less true that, in one's first approach to any composition, feelings rather than objective reading and the curiosity of discovery rather than esthetic knowledge are uppermost. As a result, the appeal of the resonance of a composition, which arises from the sum of the different significances of the elements within it, is first experienced. The perception of this resonance is inherent in human nature.

Basic elements of esthetic analysis

Everyone may appreciate the resonance of a composition to some degree because the perception of these tensional strengths is characteristic of human sensibility working subconsciously. Calmness and serenity constitute a message that, radiating from this blue composition (Fig 3-46), touches our soul and sensibility. The predominance of the blue color, expressive of calmness and relaxation, correlates perfectly with the composure of the subject, whose eyes are closed and head inclined. The contrast of this blue with red, suggesting the possibility of passion, and with the explosive quality of the yellow and the wild movements of the hair generates an esthetically pleasing tension. This resonance or "atmosphere" of the composition, which unconsciously addresses our sensibility, results from the specific qualities of each element in it and from the variety of tensions displayed by their interaction. This resonance is a primary esthetic factor.

An esthetic composition never reveals all at first glance. New elements, new aspects will always appear. One must methodically collect these feelings into a coherent whole. But human sensibility varies, and knowledge cannot substitute for it. Without it, esthetic qualities and tensions may go unperceived, and a composition may seem a mere network of color, points, lines, and shapes.

Lines arising from the destruction of the immobility of the point are at the origin of the prodigious variety of shapes. Lines design, separate, or support every material or immaterial element. Careful observation reveals that lines never identify themselves with the contour of a shape, but rather underline or encroach upon it.

Visible or invisible, our environment is exclusively constituted of lines that, in addition to the significance they display, manifest an esthetic value based on their graphic characteristics.

Lines are of primary importance in a composition by reason not only of the forces that they generate but also of the obvious fact that no element of the composition can avoid the linear system (Fig 3-47). Lines are drawn not only materially in the composition where they can hardly elude visual perception but also appear because of a purely mental phenomenon that unconsciously imposes a linear tracing between two existing or hypothetical elements. Specific perceptive conditions impose the mental tracing of lines. For example, if we try to translate with a line the first impression produced by the blue composition, we see a diagonal line suggested by the position of the subject on the canvas (Fig 3-48). The nature of this line, between the vertical and horizontal, the properties linked to its inclination, stress the characterizing duality in the composition that the initial reading has already discovered. A line, therefore, may be characterized by a specific tensional strength and

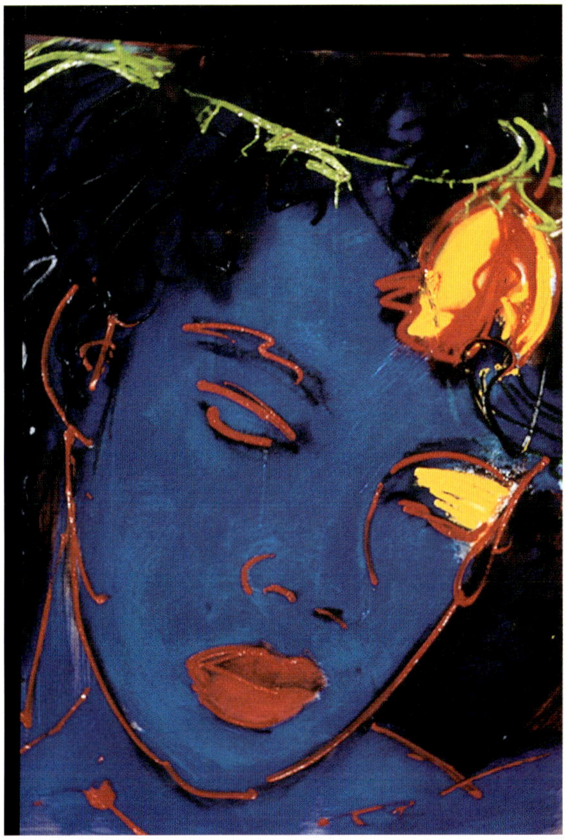

Fig 3-46 *Passion*, Luciano Castelli, 1987 (private collection). Calmness and serenity constitute a message emanating from the blue composition that touches our soul and sensibility.

Fig 3-47 The tracing of a line is not a condition for its perception. Two visible or invisible points may also impose the mental tracing of a line. In this composition the bipupillary line cannot escape notice.

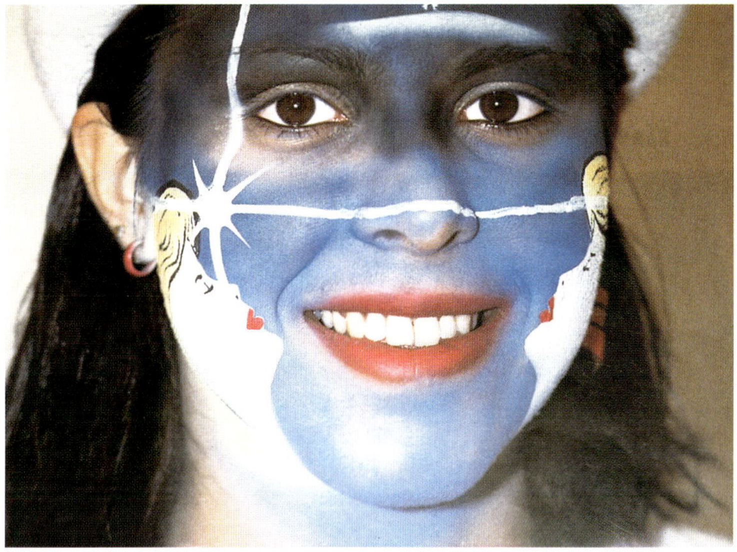

direction and does not need to be traced in order to be sensed.

Further analysis of the composition will reveal other and opposite diagonal lines, such as the eyelid-level line, eye-level line, nose line, shoulder line, and the fine green brush stroke in the upper part of the composition. They all run parallel and at right angles to the primary diagonal line suggested by the figure's head position, generating a strong feeling of equilibrium (Figs 3-48 to 3-54).

Closer observation reinforces a feeling that the directional strength of these multiple lines is generated not by the elements of the composition but by the shape of the plane-support in which they appear, which imposes the way to introduce elements into the composition in a state of equilibrium. The esthetic quality of a composition always depends on the constraining equilibrium generated by the shape of its plane. This constitutes a basic esthetic factor, which may be called "the tension of the plane."

Yet this feeling of equilibrium does not appear to be affected by the lines of the figure's mouth, which break the parallelism of the other lines and provide no counterbalance to the line implied by the figure's

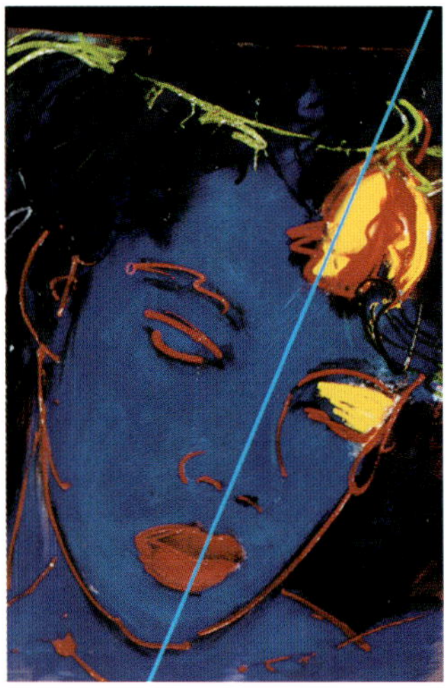

Fig 3-48 The attempt to translate into line the first impression generated by this composition results in the unconscious tracing of the diagonal line suggested by the head position.

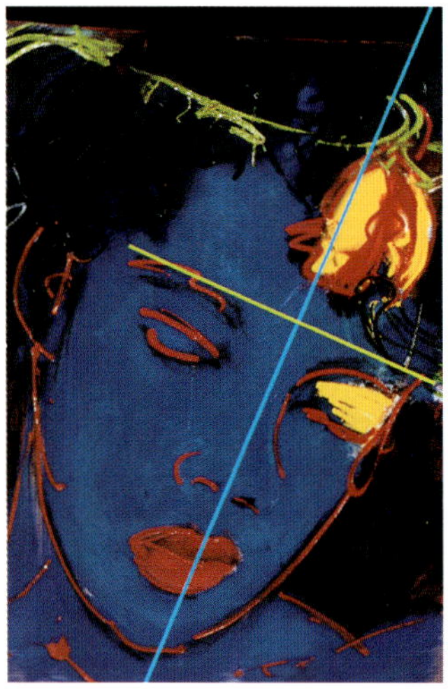

Fig 3-49 By fixing one's attention on the tracing of lines imposed by this composition, one will discover successive linear tracings starting with the tracing of the eyelid line.

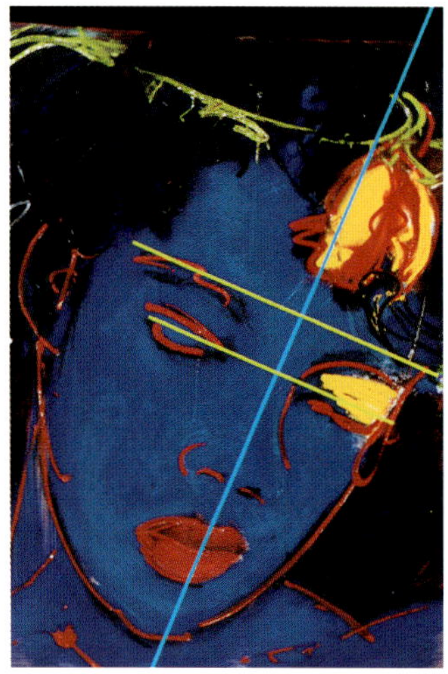

Fig 3-50 The tracing of the eyelid line will naturally lead to the tracing of the eye line.

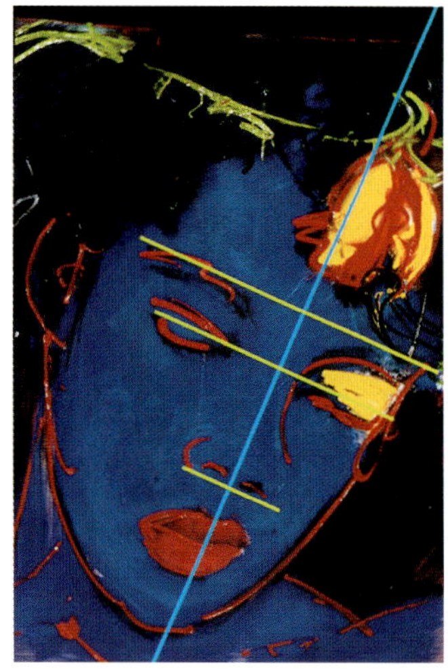

Fig 3-51 In turn, the direction of the base of the nose suggests another linear tracing.

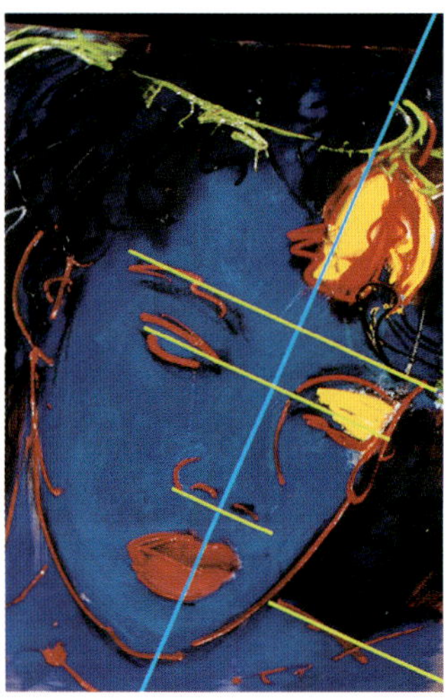

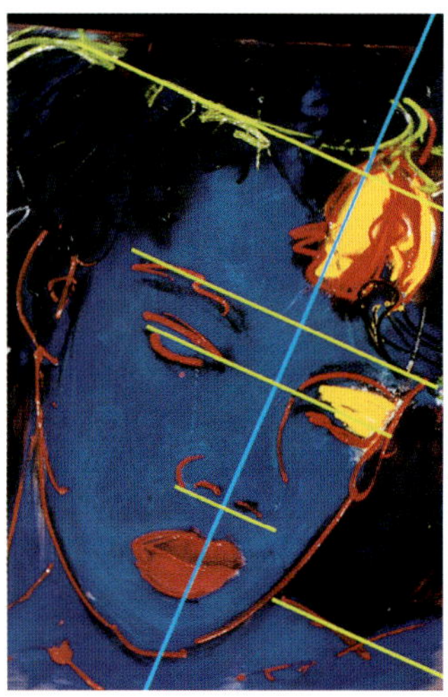

Fig 3-52 (*farleft*) The shoulder line suddenly attracts attention.

Fig 3-53 (*left*) On closer observation, it appears that the tracing of these different lines responds to specific constraints of equilibrium imposed by the shape of the whole plane, which reminds one that a green line at the upper part of the composition also runs parallel to this linear system.

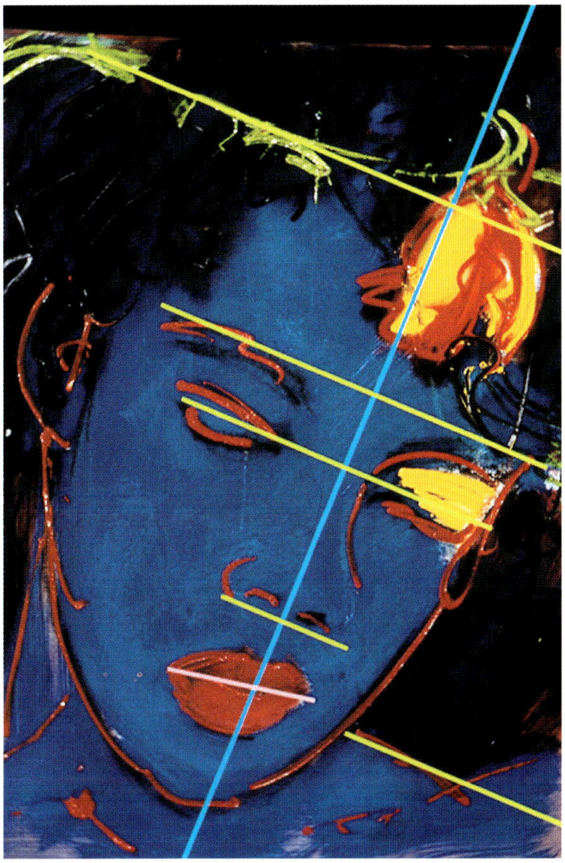

Fig 3-54 The equilibrium of this linear system, in which the multiple parallel lines seem to counterbalance the initial diagonal tracing of head position, is suddenly interrupted by the unavoidable tracing of the mouth line. However, subsequent readings of the composition do not confirm this lack of balance but rather suggest that the yellow colors in the upper part of the composition may act as an accent weighing on the commissural line, thus restoring equilibrium. The reading of lines and of the mass and colors of the elements of this composition has revealed the existence of two esthetic factors contributing to its equilibrium.

head posture (see Fig 3-58). This suggests that other factors may affect the equilibrium of the composition and provide subtle counterbalance. In this composition they apparently originate from the mass of yellow color that, placed in a line background, is felt as an accent. Since the strength and weight of this mass help prevent disequilibrium naturally, we may conclude that there is a specific esthetic factor, having to do with mass and colors, which may be called the *weight of the elements.*

This simple analysis shows that these elements of esthetic knowledge starting with a correct perception of points, lines, shapes, and colors will permit us to penetrate into the heart of the esthetic world, constituted by the three basic factors ruling the arrangement of the elements in a composition:

- Tension of the elements
- Tension of the plane
- Weight of the elements

In addition to these elements of constraint, weight, and tension, basic esthetic factors common to any beautiful composition, the geometric characteristics of each single form should also be analyzed with respect to the psychological connotation that determines its significance.

Once again it needs to be stressed that the ability to perceive the significance of a form depends upon the individual human sensibility, which defies intellectual understanding. However, in this approach to esthetic knowledge, sooner or later guided repetitive training will help develop and improve this sensibility and with it the ability to integrate dental elements into the facial map in a state of harmony.

Tension of the plane

With its four identical sides and four identical angles, the square can be regarded as the most primitive plane, the simplest geometric figure. The introduction of a large material point close to one or another corner of the square will generate in the observer a phenomenon of optico-psychological instability. This can be relieved only by moving the point to the center of the square or by introducing along the same diagonal another point in the opposite angle. We are faced with a phenomenon generated by the effect of the shape of the plane on our sense of equilibrium (Figs 3-55 and 3-56).

Each geometric plane generates lines of force whose power of attraction varies according to its specific design. These lines are easily detectable in the simplest geometric shapes like the square or the rectangle as they develop in diagonal from one corner of the plane to the other. In crossing each other, these lines determine secondary lines of constraint that, running parallel to the sides of the plane, can undergo infinite multiplication. These diagonal, vertical, and horizontal lines running from the center to the

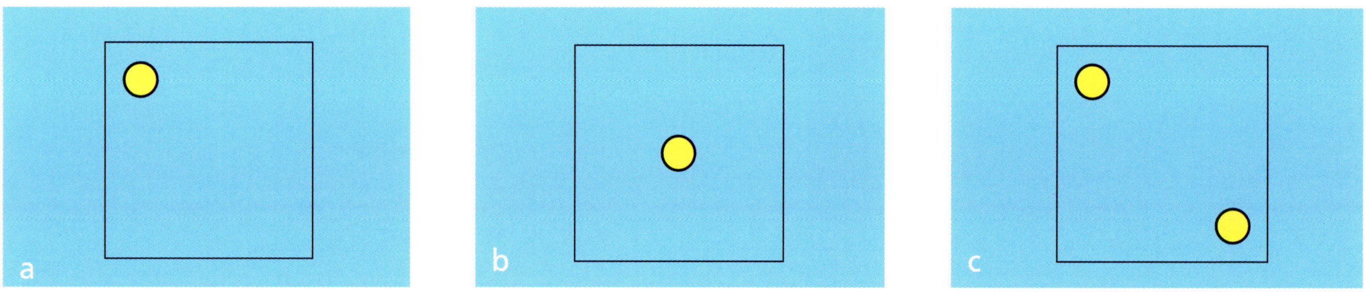

Figs 3-55a to 3-55c (a) The introduction of a round element in an angle of a square plane provokes a strong feeling of instability. (b) Stability can be achieved by moving the round shape to the center of the plane or (c) by introducing a similar element in the other corner of the plane, using as a guideline the virtual and constraining diagonal line running from one corner of the square plane to the other.

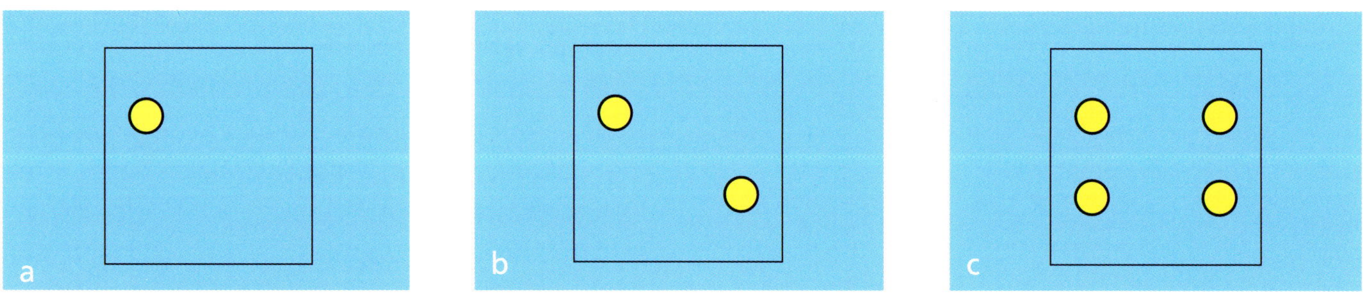

Figs 3-56a to 3-56c (a) Placed along the borderline of the square plane, the same round element generates a more impressive feeling of instability. (b) Equilibrium can yet be obtained by introducing a similar element into a comparable position along vertical and horizontal lines running parallel to the sides of the plane. (c) The intersection of these lines even allows for the placement of four identical elements, which definitely break this feeling of equilibrium.

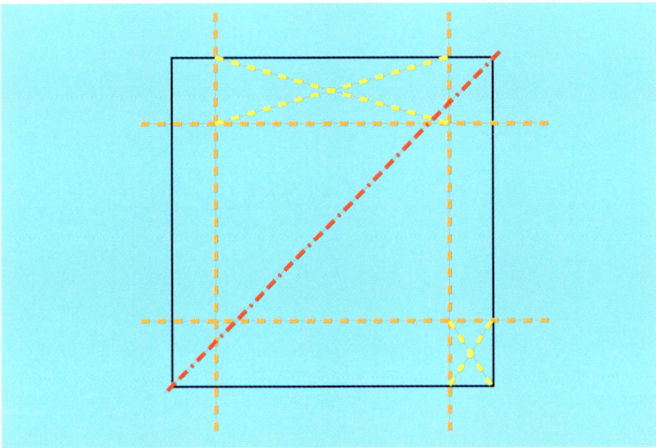

Fig 3-57 Each plane generates lines of constraint of variable strength that determine the introduction of new elements in a state of equilibrium. Overall equilibrium will be achieved when all the elements of a composition conform to the lines of constraint dictated by the shape of the basic plane. In this organization, the diagonal lines running from one corner of the plane to the other appear to be the most constraining, but the absence of subsidiary lines of constraint more difficult to approach may also ruin the equilibrium of a composition.

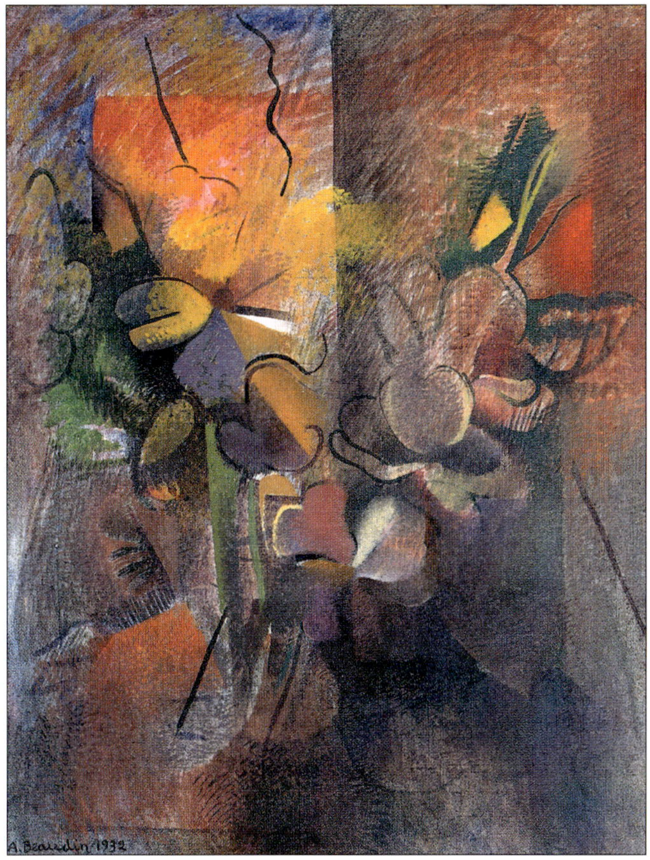

Fig 3-58 According to cubist theory, the main element of the subject has been exploded into parts that have been placed along the lines of constraint of the plane. The rhythm of the composition is marked by transitional zones of color placed along secondary lines of tension, stressing the equilibrium of the composition. (A. Beaudin, 1932, private collection.)

corners of the plane, or along and parallel to the sides of the plane, build a network of constraints of variable intensity. They determine the way to introduce new elements into a composition in a state of harmony (Fig 3-57). This notion of equilibrium, most familiar to sculptors and painters, has influenced a number of artistic movements (Figs 3-58 and 3-59).

It is left to our sensibility to determine the lines of constraint in a plane that lacks the simple geometric design of a square or a rectangle. This may be easy, or, when the determination of the supporting plane or esthetic support is not seen immediately, it may be difficult. In our field of interest it is often difficult.

If we consider the oral plane as the spatial limitation of what has been called the dentofacial compo-

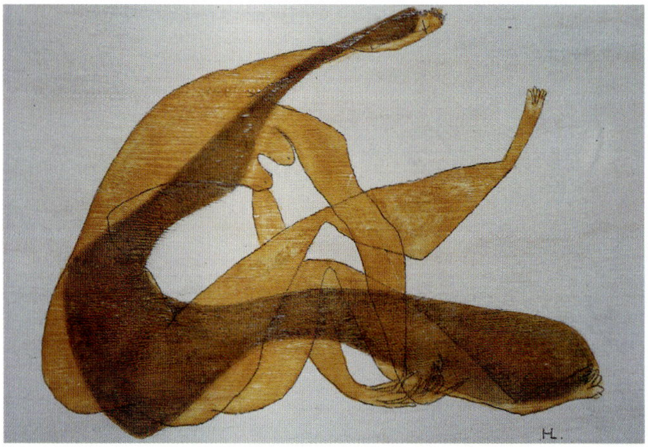

Fig 3-59 A main diagonal line of tension crossing the subject and picture plane and compensated by two secondary tensional strengths, one vertical and another horizontal and parallel to the sides of the picture plane, contributes to the feeling of stability displayed by this composition. (H. Laurens, 1951, private collection.)

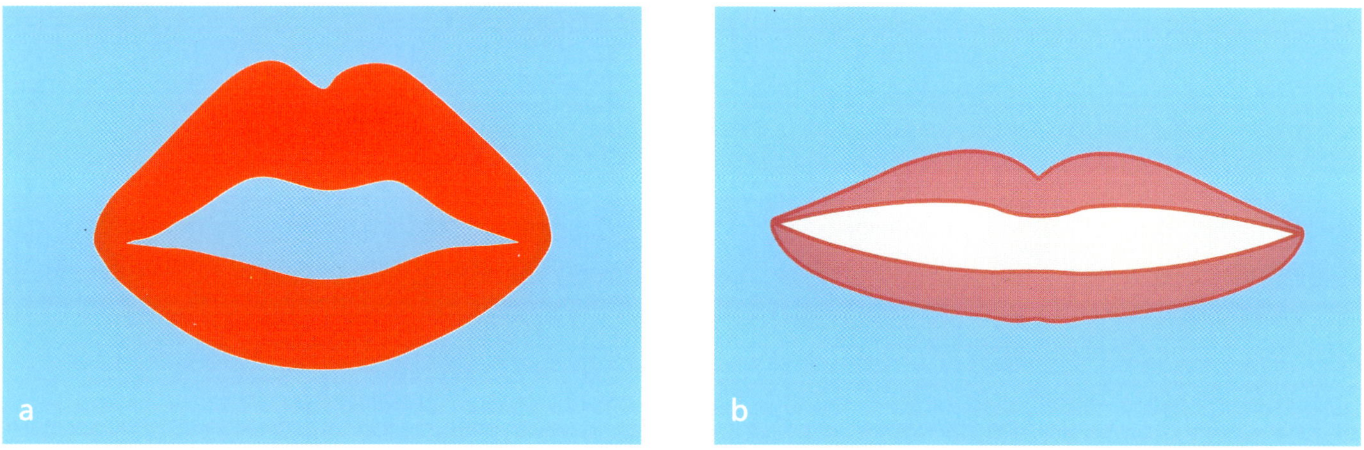

Figs 3-60a and 3-60b Like any other plane, the mouth generates lines of constraint, running from one corner to the other, whatever its shape, whether closed or open.

sition, its horizontally elongated shape is determined by a line that runs from one corner of the mouth to the other (Fig 3-60). This tracing line will be repeated indefinitely in the horizontal plane, whatever the variations of shape and dimension of the oral frame. For ages this line has served as the basis for the construction of the anterior dental segment. Though it may seem exclusively important from a distance of focus that suits the dental profession, in reality one must also consider, in all circumstances, a larger component: the facial plane.

A major vertical line of force, crossing the mouth line at right angles, appears immediately to anyone who looks at the whole face (Fig 3-61). Too often, from habit, we ignore this and project the whole facial picture by considering only a part. The facial plane

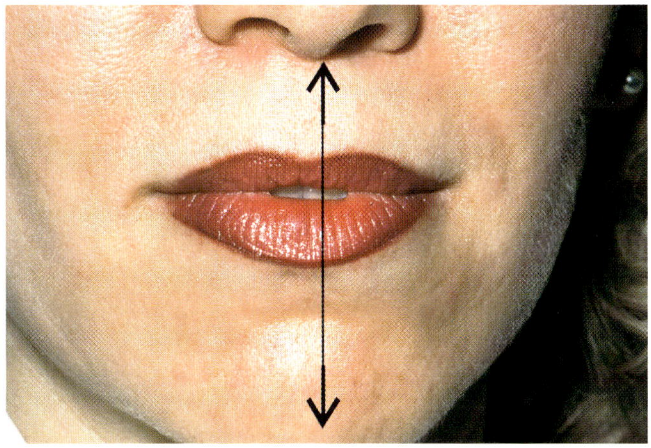

Fig 3-61 On the other hand, the facial composition, whatever its ethnic origins, balances the horizontal line of constraint generated by the mouth with a main vertical line of constraint, even if only part of the facial composition is visualized.

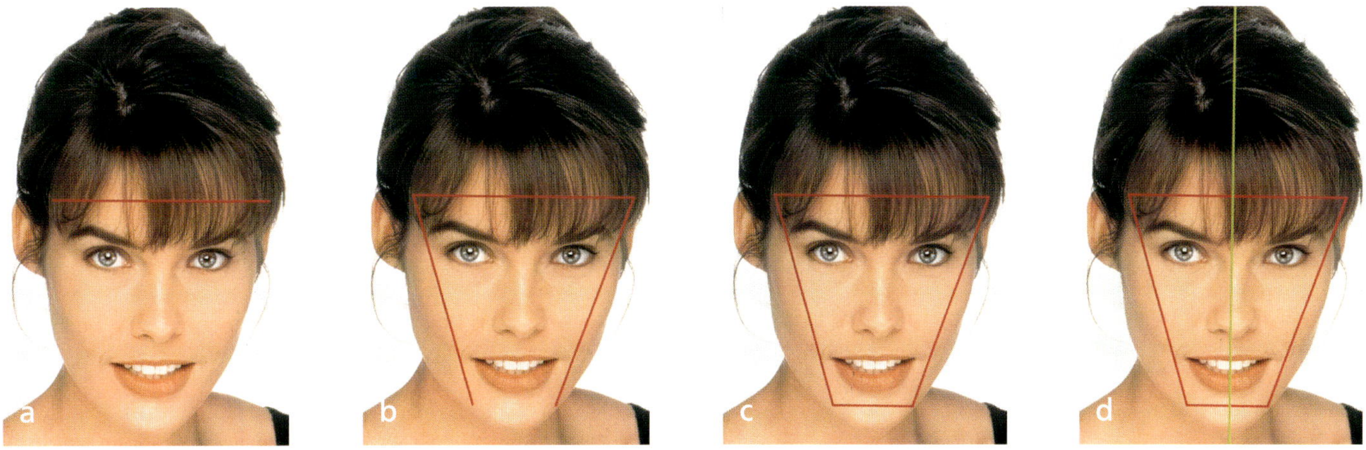

Figs 3-62a to 3-62d The morphological concept has divided the face into a vestibular frame containing the facial receptors—eyes, nose, and mouth—and the general frame resulting from the expansion of the osseous framework. (a,b,c) In surrounding the receptors with straight lines in a geometric design that more or less duplicates the facial pentagon proposed by the Italian Renaissance and (d) in imposing a vertical line of constraint, we appeal to the human tendency for mathematical order.

is the plane of reference in evaluating esthetically the integration of restored elements, the whole facial plane, confronted with ethnic and individual differences. This, however, has been too often ignored in favor of the particulars of the dental composition. We need to consider the facial plane as an entity in which all the elements relevant to esthetic interaction with the dental composition can be taken in at a glance.

Morphopsychology has long made a distinction between the general facial frame, easy to appreciate but subject to change according to circumstances or the progression of age, and the vestibular frame, more restricted but less mutable. The vestibular frame, a delimited geometric plane surrounding the facial receptors—eyes, nose, and mouth—remains stable with advancing age (Fig 3-62).

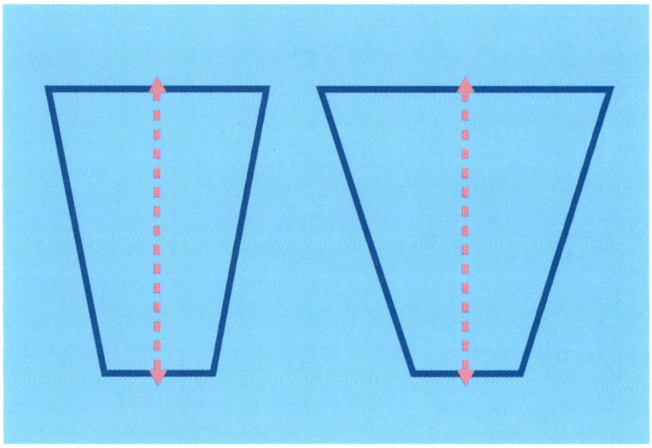

Fig 3-63 It can also be stated that, whatever the individual or ethnic morphological differences, not only the facial frame but also the resulting vestibular frame generates a vertical line of constraint. Facial and vestibular lines of constraint are not necessarily coincidental. This observation answers the perennial question relating to the placement of the interincisal line, which should run coincidental to the main line of constraint of the vestibular frame.

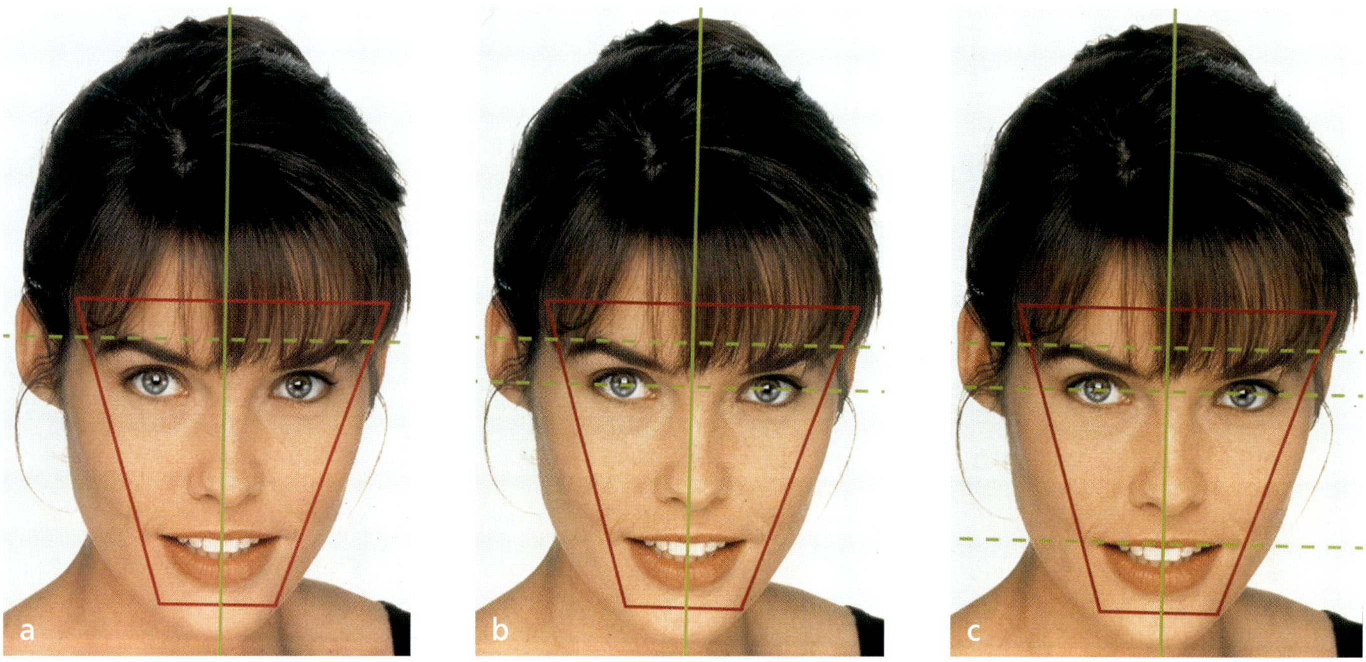

Figs 3-64a to 3-64c As in the blue composition, analysis of the linear system of this composition naturally generates the tracing of the eyebrow line, bipupillary line, and commissural line. We know that nature has located facial receptors along the secondary lines of constraint of the vestibular frame, running parallel to the horizontal upper and lower sides of this plane support.

This vestibular frame permits a perfect visualization of the dental elements. In response to the human inclination for mathematical order, this plane of reference has been traced with straight lines and reduced to a geometric figure, resembling part of the facial pentagon promoted by many authors of the Italian Renaissance, to help in the determination of ideal facial proportions. This schematic geometric shape is perfectly defined by physical evidence. Whatever the individual, the trapezoidal design of the vestibular frame invariably produces a vertical central tensional strength and projects this tension with a variable intensity (Fig 3-63). Consequently, all the elements of vertical integration will articulate around this line of force, including the placement of the eyes, nose, and mouth. At the same time the eyebrow line, bipupillary line, and commissural line run parallel to each other in most faces. These lines, running parallel to the outer borders of the vestibular frame, represent secondary lines of tension generated by the shape of the facial plane (Fig 3-64).

Further analysis demonstrates that the outer vertical lines of constraint generated by the vestibular frame run, in smiling, parallel to a line drawn from

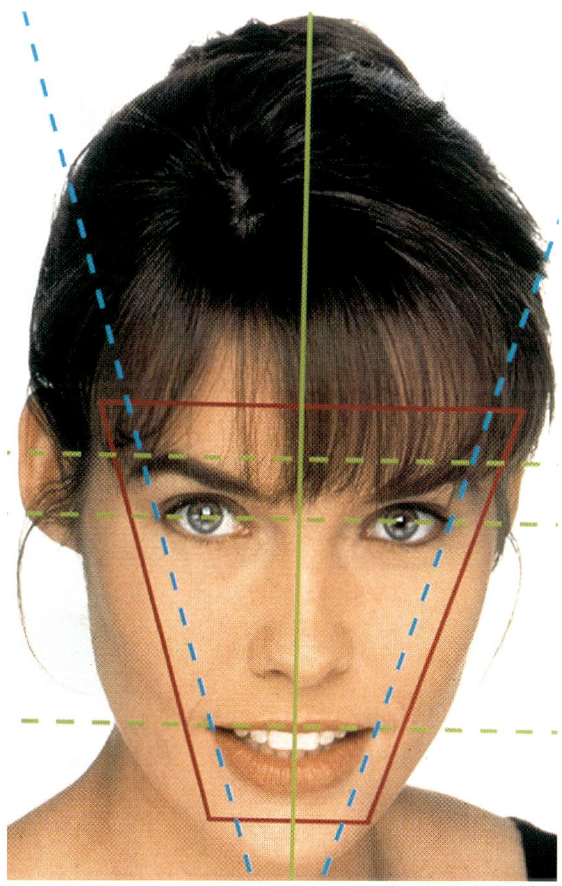

Fig 3-65 It is hard to believe that in a composition only the horizontal secondary lines of constraint should receive consideration. Sharper perception shows that a line drawn from the outer border of the eye to the outer border of the lip takes, in smiling, a coincidental direction to the vertical outer border of the plane, stressing the importance of considering the various aspects of facial dynamics in esthetic analysis.

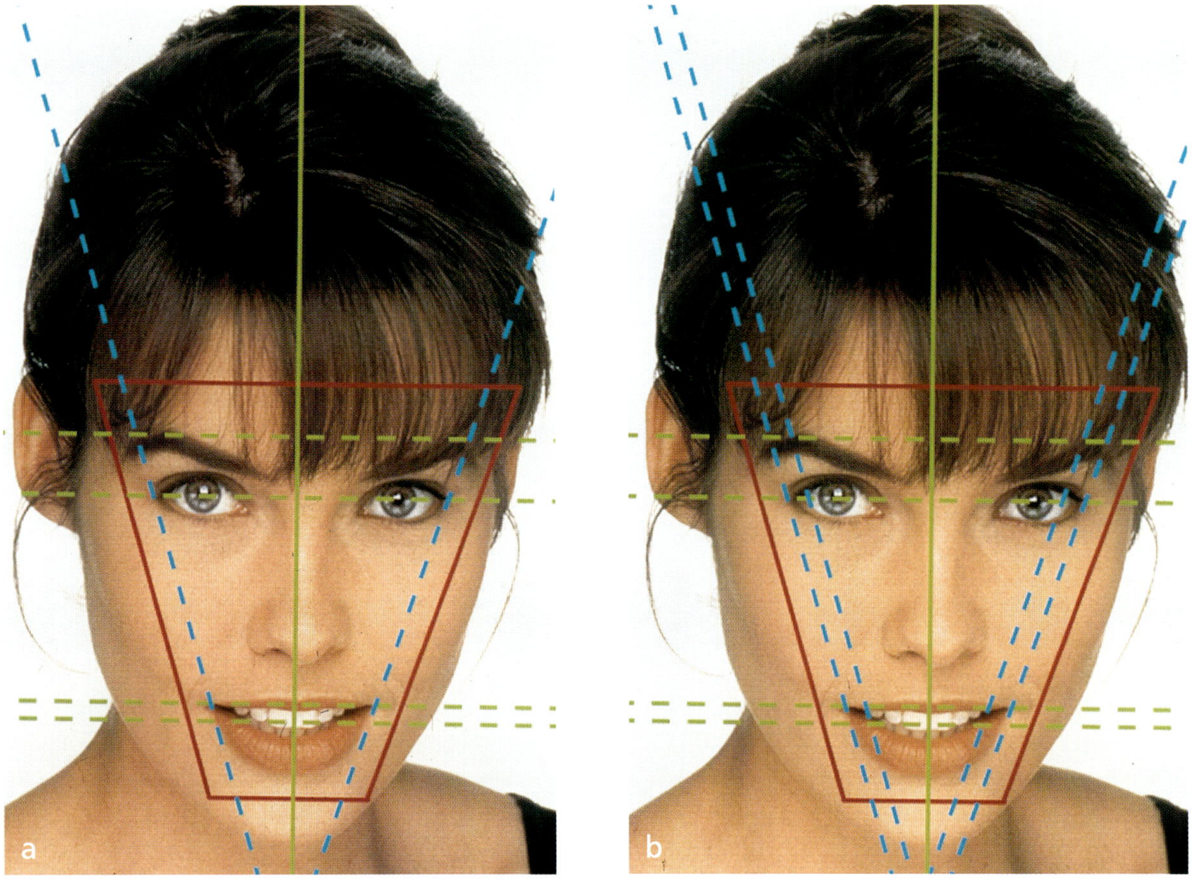

Figs 3-66a and 3-66b (a) The confrontation of the upper occlusal plane with the horizontal lines of constraint of the vestibular frame has long been recognized as coincidental to the commissural line. There is no reason to exclude the lower occlusal plane from this constraining location at mouth opening. (b) Yet, in the vertical plane, the frontal perception of the canine axial direction, dictating the whole front-back progression, should be acknowledged as one of the elements permitting the integration of the dental composition into its facial support.

the side of the eye to the corner of the mouth. This both explains and fixes the axial direction of the corner tooth canine or first premolar, which dictates that the front-back progression of the posterior segment should run parallel to the vertical sides of the vestibular plane (Figs 3-65 and 3-66).

Prosthodontists have long used the bipupillary line to construct the frontal occlusal plane. The parallelism of lines, which can be extended to the commissural line, runs coincidental to the outer horizontal linear constraints of the vestibular frame. This parallelism can be considered a constant in dentofacial esthet-

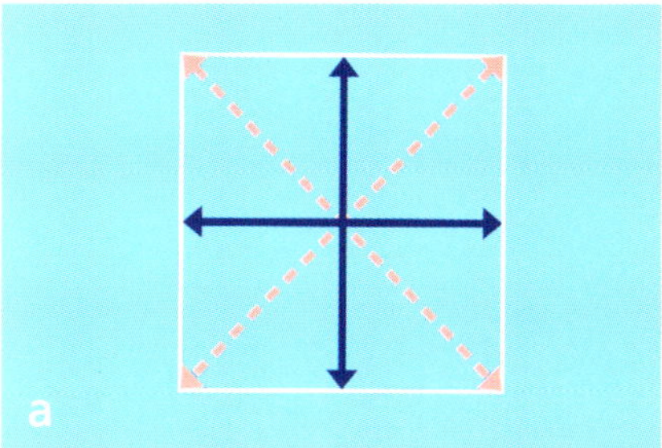

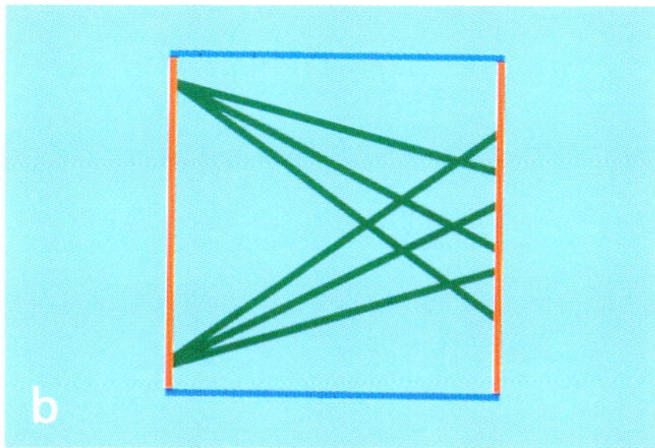

Figs 3-67a and 3-67b (a) Each plane support, like the square, generates lines of constraint dictating the way to introduce new elements into a composition in a state of harmony. (b) When these constraints are not respected and elements are introduced along fantasied linear tracings, they can relate only very loosely with the plane, and the esthetic value of the composition will be affected.

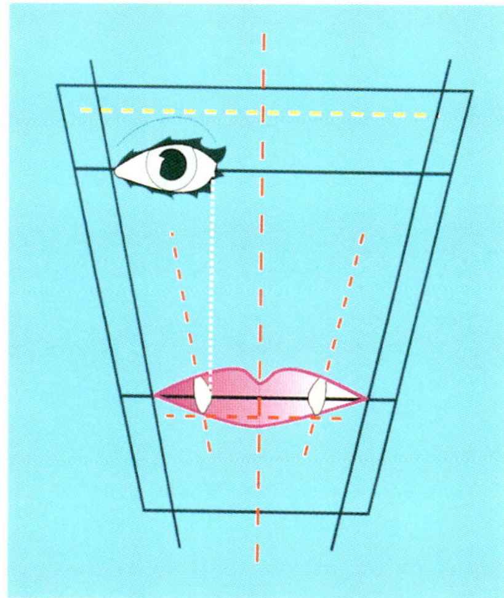

Fig 3-68 As with tooth-gingival relationships, whose nature will permit the biological integration of dental restorations into their dental support, the linear tracings of the constraints generated by the vestibular frame must remain foremost in the prosthodontist's mind and be frequently queried and evaluated during the setting up of any type of rehabilitation, since it constitutes a prerequisite for the esthetic integration of dental elements into the facial support.

ics. The multiplication of parallel lines—eyebrow line, bipupillary line, intercommissural line, upper and lower occlusal lines, gingival line, incisal line—is typical of the rhythmic properties at the origins of facial esthetics. It can be added that the appearance during oral movements of lines that are not only part of the dental composition but also run parallel to the lines of force of the vestibular facial frame introduces a cohesion that helps integrate the dental composition into the dentofacial and facial compositions (Fig 3-66).

The lines of force generated by a plane stipulate the way new elements may be introduced into a composition in a state of equilibrium (Fig 3-67). Usually the elements of the dentofacial and facial composition naturally respond to this architectural requirement. The position of these elements is not accidental and the integration of the restorative dental elements is naturally subjected to the same constraints imposed by the nature of the vestibular frame support, both in the horizontal and vertical planes (Fig 3-68).

It can be added that any type of facial distortion of genetic origin requiring orthognathic or orthopedic therapeutic measures (Fig 3-69) displays a lack of coordination in the parallelism between facial lines, whereas a dislocation from the constraints of the vestibular frame, affecting the anterior occlusal plane, usually results either from failure in prosthodontic reconstitution or orthodontic arrangement or

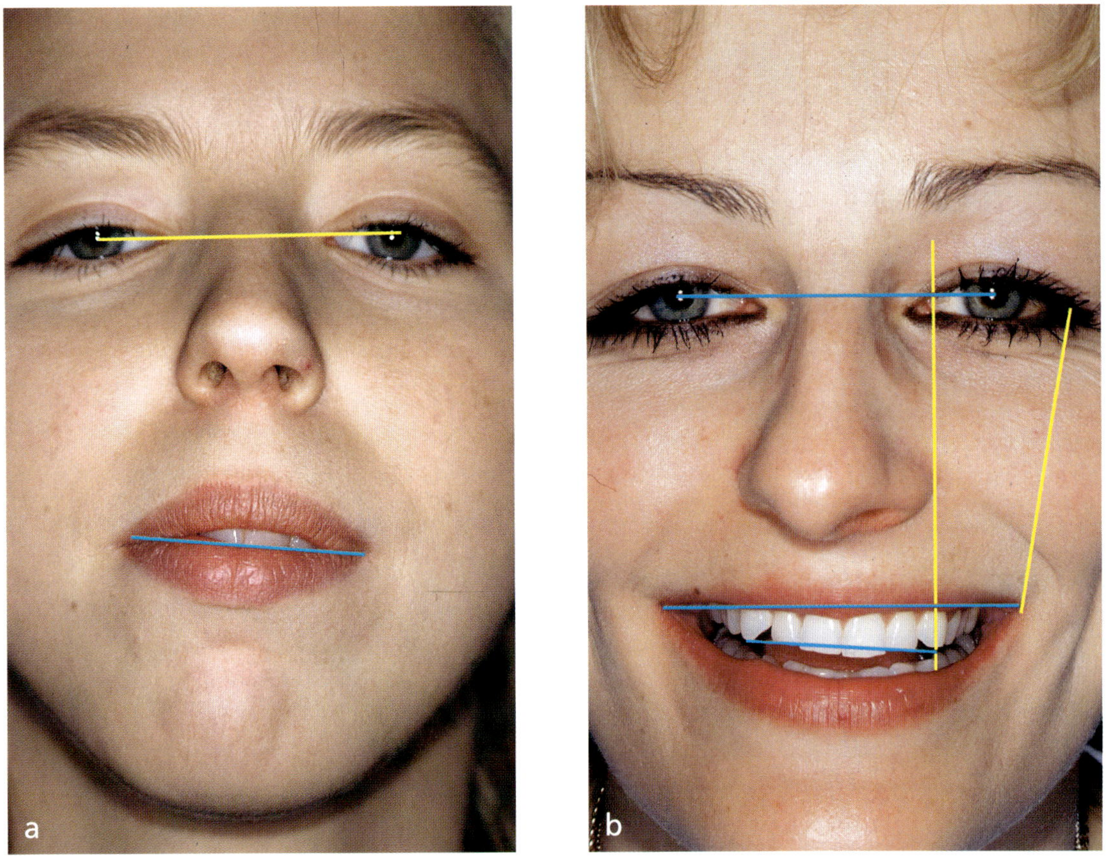

Figs 3-69a and 3-69b Clinically, reference to the linear constraints of the vestibular frame allows for an early detection of esthetic deficiencies. (a) In this particular case, a noncoincidental linear parallelism affecting the bipupillary and commissural lines stresses a deviation of the lower facial third, requiring orthognathic surgery. (b) A lack of coordination between the line running from the corner of the eye to that of the mouth and canine axial direction affects the vertical cohesion of the composition and should have been corrected in the usual orthodontic approach, whereas a lack of coordination between the occlusal plane and the horizontal sides of the vestibular frame stresses functional problems.

from functional problems affecting the natural dentitions (Figs 3-70 to 3-72). The identification of functional problems based on linear dislocation from the constraints of the vestibular frame underlines the often close relationship between esthetics and function.

These pathologies, born of loosened relationships with the plane support and breaking the rhythmic particulars of the facial plane, deeply impair the esthetic worth of the composition. In the arrangement of the anterior segment, however, the constraints imposed by the geometric schema of the vestibular

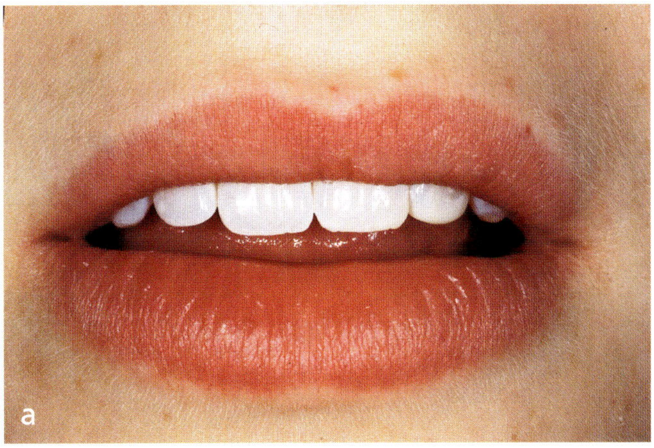

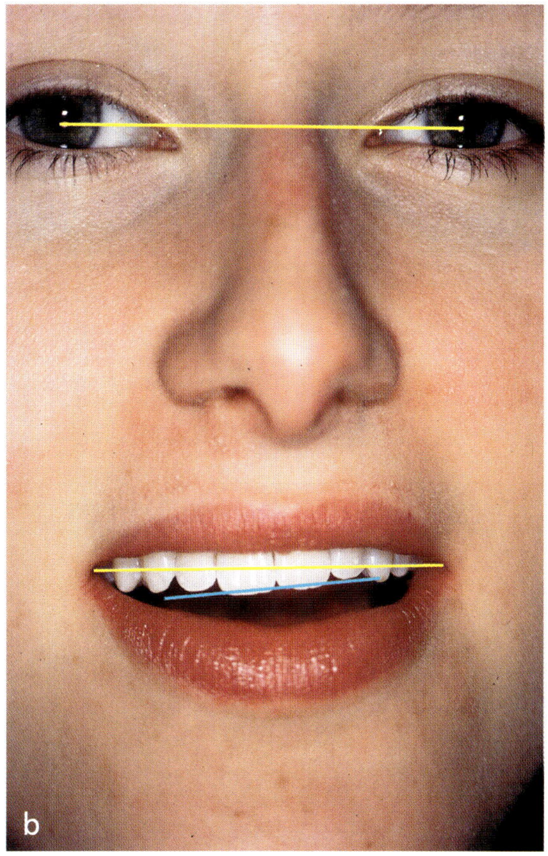

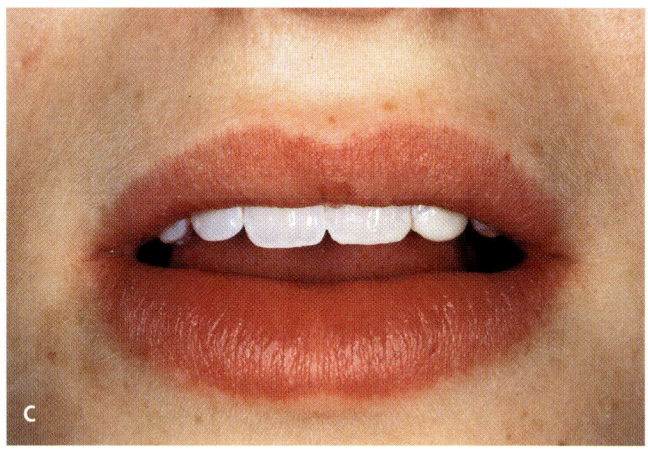

Figs 3-70a to 3-70c (a) Orthodontic setup of the anterior dental segment ignoring the constraints of the vestibular frame. This represents a common mistake in orthodontic treatments. (b) The maxillary anterior occlusal plane does not run parallel to the commissural line, which jeopardizes dentofacial cohesion. (c) In lengthening the left lateral incisor, we tried to create the illusion of line parallelism and equilibrium, using another esthetic factor called "weight of the elements."

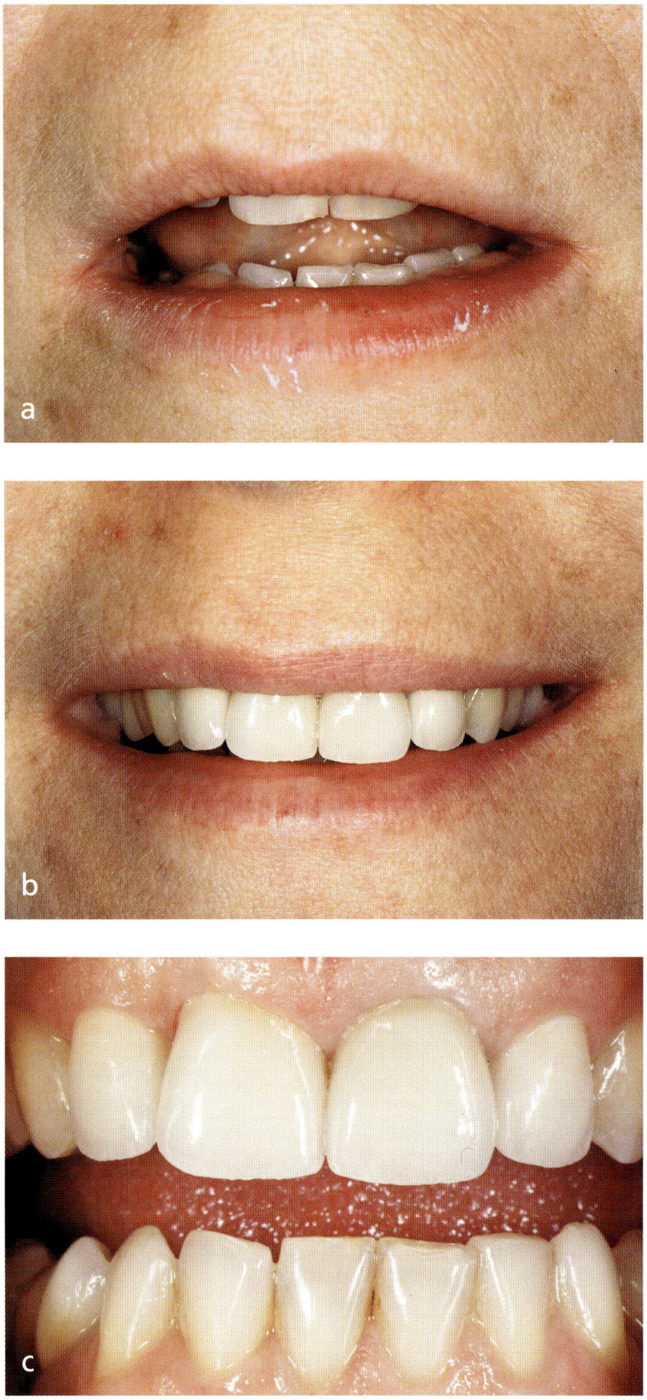

Figs 3-71a to 3-71c (a) A linear discord between the incisal and commissural lines, which took place with advancing age, underlines functional disturbances and affects dentofacial cohesion. In this case treatment planning has consisted of (b) restoring dentofacial linear parallelism and (c) establishing consistent anterior occlusal relationships.

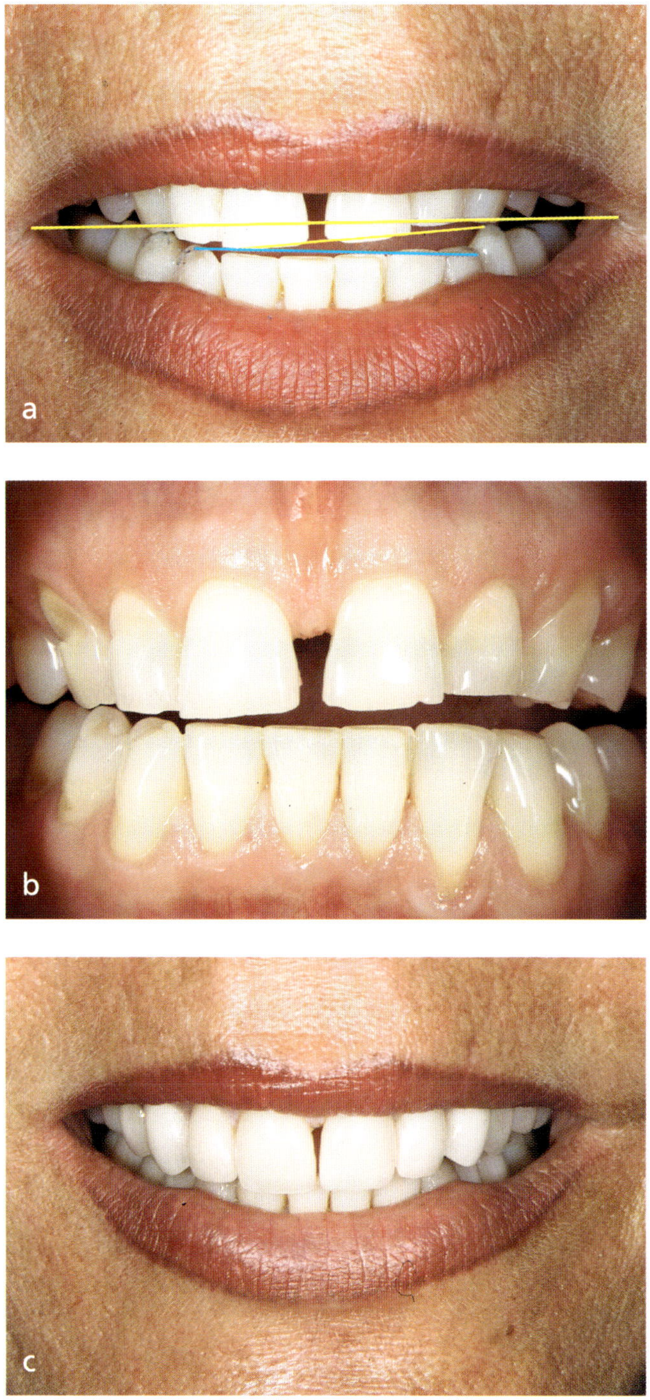

Figs 3-72a to 3-72c A direct relationship exists between esthetics and function. (a,b) When occlusal trauma generates a morphological destruction of original dental elements, the lines of constraint are dislocated and the esthetic quality of both dental and dentofacial compositions is severely affected. The rehabilitative process involves a restoration of tooth anatomic integrity in line with functional and esthetic linear requirements. (c) The multiplication of lines and linear parallelism (gingival line, upper and lower; occlusal line; commissural line; bipupillary line) strengthens the cohesion of the composition.

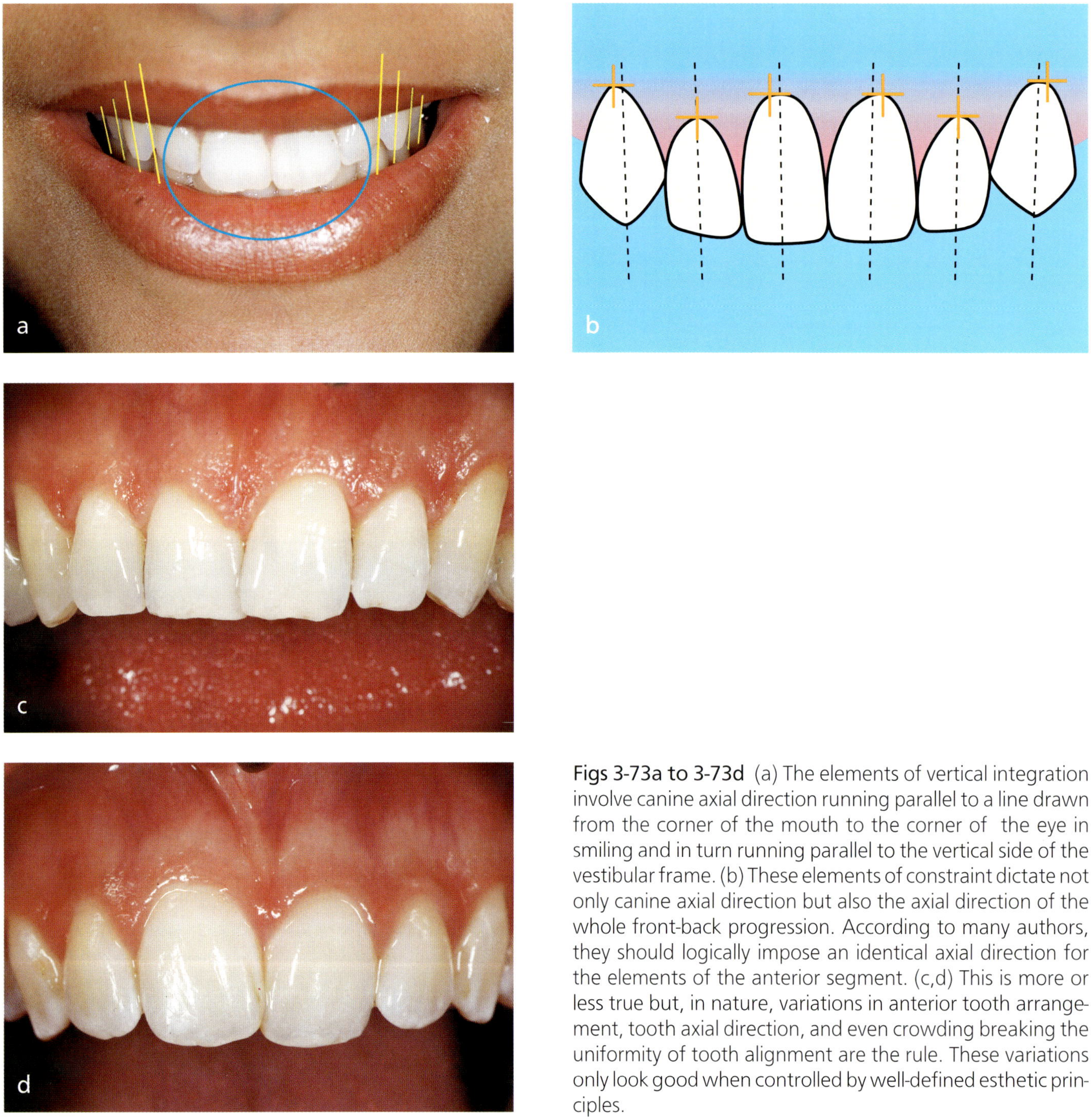

Figs 3-73a to 3-73d (a) The elements of vertical integration involve canine axial direction running parallel to a line drawn from the corner of the mouth to the corner of the eye in smiling and in turn running parallel to the vertical side of the vestibular frame. (b) These elements of constraint dictate not only canine axial direction but also the axial direction of the whole front-back progression. According to many authors, they should logically impose an identical axial direction for the elements of the anterior segment. (c,d) This is more or less true but, in nature, variations in anterior tooth arrangement, tooth axial direction, and even crowding breaking the uniformity of tooth alignment are the rule. These variations only look good when controlled by well-defined esthetic principles.

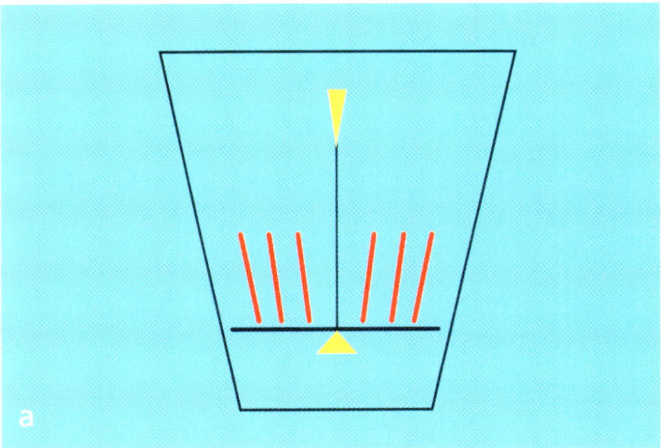

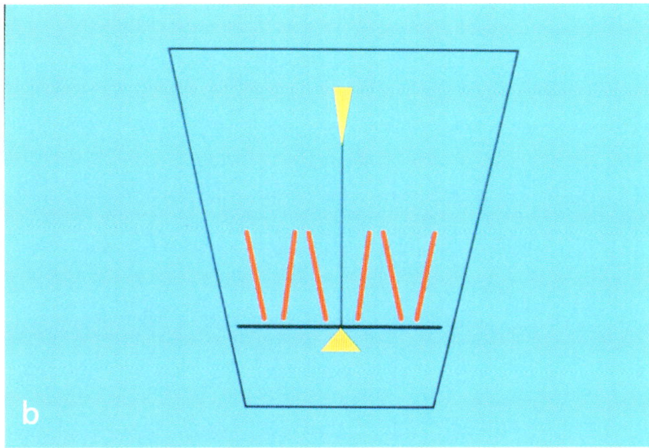

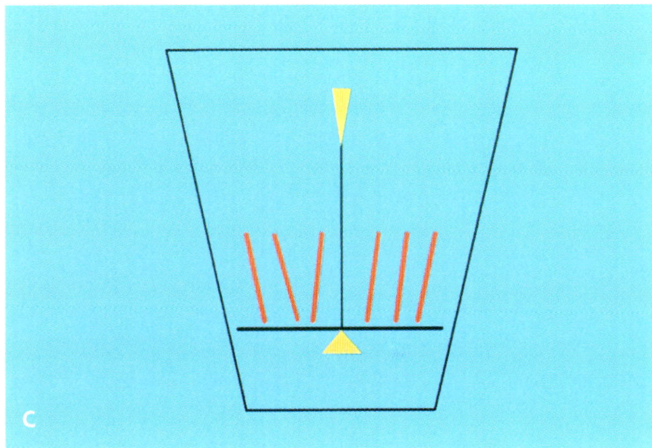

Figs 3-74a to 3-74c It can be observed that the elements of vertical integration articulate around the main line of constraint of the vestibular frame, which develops in its center and so acts as a fulcrum. Consequently, all the elements located on each side of this line should appear in balance. This notion not only finds a practical application in the vertical setup of the posterior segment but also rules the axial arrangement of anterior teeth, according to the basic principle that elements far away from the fulcrum grow in importance. (a) Frontal axial equilibrium, described as ideal by many authors. (b) Frontal axial equilibrium with bilateral axial compensation of divergent lateral incisors. (c) Compensation of the axial divergence of a maxillary central incisor by a weaker divergence of the collateral lateral incisor.

frame, far from presenting restrictions, open a range of clinical possibilities extending from a mathematical rigorism to a controlled artistic creativity. Indeed, the arrangement of the anterior segment can only be judged esthetically appealing when anterior tooth axial direction is determined in such a way that all the teeth are perfectly aligned, according to a rule of order proposed by different authors (Fig 3-73). An esthetic result can also be achieved when malpositioning affecting one tooth or another is controlled by the equilibrium that can occur around the central midline, the primary line of constraint of the vestibular frame. The use of the principle of balance of tooth axial direction finds here an ideal field of clinical application, permitting the individualizing and enhancing of dentofacial esthetics according to principles simulating the laws of nature (Fig 3-74).

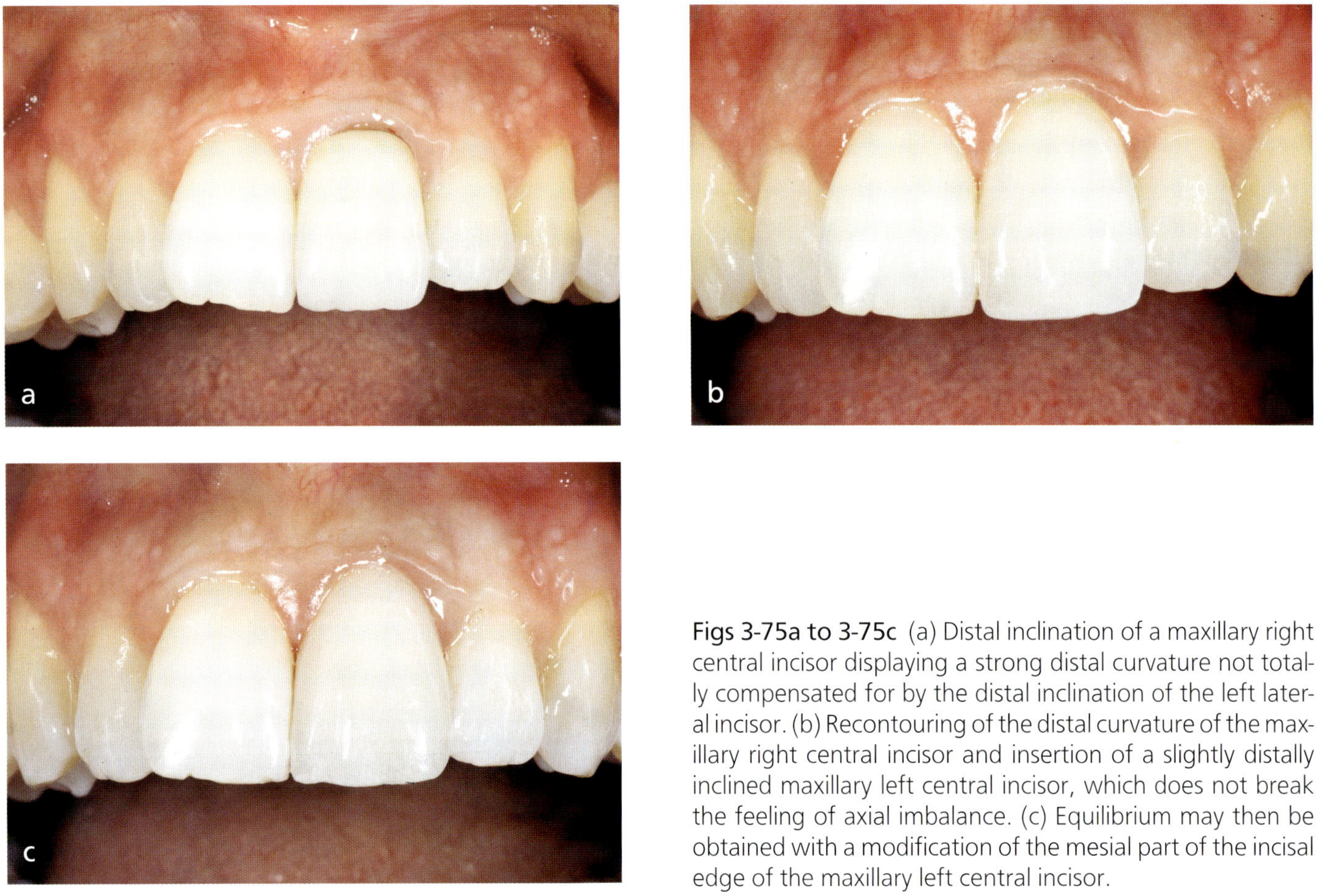

Figs 3-75a to 3-75c (a) Distal inclination of a maxillary right central incisor displaying a strong distal curvature not totally compensated for by the distal inclination of the left lateral incisor. (b) Recontouring of the distal curvature of the maxillary right central incisor and insertion of a slightly distally inclined maxillary left central incisor, which does not break the feeling of axial imbalance. (c) Equilibrium may then be obtained with a modification of the mesial part of the incisal edge of the maxillary left central incisor.

When considering this esthetic factor, which was identified as an objective in a previous publication, one should remember that elements placed far from the fulcrum grow in importance, which means that the mesial inclination of the right central incisor, for example, will be easily counterbalanced by a slight mesial inclination of the left canine, or even a lesser mesial inclination of the left first premolar (Figs 3-75 and 3-76).

Theoretically, the manipulation of this parameter is not restricted as long as it responds to a controlled equilibrium. Yet in practice, the controlled equilibrium that should appear in the dental composition remains extremely difficult to realize at the laboratory level and is best visualized clinically, where the perception of the nature and location of gingival level, of the gingival zenith, influences tooth axial inclination.

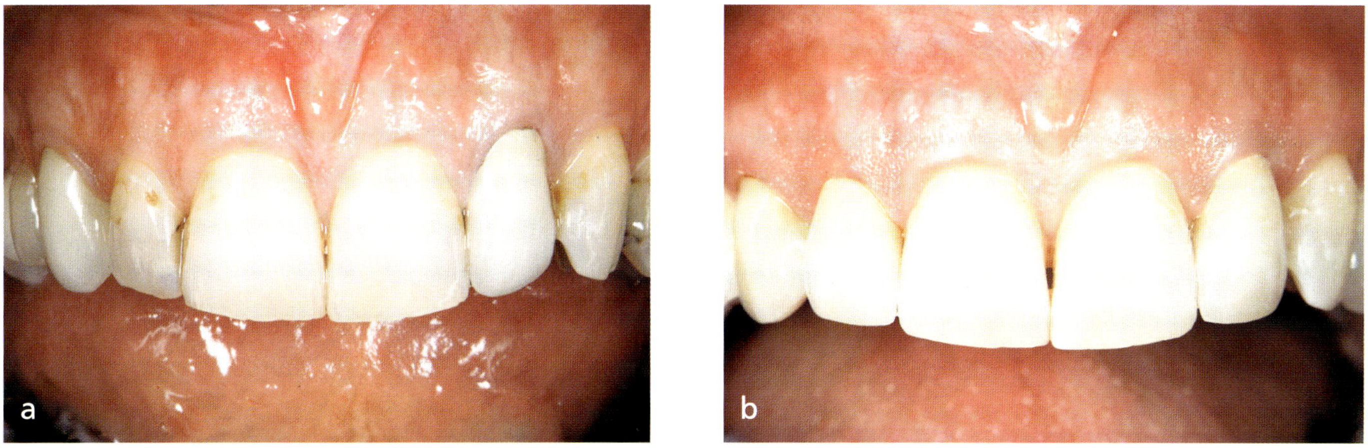

Figs 3-76a and 3-76b (a) Axial disequilibrium of the anterior segment with a general feeling of axial deviation toward the left (b) restored by means of a mesial inclination of the maxillary left lateral incisor over the central.

At this point, one has to keep in mind that the restorative elements of the dental composition should attain in their placement in the horizontal and vertical planes adequate coordination with the lines of constraint generated by the vestibular frame. Indeed, the perception of the lines of force generated by the vestibular frame represents a key factor in restorative procedures, as these lines not only constitute an unavoidable and constraining guideline to introducing new elements into the facial composition in a state of equilibrium but also assure the cohesion between the dental, dentofacial, and facial compositions and, as such, join in the rhythmic patterns that individualize the facial composition.

Visual weight

The notion of weight can be considered an adaptation of a notion of physics, which needs to be explained in the light of natural experience.

We are constantly influenced by an empirical sense of the earth's attraction. Should we have to fix the center of an upright square shape, we invariably position this center slightly higher than its geometric location, unless the square is placed on the ground or the ceiling, in which case the determination of its center will respond to geometric evidence. When a white and a black shape are placed in a plane provided with a clear background, we feel that the dark could be heavier. However, in a complicated and dark composition, a unique white or clear color is perceived as an accent and experienced as relatively heavy (Fig 3-77).

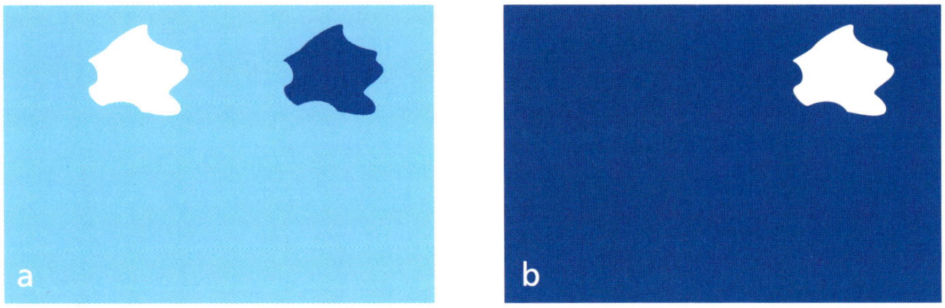

Figs 3-77a and 3-77b (a) When a white and a dark shape are placed on a clear background, the dark seems heavier (b) while in a dark background a unique clear element is felt as an accent and as relatively heavy.

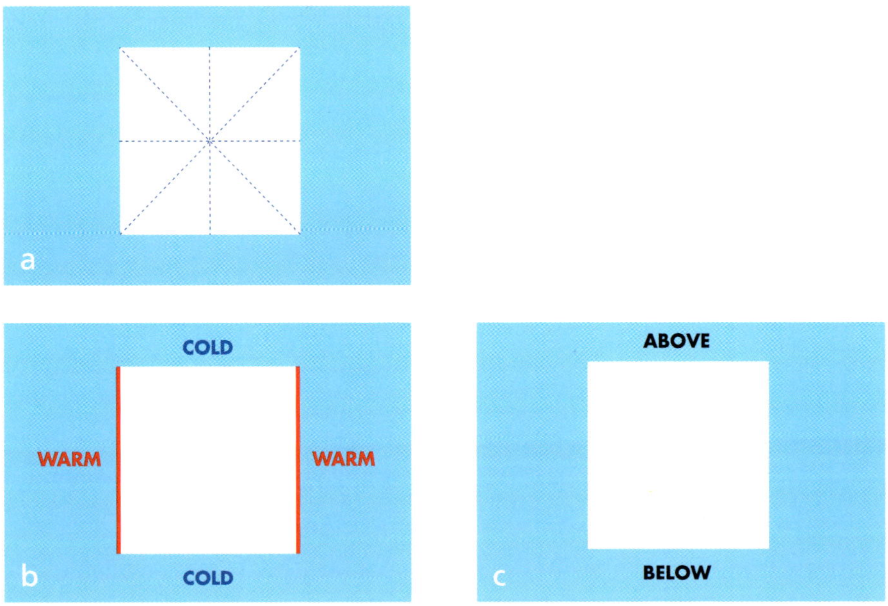

Figs 3-78a to 3-78c (a) In esthetic science, dominated by perceptive capabilities and subjective feelings, everybody can experience the tensions generated by a properly designed basic plane, which determines how new elements may be introduced in a composition in a state of balanced harmony. (b) However, the basic plane can be felt in a totally different way. In its significant qualification, the calm aspect of the basic plane is created by two horizontal lines of coldness and two vertical lines of warmth. This resonance will be transformed into a colder or warmer atmosphere by the extension of the width or height of the basic plane. (c) In its physical qualification, the basic plane can be understood by adopting a more pragmatic approach. Influenced by the phenomenon of gravity, we will perceive the upper and lower parts as the "above" and the "below."

The notion of visual weight adds to the notion of constraints generated by the shape of a plane a notion of tensional strength, which originates from the specific relationships between the mass, the color, and the position of the elements contained in the basic plane. By the term *basic plane* we mean the material plane or esthetic support that holds a composition. In fact, all the elements contained in a composition institute with the basic plane specific relationships which generate tension. These tensions are basic esthetic qualities; variations in their nature and intensity result from the different ways they interact with the basic plane.

While the "tensional" quality of the basic plane, which generates lines of constraint, is the most easily understood, the "physical" quality of the basic plane that will be covered in this chapter needs to be clarified and differentiated from a quality that could be termed "significant" (Fig 3-78). The square's "significant" quality is the two horizontal and two vertical lines of the same dimension that define it.

The qualities of horizontals and verticals have been specified in a previous section. Two elements of cold balanced with two elements of warm determine the objective and tranquil significance of this plane. But whenever the warm or cold predominates, in a rectangular plane for instance, this preponderance determines the significance of the plane. In the trapezoid shape of the vestibular plane, for example, which develops in height, the warm predominates while in the rectangular plane the cold or the warm predominates according to the vertical or horizontal position of the rectangle. What determines its resonance is the spatial position of the shape of the plane.

As a result, the warm atmosphere of the facial plane will never be completely eliminated, no matter what opposing elements are introduced into it. A horizontal in such a plane will always generate a more or less accentuated tension by simple opposition. The esthetic quality of a composition, and the appeal that it generates, is always based on the tensions between predominately opposite natures. These tensions are perfectly realized in the facial plane with marked horizontal elements like the eye line, the bipupillary line, and the commissural line. However, when these oppositions become too strong, for example, with an oversized mouth or eye, the tensional sensation may become unbearable.

In its physical qualification, the basic square plane can be understood and analyzed more pragmatically as its two horizontal lines can be classified as high and low, or more precisely as "above" and "below." Influenced by the empirical properties of gravity, "above and below" have always conditioned every living thing (Fig 3-78). This relationship is also true for the plane, which therefore can also be considered a living thing. Though this assertion may appear strange to someone who has no artistic bent, everyone knows of things that gain in credibility with persistent observation. The "above" and "below" naturally appear to generate opposed tensions (Fig 3-79). Because of the phenomenon of gravity, the "above," which characterizes this part of the plane, seems loose, light, emancipated and free, properties that find their expression in a "warm" atmosphere. On the contrary, heaviness, constraint, condensation characterize the "cold" environment of the "below."

Looseness is the negation of density. The nearer to the upper border of the plane, the smaller individual shapes seem and the more separate they appear. But they are not only farther removed from each

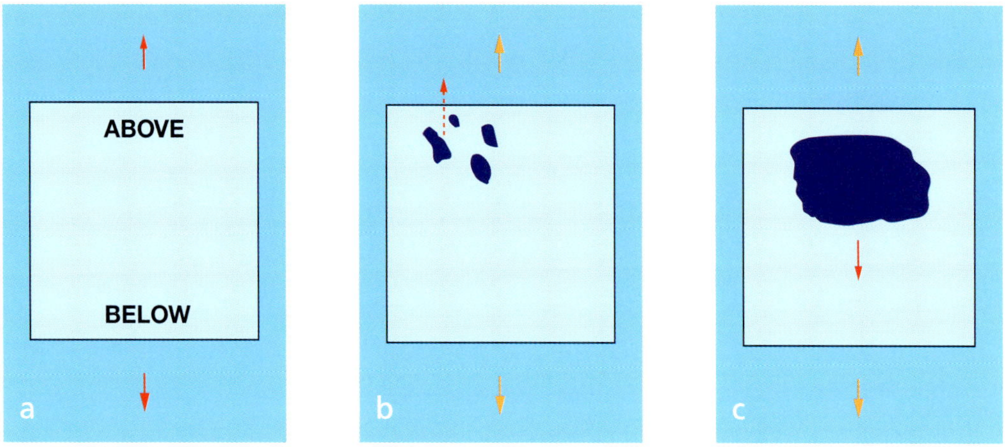

Figs 3-79a to 3-79c (a) The above and below naturally seem to generate opposed tensions. Under the phenomenon of gravity, low density characterizes the above, which gives the impression of looseness, while heaviness and constraint characterize the below. (b) In the above, light and small elements lose weight and increase upward tension while (c) weighty forms grow heavier and generate opposed downward tension.

other; liberty and lightness also increase their inner properties and upward tensional strength. In the "above" part of the plane, light and small elements lose weight and thereby the capacity to support while, as a corollary, weighty forms grow heavier, and this notion of heaviness generates a compensatory downward tension (Fig 3-79). In this atmosphere of freedom, tensions can express themselves more easily. Notions of climbing or falling, which have to be understood as the tensions active within the elements and modified by the tensions of the plane, gain in intensity.

On the other hand, the closer one approaches the lower border of the plane, the denser the atmosphere. Freedom of movement becomes more and more limited and restraint increases. As a result, the smallest shapes lie nearer together and lose weight (Fig 3-80). The downward tensional strength of the plane is reinforced and can only be subjected to tensional compensation with specific opposing directional designs.

The properties of these areas "above" and "below" create the greatest possible tensional contrast. These opposing tensions can be strengthened in a natural way by the accumulation of heavier forms below and lighter ones above. Reciprocally, these characteristics can be neutralized, or at least modified, by the accumulation of heavy forms above and lighter ones below (Fig 3-80).

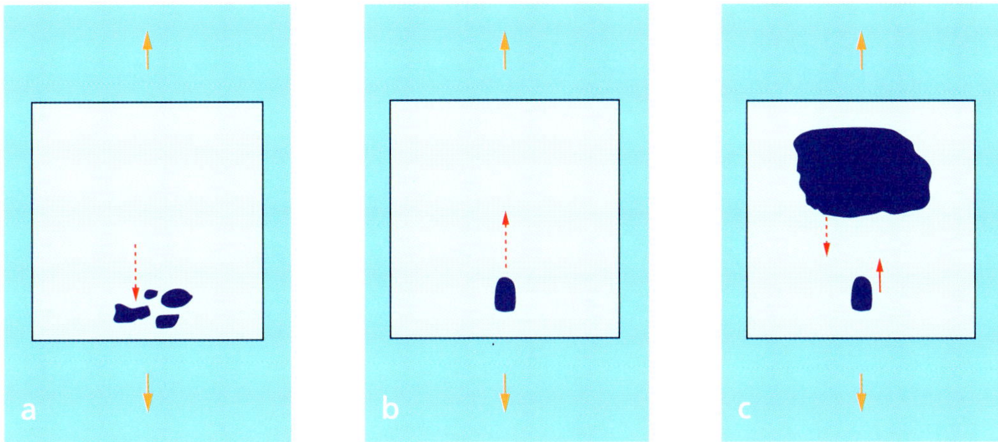

Figs 3-80a to 3-80c (a) In the below, freedom of movement becomes more limited, restraint increases, and the presence of a single or multiple element increases the downward tension. (b) In the below, only specifically designed elements like arrows or sharp incisal edges may create opposed directional tensions. (c) The tensions created by the above and below can be compensated for by the presence of weighty elements in the above and specific designs in the below. This compensatory play of successive opposed tensions creates rhythmic qualities that generate esthetic appeal.

These differences in the placement of simple elements in the basic plane have no impact other than creating subsequent modifications in the rhythmic quality of the plane. This rhythmic quality originates in the position and the nature of its elements and their visual weight. This visual weight, in which colors are of key importance, depends on the subconscious appreciation of a play of tensions which can in turn be accentuated, compensated, or eclipsed.

Like any other plane, the facial and dentofacial planes cannot escape the phenomenon of visual weight. It can be stated that the character, nature, and dimension of the elements of the facial plane—eyes, nose, and mouth, or "facial receptors"—are unlimited. Opened or closed, they represent variables in the play of tensions that, influencing the visual weight of the facial plane, must be considered important factors in esthetic evaluation.

With the advancement of age, the facial receptors, whatever their individual or ethnic particularities, do not undergo profound modifications, with the exception of the mouth, whose spatial position is submitted to the influence of infraorbital soft tissue laxness generating variations in upper and lower tooth display. In practice, it is in this area, defined as the dentofacial composition and characterized by the "above" of the upper lip and the "below" of the lower lip, that the various manifestations of visual weight will demand our attention.

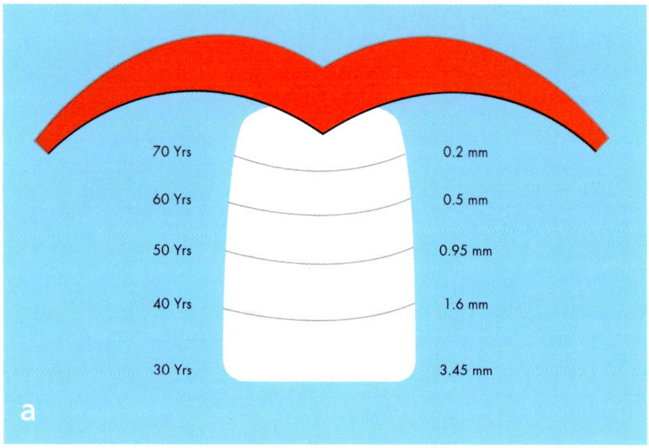

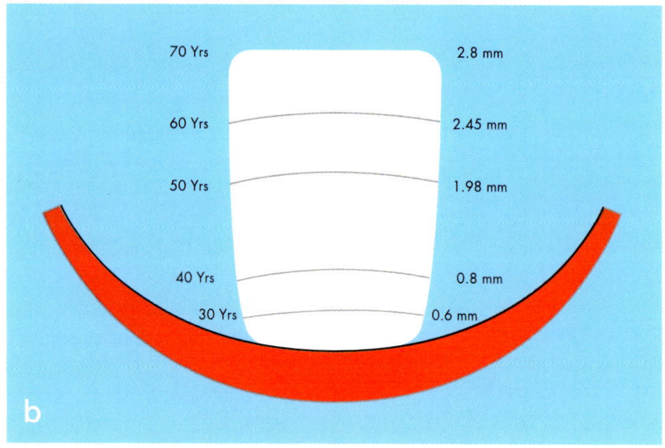

Figs 3-81a and 3-81b A diagram of (a) maxillary and (b) mandibular tooth exposure in rest position as a result of aging.

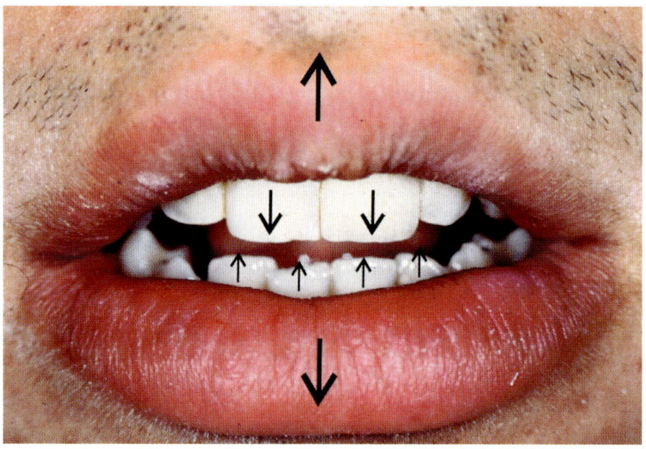

Fig 3-82 A young person displaying, at mandibular and lip-rest position, a large amount of maxillary tooth and minimal mandibular anterior dental elements, creating in the dentofacial plane successive upward-downward tensions that result in an appealing visual and psychological pull and push.

We know that at 20 years of age, mouth slightly opened, maxillary tooth display reaches an average of 3.5 mm while lower teeth remain barely visible, a situation generating interesting rhythmic qualities in the dentofacial composition (Figs 3-81 and 3-82). With the advancement of age, the increase of muscle laxness affecting the infraorbital muscles will progressively diminish maxillary incisor tooth display, insidiously causing mandibular incisor visibility and loading excessively the lower part of the dentofacial plane (Figs 3-83 and 3-84). As a result, the rhythmic quality of the dentofacial plane that characterizes the average individual in youth is irreversibly affected. Individual variations are multiple but never really bring in doubt the irreversibility of this degrading process (Figs 3-85 and 3-86).

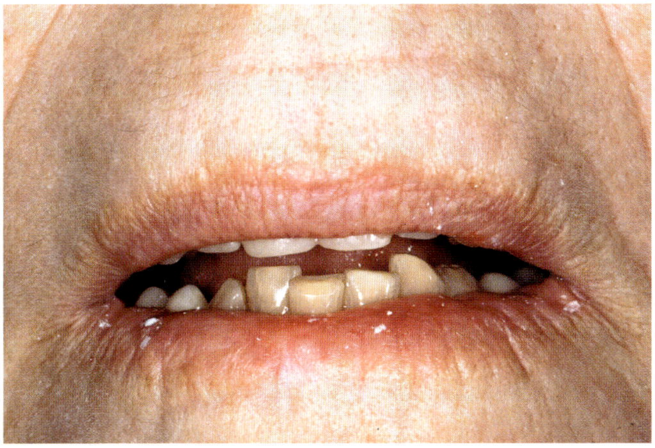

Fig 3-83 With the advancement of years, maxillary tooth display decreases while mandibular tooth display increases. In this composition, maxillary teeth are still visible, but they increase the upward tension of the above while mandibular tooth visibility increases the downward tension of the below. The composition is reduced to two opposed tensions dominated by the tension of the below, a situation disturbed by punctual upward tensions from erupted mandibular elements.

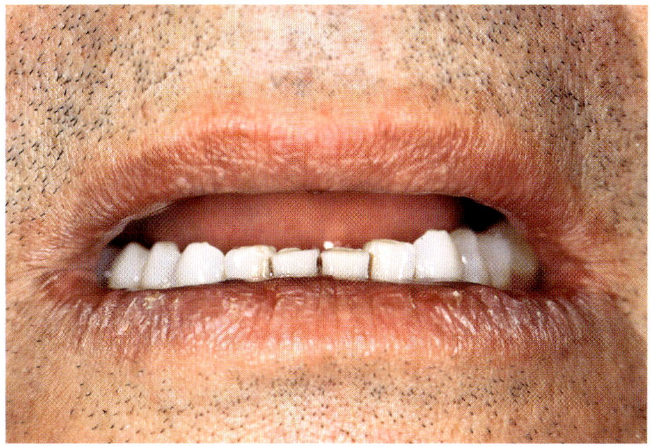

Fig 3-84 The increase of muscle laxness starts to become obvious between 30 and 40 years of age and never ceases its debilitating effects, characterized by tooth display in rest position and by the dynamic of speech limited to the lower segment.

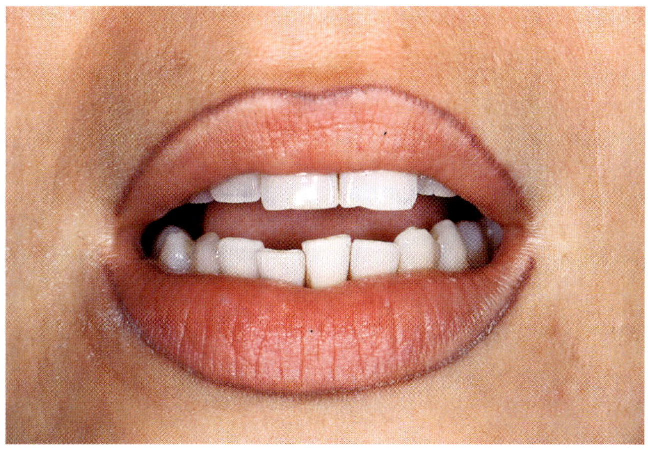

Fig 3-85 The significant mandibular tooth display of this woman in her 30s may contravene the norm of average tooth display related to age yet conforms to that related to ethnic origins. Note that the raised upper lip, generating the strong upward tension of the above, requires as counterbalance the full quantity of the downward opposite tension of maxillary central incisors, unfortunately eroded by the abrasion process. As a result, the downward load of the below, stressed by low lip width and design, which has achieved some type of equilibrium in the sharpness of badly positioned incisors, cannot be totally compensated for.

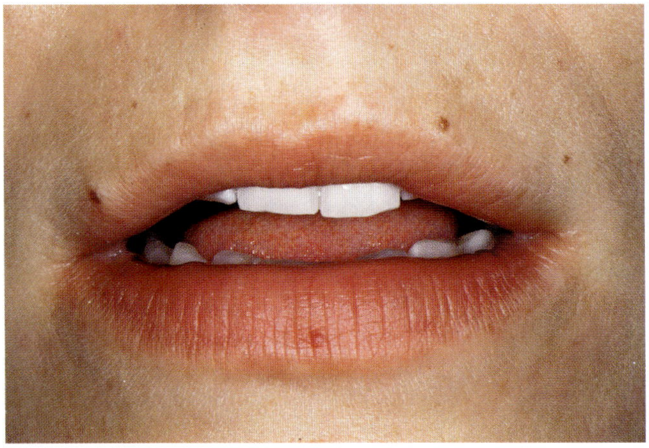

Fig 3-86 Worn maxillary incisors can no longer provide the compensatory downward tension required by the above for this woman in her 30s. Mandibular tooth display is reduced to its most lateral elements by reason of ineptly posed mandibular incisors. The play of tensions in the dentofacial composition is restricted to the opposition between the above and the below and generates nothing more than weak and undefined rhythmic properties.

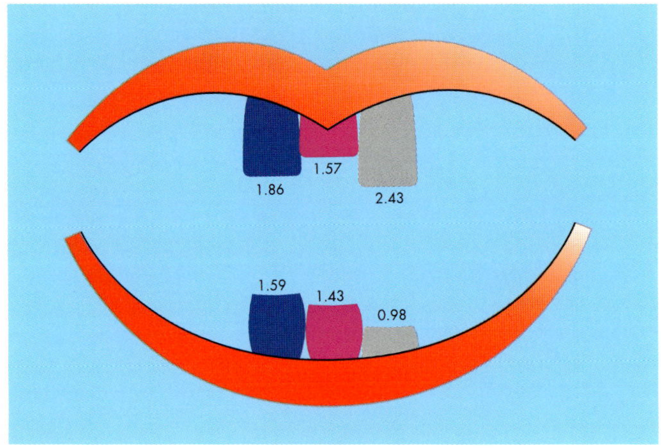

Fig 3-87 A diagram representing tooth display according to ethnic origins, showing that evaluation and treatment have to be adapted to individual conditions: blue = Asian; pink = African; gray = Caucasian.

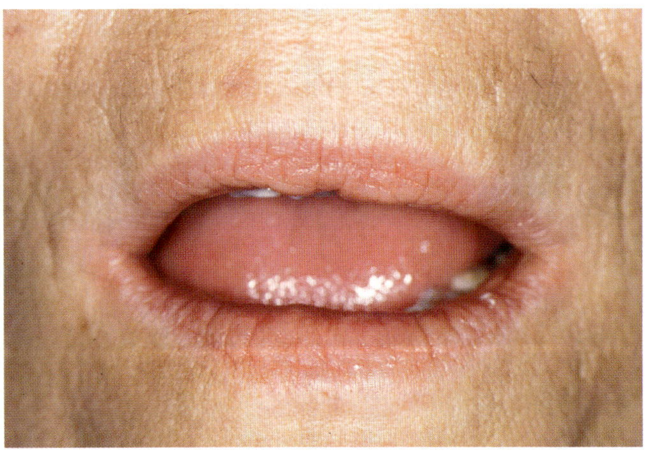

Fig 3-88 When both wear patterns have succeeded in totally eliminating maxillary and mandibular tooth morphology, tooth display may still not be absent in rest position. Dentofacial equilibrium is restricted to the opposed upward and downward tensions of the above and the below.

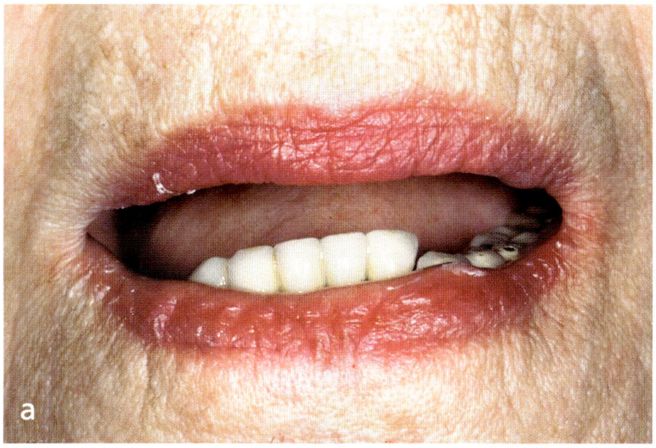

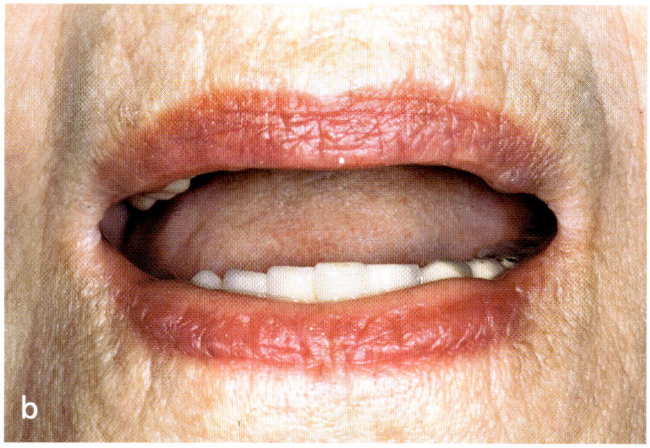

Figs 3-89a and 3-89b (a) The eruptive process of the mandibular anterior segment invading the oral cavity, originating from an absence of interocclusal relationships. (b) Restoration of mandibular tooth visibility without much benefit for the rhythmic qualities of this composition, yet improving facial cohesion by the addition of a supplementary parallel linear tracing.

It must also be mentioned that not only age but gender and race affect tooth exposure. Indeed, the average tooth exposure in rest position increases from African to Asian and Caucasian for the maxillary central incisor and decreases from Asian to African and from African to Caucasian for the mandibular incisor (Fig 3-87). These elements show that the restoration of ideal rhythmic qualities in the dentofacial composition are not fixed but must be adapted to each particular case. Therefore, the restoration of interesting rhythmic qualities constitutes a very real challenge for the restorative dentist when the advancement of age has made visible the impacts of successive accidental events.

In fact, one can frequently notice an absence of any tooth visibility in mandibular and lip-rest position when infraorbital muscle laxness and tooth wear advancement have combined their degrading effects. This absence of tooth visibility leaves visual weight only to the two opposed tensions of the "above" of upper lip design and the "below" of lower lip design. Yet this hardly draws visual attention and never receives esthetic appreciation (Fig 3-88).

When, with advancing age, progressive muscle laxness afflicts an individual with various degrees of intensity, we are faced not only with the combination of various functional manifestations of tooth wear but also with migratory movements originating from unstable anterior occlusal relationships, another cause of reduced esthetic appeal in the dentofacial composition and, by extension, the whole facial composition (Fig 3-89).

The determination of the mandibular frontal occlusal plane, and the clinical modifications of this

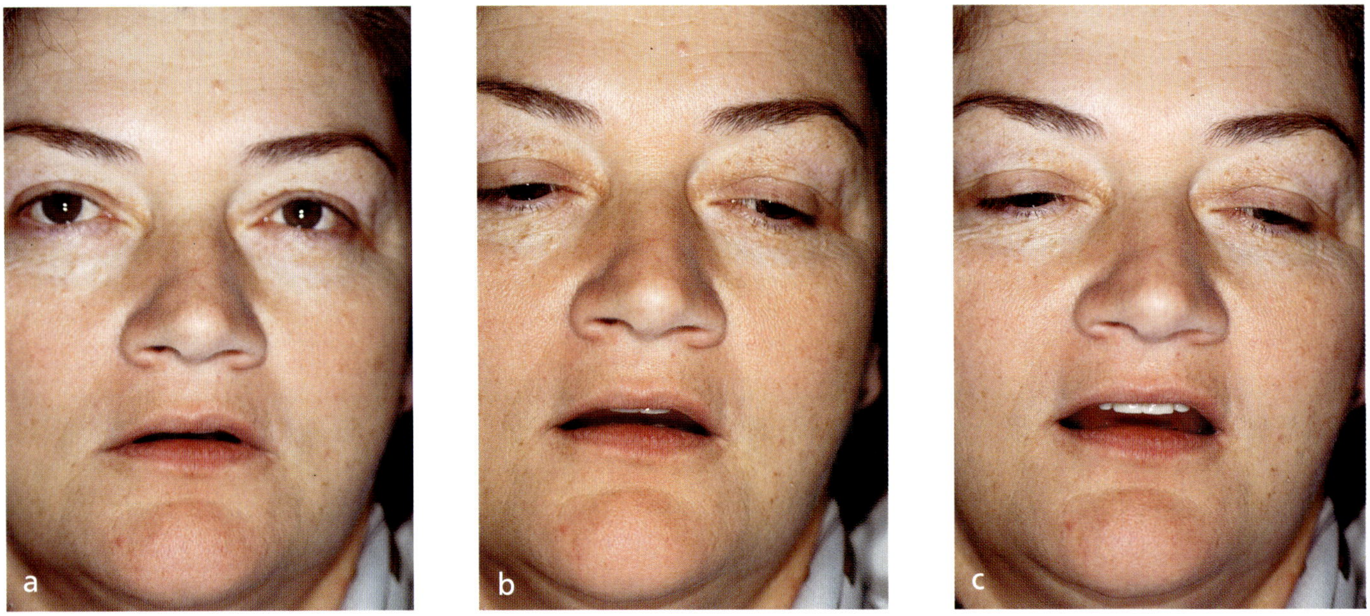

Figs 3-90a to 3-90c Progressive and temporary setup of maxillary tooth display in rest position in the initial phase of full-mouth rehabilitation. These conditions will be provisionalized and finalized in the ultimate phase of the treatment.

plane with respect to tooth visibility, must be considered a prerequisite to any rehabilitative procedure. Indeed, the rhythmic properties of the dentofacial composition arising from this determination will deeply influence and condition the esthetic quality of a rehabilitation, the purpose of which is the duplication of the original rhythmic characteristics of a young dentofacial composition.

Clinically, we should take here a sequential approach beginning with an evaluation of mandibular tooth display, though the establishment of the maxillary central incisor's visibility in rest position by means of repetitive interrogations must be considered coincidental (Fig 3-90). One to three millimeters of maxillary tooth display can be considered ideal, with appropriate variations according to age, gender, and tooth coloring. Tooth color demands care in aging patients even if they express some inclination for exaggeration since colors, white in particular, influence the esthetic quality of forms (Fig 3-91). However, while clinically the evaluation of maxillary tooth display is practically coincidental with mandibular tooth display, the setup of the mandibular anterior segment always precedes the finalization of the maxillary segment since this sequential setup permits the fulfilling or refining of esthetic and functional requirements.

The increase of mandibular tooth display with age

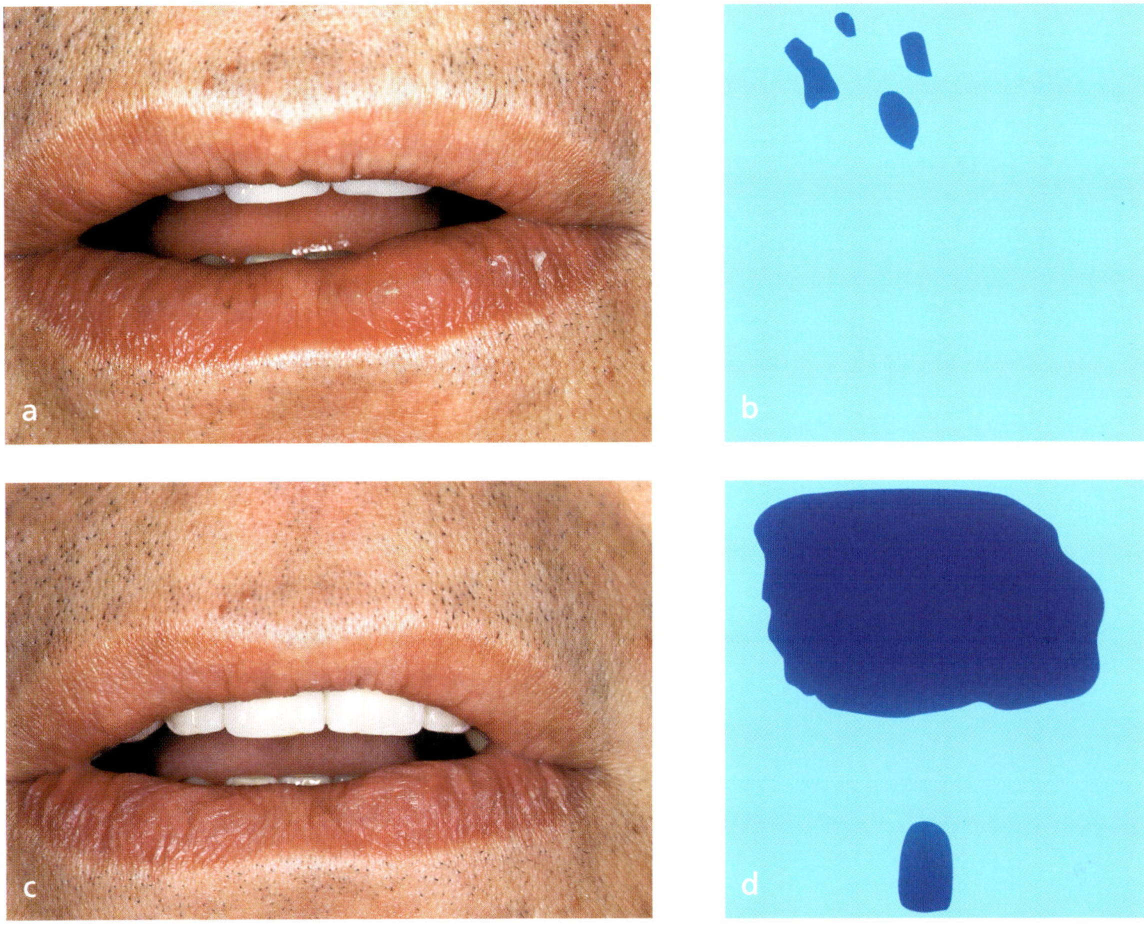

Figs 3-91a to 3-91d (a) Limited maxillary tooth display in rest position in a zone of low density, promoting a climbing effect or (b) an upward tension coincidental to that generated by the above of the plane. Practically no mandibular tooth display can be seen, which means no tensional impact. (c) Restoration of a limited mass of excessively white maxillary incisors, compensating for the upward tension of the dentofacial plane. In the mandibular area this excessive tooth coloring already promotes a perceptive upward tensional strength that compensates for the downward tension of the below. (d) These conditions mirror the rhythmic qualities displayed in young adults.

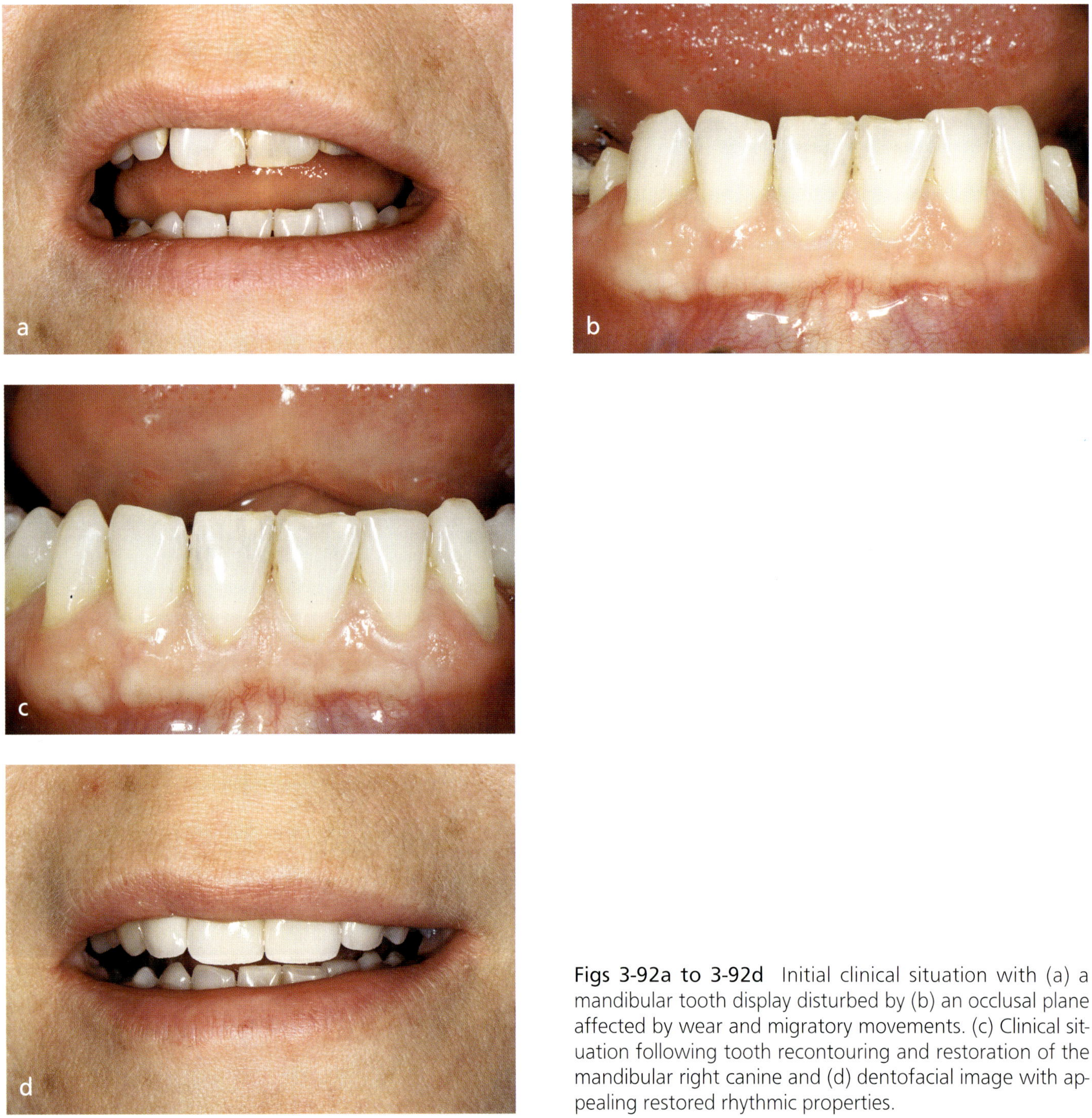

Figs 3-92a to 3-92d Initial clinical situation with (a) a mandibular tooth display disturbed by (b) an occlusal plane affected by wear and migratory movements. (c) Clinical situation following tooth recontouring and restoration of the mandibular right canine and (d) dentofacial image with appealing restored rhythmic properties.

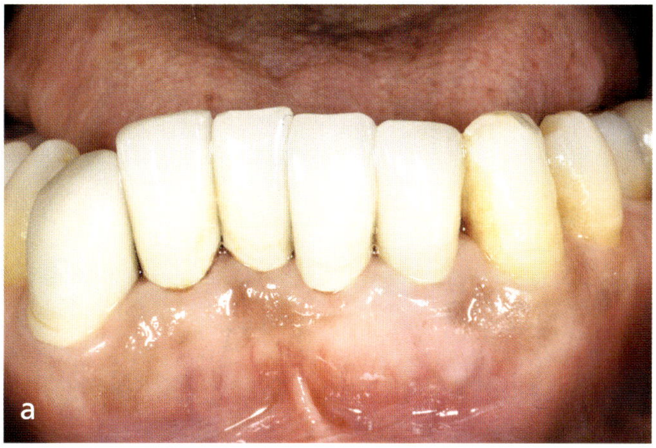

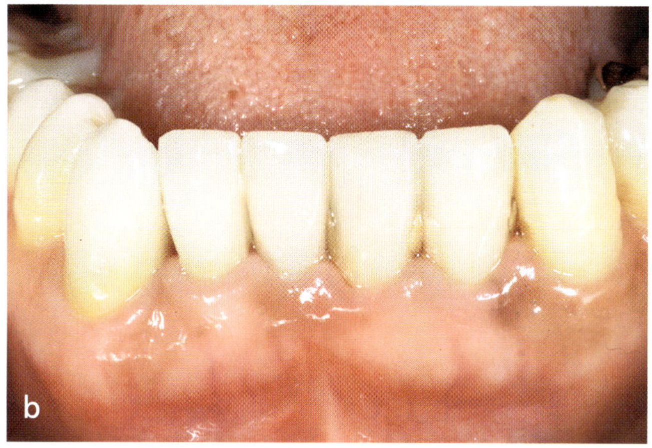

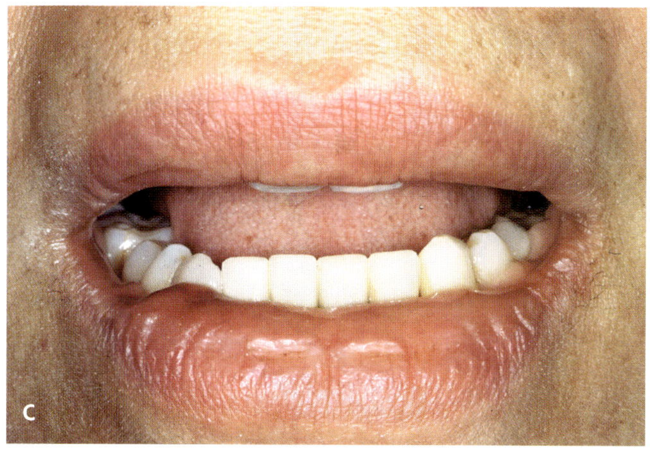

Figs 3-93a to 3-93c (a) Mandibular anterior segment with right malposed canine and incisors erupting in the below of the dentofacial plane. (b) Clinical situation following periodontal tooth elongation and subsequent prosthodontic restoration. (c) The confrontation of the restored dental composition with its dentofacial plane environment does not really call into question the validity of such a treatment but shows that each individual detail has its importance in achieving esthetic objectives. Sharp incisal edges could have provided the means to introduce contradictory upward tensions in the downward tensional loading of the below, whereas in this case maxillary tooth elongation was necessary to restore ideal rhythmic properties.

imposes, with few exceptions, a systematic lowering of the mandibular anterior occlusal plane, which involves three different types of approach: (*1*) tooth recontouring procedures when a minimal reduction of tooth exposure is sufficient (Fig 3-92); (*2*) periodontal elongation with a reduced restored tooth length at a lower level, which usually satisfies most of the compromised cases (Fig 3-93); and (*3*) extraction of the lower anterior segment, with or without reduction of osseous height, and consequent restoration of these teeth at a lower level when occlusal conditions have permitted an eruptive movement of teeth and supporting structures (Fig 3-94). In extreme cases, presenting simultaneously an eruption of the lower anterior segment and TMJ problems, usually occurring in Class II, division 2 cases as a result of repetitive protrusive-retrusive centric precontacts, it must be admitted that the final approach, however brutal, is the best for both functional and esthetic reasons.

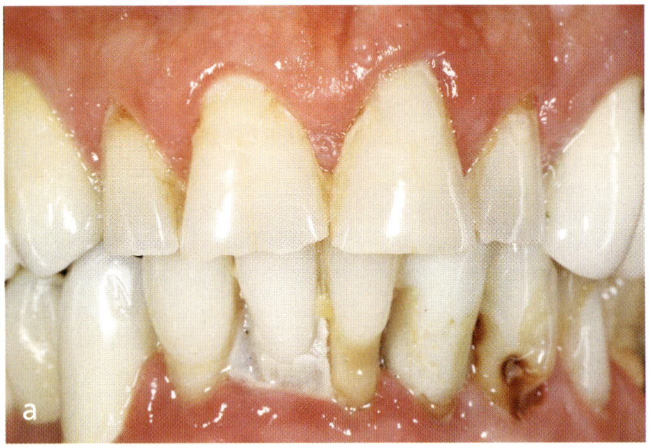

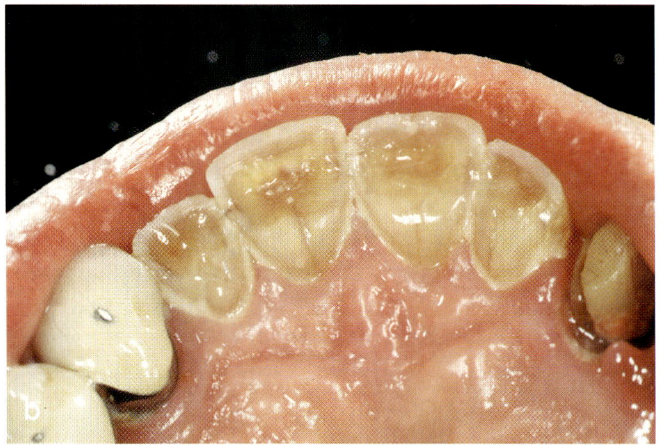

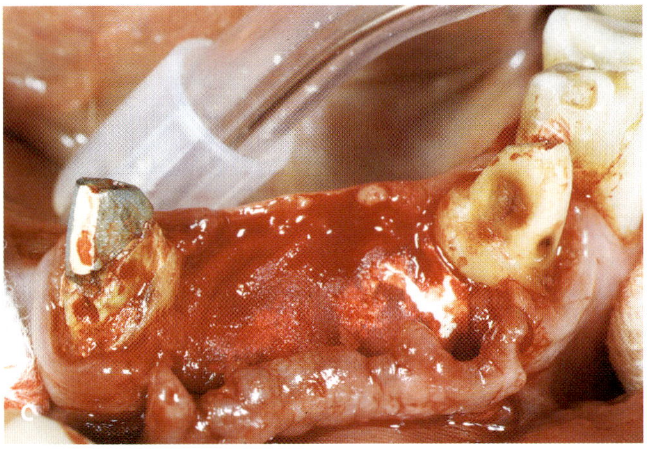

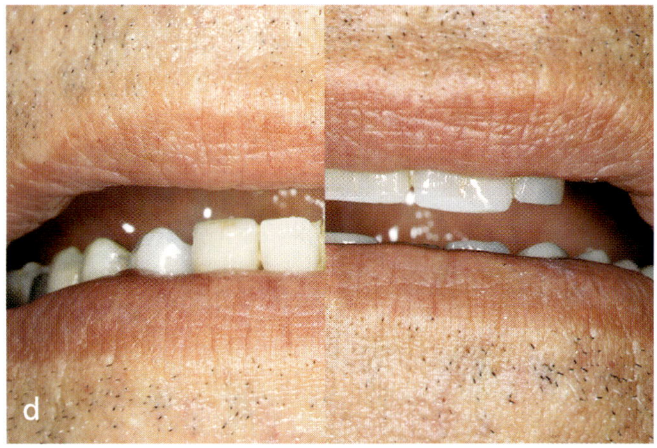

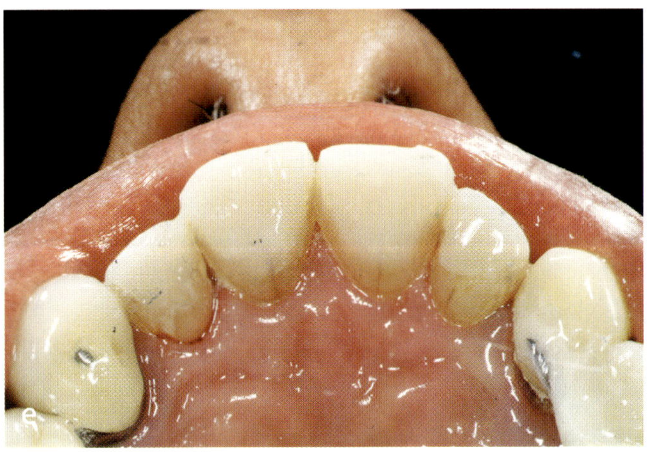

Figs 3-94a to 3-94e (a) Interocclusal relationship with periodontally compromised dental elements. (b) Lingually abraded maxillary segment. (c) Extraction and surgical reduction of the level of the mandibular anterior osseous base. (d) Comparative tooth display at rest position before (*left*) and after (*right*) lowering of the mandibular occlusal plane. (e) Anterior occlusal stabilization by addition of provisional composite restorations on the maxillary lingual antagonist surface.

To start any rehabilitative procedure with the restoration of the maxillary anterior segment is a major clinical error. When the location of the lower occlusal plane and tooth display have been determined as an initial therapeutic measure, the adaptation of the maxillary segment by the modification of tooth length and lingual morphology permits the fulfillment at the same time of functional and esthetic needs. Any other approach would impair both function and esthetics.

The purpose of a correct placement of the maxillary and mandibular occlusal planes is to restore the most appealing tooth display, both in the rest position and during the dynamic of oral movements, and to duplicate the rhythmic properties that are seen in the young and characterized by a succession of opposed tensions, generating an appealing movement of eye and mind, a "pull and push" suggesting elements of the esthetic doctrine of Hans Hofman, who has so greatly influenced the movement of American abstract expressionism.

The determination of maxillary and mandibular occlusal planes will be useless if it ignores such basic functional requirements as the restoration of ideal maxillomandibular teeth relationships, specific parameters linked to the vertical dimension of occlusion and a coordinated adaptation of posterior occlusal planes. When the proper determination of anterior occlusal planes generates and restores the rhythmic properties of the dentofacial composition, specific oral parameters such as maxillary tooth length and position can then be reappraised according to environmental conditions. This involves modifying tooth display and tooth length with regard to the tensional strength originating from the "above" of the dentofacial plane, that is to say, the upper lip. A thin, straight upper lip does not generate the same upward tensional strength as a raised, firm, thick upper lip, which requires longer or more massive dental elements that generate a downward tensional counterbalance. None but the trained practitioner can evaluate these parameters, all too often the cause of esthetic failure when left to the laws of chance.

Tension of the elements

The tension of the plane and the weight of the elements together constitute a framework, a guideline for introducing elements into a composition so as to attain an equilibrium of weight and position. They are the obligatory organizational factors of a composition. But they are affected by the emotional resonance of a composition, which helps generate its esthetic appeal. This resonance results from an esthetic language composed not of words but of forms and colors.

Each esthetic element has been described as the outward expression of inner tensions. The resonance of a composition must be considered the result of, or the sum of, the tensions inherent in every element, the tensions between the elements, and those between each element and the whole. These tensions, which are key factors in our esthetic response, must be made intelligible and perceptible.

The esthetic science consists in discovering among straight lines, curved lines, and shapes a potentially infinite network of mutual relationships that requires a constant action of the eye and mind. Within this inextricable network, one must identify the phenomena that attract the eye and stimulate the mind. These

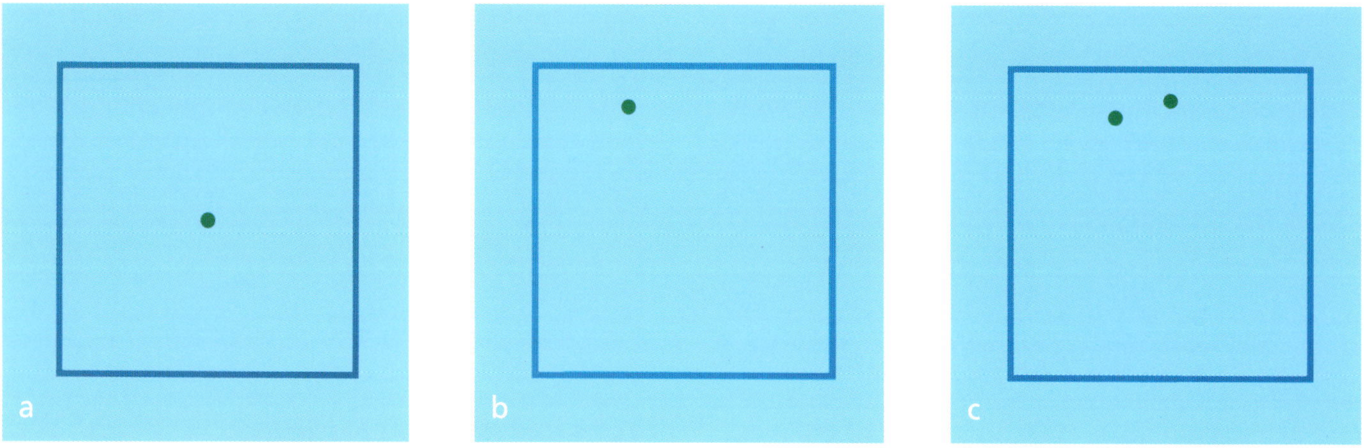

Figs 3-95a to 3-95c (a) When placed in the center of a square composed of two elements of cold and two elements of warm (which together negate its expressivity) at the crossing point where tensional strength is relieved, the point loses its concentric and intrinsic qualities. (b) If we were to move this point in another direction, these qualities would again become perceptible, vibrating on the whole plane. (c) The introduction of another point reinforces its intrinsic qualities while at the same time its extrinsic qualities become suddenly perceptible.

are generated by the excess of tension displayed by one or two elements, by the tension between elements, by the material accumulation of elements on a privileged surface, by the specific arrangement of elements according to character—for example, by contrast—and by the sensation of possible disequilibrium.

Dominance factor

So far the basic elements of esthetic language—points, lines, and shapes—and the various morphological developments of facial structures have been presented here in isolation from any type of environmental influence. Yet the esthetic reality of a composition is never so restricted.

We have defined the origin of any esthetic composition as the moment a point finds materialization on a plane, stressing the fact that these two elements are inseparable. Point and plane alone constitute the simplest composition and the point in the center of the square its most concise manifestation (Fig 3-95).

From this composition, we might expect a specific resonance given the inherent tension between point and square. But two elements of cold and two of warm that constitute the geometric square negate its expressivity and reduce the resonance of the composition to that expressed by the only element it possesses, the point. Yet that point's intrinsic and concentric qualities, placed in the geometric center of the basic plane, at the crossing point of the lines of constraints, at the key point where tensional strengths are relieved, are suddenly reduced to silence (Fig 3-95).

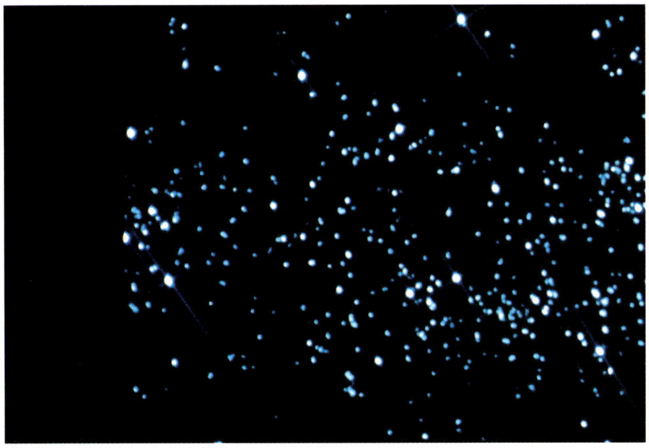

Fig 3-96 Each shape radiates its qualities to the surrounding structures. Thus the intrinsic qualities of an element may be tempered, eroded, or augmented by contact with other forms.

Should we move the point away from the center, its significance becomes perceptible again because of vibrations or exterior tensions that influence the whole plane, and the resonance of the composition is increased. This movement has reinforced the primary concentric qualities of the point, which now become predominant (Fig 3-95). Apart from the restored perception of the significance of the point, every similar movement in various directions generates different sonorities that the previous construction had reduced to silence. Apparently minor modifications of the composition may result in rather complex consequences, generating a specific resonance each time.

Again we are dealing here with a composition connecting a single primary element with the simplest basic plane. If we introduce another point into the basic plane, not only will the concentric qualities of the point be reinforced but also, at the same time, its eccentric qualities will appear.

The resonance of a composition is generated by the interaction of its outer form and the elements it contains. A primary element of the esthetic composition, the point, whatever its location and its static characteristics, can either overpower or be overpowered by exterior forces that may draw it in one direction or another.

Each element radiates its qualities to the surrounding structures (Fig 3-96). Though its primary tension may well remain predominant, that tension may be either weakened or reinforced by exterior tensional strengths produced by other elements of the composition. The tensions inherent in each element are affected by contact with other elements, and may be either tempered or augmented by such contact. It may be destroyed or flourish; it may multiply or disappear.

As a result, a form more potent than those which surround it may take over the whole picture and imprint its own image on everything. This dominance factor is crucial to the esthetic effect of a composition. It is this that determines its final resonance.

The criteria that influence the evaluation of the facial resonance are extremely complex. The dentofa-

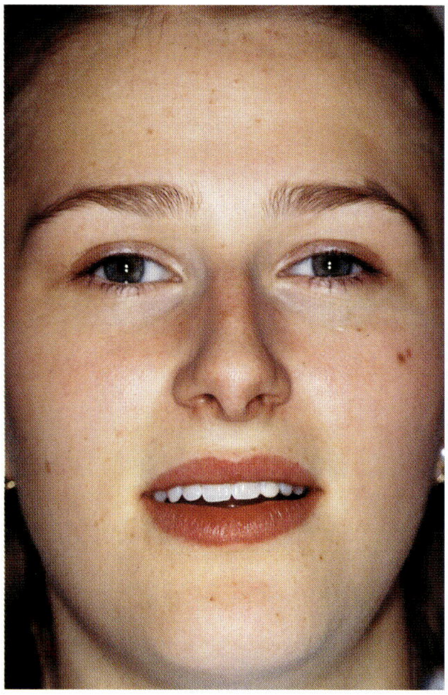

Fig 3-97 A facial composition with perfect oval shaping, apparently imposing multiple facial and dentofacial curvatures, among them upper and lower lip design, incisal line, and well-designed rounded dental elements. The constraint of the suggested eyeline and commissural line breaks and, at the same time, realizes the prevalence of these curvatures.

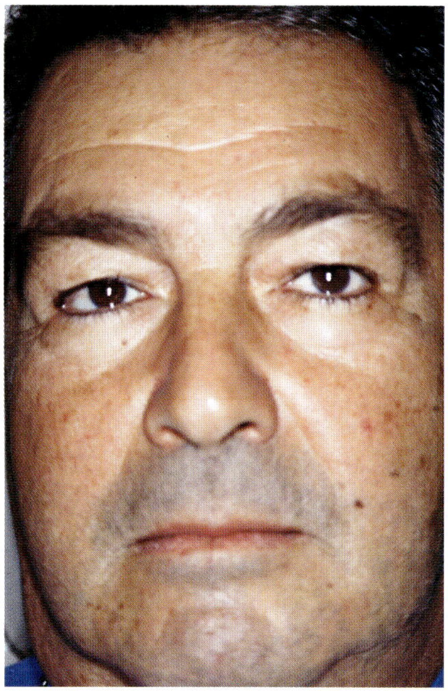

Fig 3-98 A facial composition characterized by multiple square components and straight lines, conveying the characteristics of maturity, calmness, and rigor. Could the dental composition present anything other than a straight linear design and square dental elements?

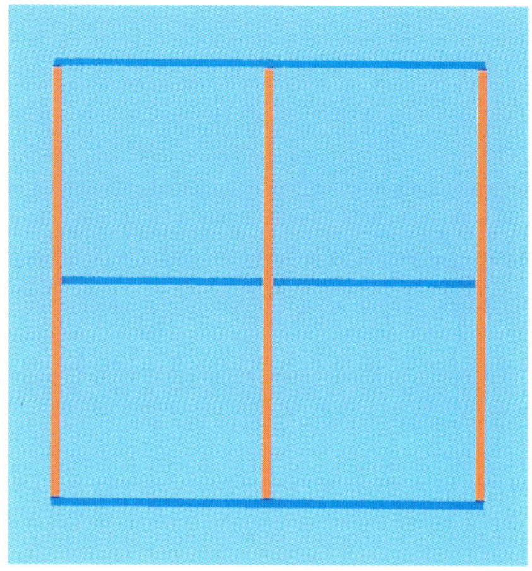

Fig 3-99 In comparison with a composition presenting a single sonority, the introduction of these two lines is accompanied by an increase to 12 sonorities. The multiplication of more or less identical tensions gives the composition its resonance.

cial composition may present elements of such dominance that they will overpower the new elements or impose their own character on them (Figs 3-97 and 3-98).

But a composition may elude the power of a specific character and display a resonance of a weaker nature. For an example, let us take again the same basic square plane. Instead of placing a point in its center, or two, or multiple points on its surface, we draw two lines, one vertical, one horizontal, crossing each other in its center. A new and complex composition is now created (Fig 3-99). These two lines, which can be considered isolated by reason of the impossibility of repeating them, display a strong resonance. The opposition of significance attributed to each of these lines should logically destroy this resonance. However, esthetic logic does not conform to Cartesian logic, and this resonance remains perceptible through the reciprocal action of simple elements in elementary combinations. In reality this composition,

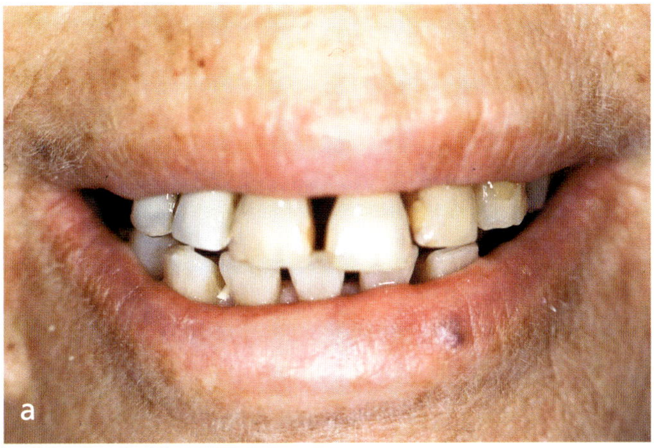

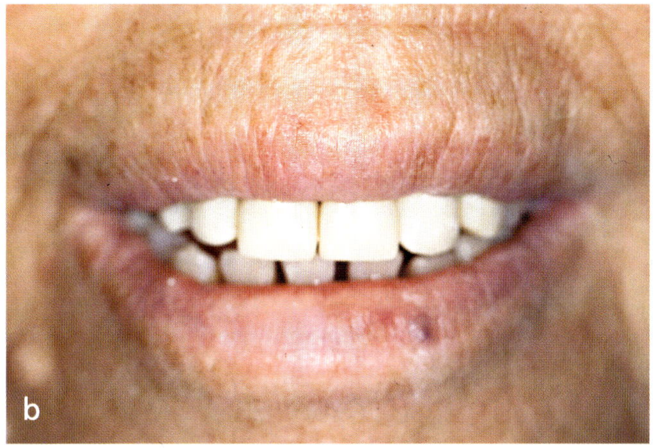

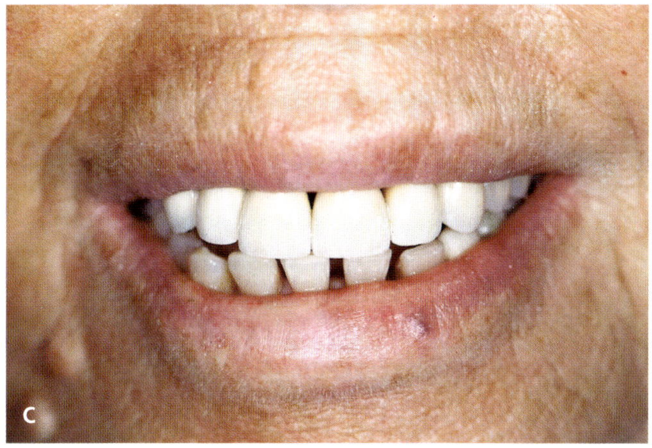

Figs 3-100a to 3-100c (a) Physical and psychological laxness, volumes, and depressions characterize this dentofacial composition. Yet square maxillary lateral incisors and broken and straight lines in lower lip design suggest that a natural modification of these characteristics has taken place. (b) A provisional setup with square maxillary central incisors and correction of the anterior flare. (c) Final restoration with more rounded dental elements and breaks in the incisal line, the dotted line optically reducing anterior segmental width. Observation shows that any type of physical or psychological modulating element can be introduced into this composition. This is an example of a dominant factor of a relatively weak nature.

made up of a square divided in four squares, represents the simplest division of a schematic plane. Six horizontal elements of cold and 6 vertical elements of warm bring the sum of the perceptible tensions to 12. If the composition with a unique point in its center has one sonority, this one has 12 sonorities. These 12 sonorities involve 4 sonorities of the plane and 2 of the line, making a total of 6, doubled by the juxtaposition or combination of elements. Yet the multiplication of more or less identical tensions has achieved the resonance of the composition (Fig 3-99).

Identical situations may surface in rehabilitating the dentofacial composition, leaving various possibilities for modifying, modulating, or confirming its resonance (Fig 3-100). The principle of dominance is especially important since it introduces a privileged element of tension that will first attract our attention and sensibility.

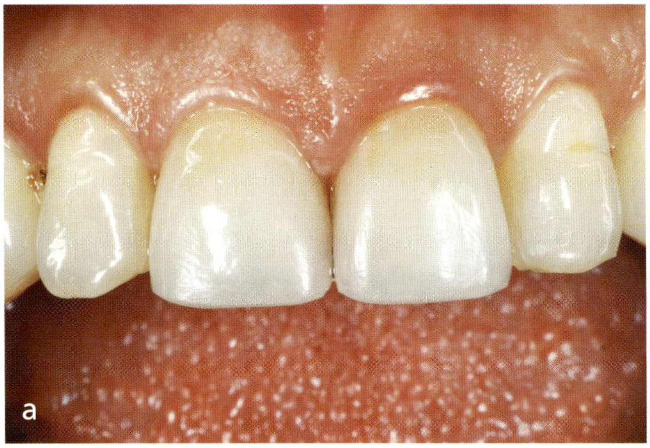

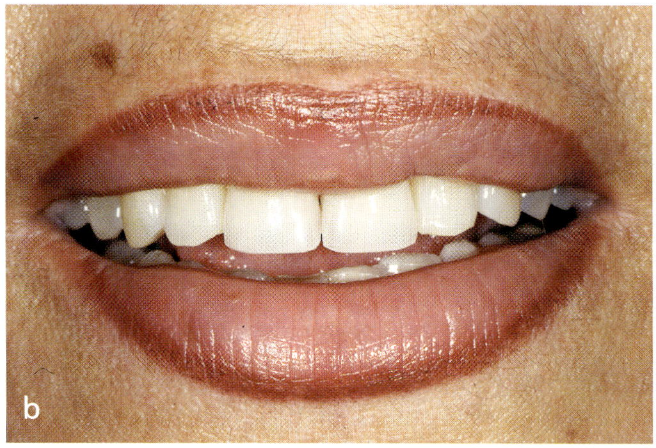

Figs 3-101a and 3-101b (a) The introduction of two maxillary central incisors, exceeding in length the lateral incisors, generates what has been called an individual dominance. (b) This definition loses sense when the composition is seen from another vantage point where the dominance is appreciated as segmental.

Strength and quality of the dominance factor

In a composition, each element radiates its qualities to the surrounding structures. The resonance of a composition results from the psychological impact either of all the elements in it acting in concert or of the prevalence of one of its elements. No absolute criteria can determine which, if any, element is dominant. Each element is subject to the nature of its environment and to the various kinds of interference taking place in this environment, as perceived by a human individual influenced by physiological and psychological reactions.

As we have seen, a point in the center of a square loses expression. But if it is moved away from the center, the concentric and intrinsic qualities of the point are suddenly restored, influencing the whole plane, individual elements of which are either relieved of or impose their dominance. An accumulation of points in a square surface may well release multiple eccentric tensions; however, the concentric qualities of the point remain predominant, and the multiplicity of the elements only reinforces their impact.

The dominance factor can be considered the materialization of disequilibrium, an unavoidable and essential element of esthetic appeal. In dentofacial esthetics the dominance factor implies a concerted disequilibrium of shape, color, or character radiating from the expansion or reduction of facial zones, from each facial receptor or element of the facial structure (Figs 3-101 to 3-104).

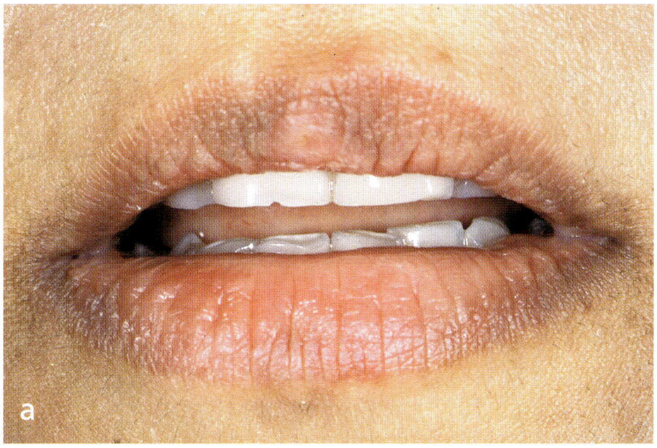

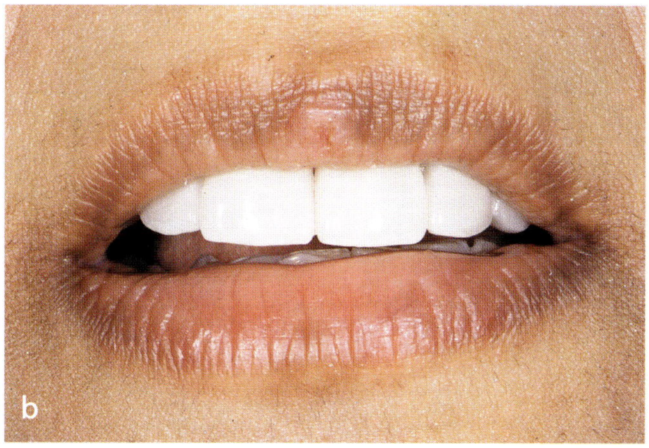

Figs 3-102a and 3-102b The restoration of a dentofacial composition may well promote interesting elements of physical or character dominance and, like the extroversion and ambition displayed by a thick and raised upper lip, these characteristics have to find confirmation in a confrontation with the whole facial composition. At the same time, these elements need to be stressed by parameters of a purely esthetic nature, such as the sensitive introduction of opposing tensions in the shape of the "above," the pronounced upper lip curvature, achieved in this case by the mass and design of maxillary incisors.

This point of view also encourages us to consider the patient's personality as an essential element of dentofacial esthetics. Respect for the patient's facial resonance or its improvement is the ultimate objective of dentofacial rehabilitation. Such facial harmony can only be achieved when restorative elements are perfectly subordinated to this resonance.

This subordination requires the following:

1. Promoting the predominance of a main tension
2. Using subsidiary elements to lessen or intensify the main tension
3. Avoiding the repetition of identical tensions that generate monotony.

The apparent disequilibrium generated by the dominance principle is rectified by a continuous action of the eyes and mind, which generate what has been termed a "dynamic equilibrium." In esthetics, this factor of dominance is characterized not only by its strength, which implies a concerted disequilibrium of size, number, and character, but also by its quality.

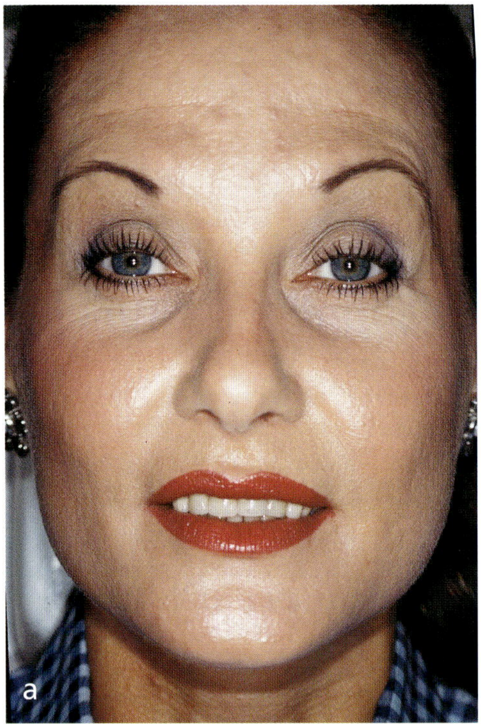

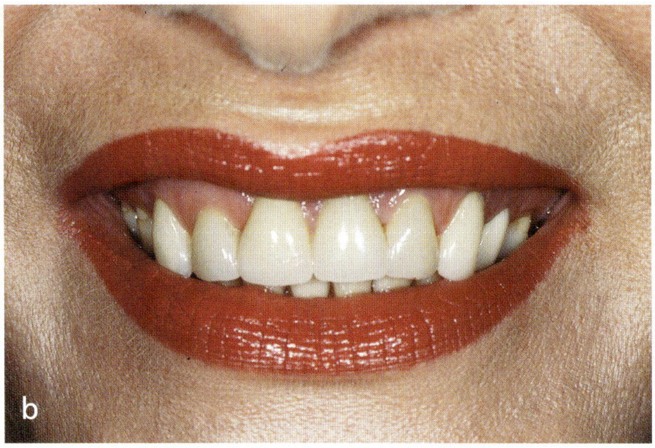

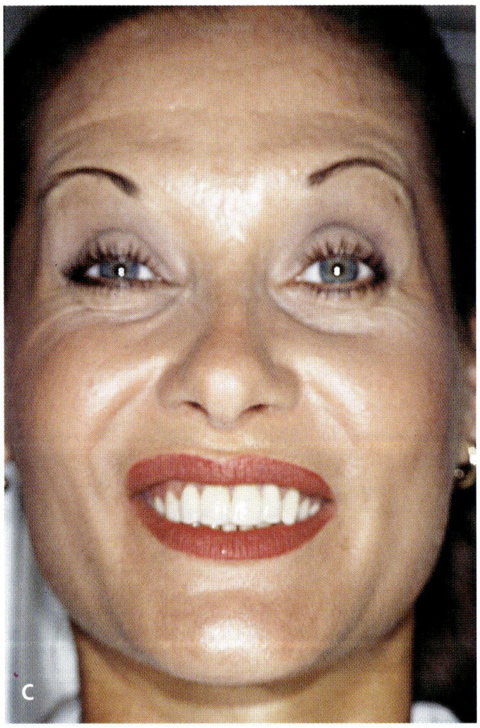

Figs 3-103a to 3-103d Two elements have to be considered in the evaluation of the dominance factor as displayed in the facial composition: (*1*) The extension of the facial zones (a) and (*2*) The nature of the receptors, either closed or opened (b). In the absence of any type of dominating element, the facial composition remains dull and loses attraction. In increasing tooth length, the dental restoration has promoted both the virtual expansion of the lower facial third and the prevalence of the mouth, emphasizing character traits linked to this facial zone. Analysis of the dentofacial composition (c,d) provides only limited information about its participation in the whole facial composition.

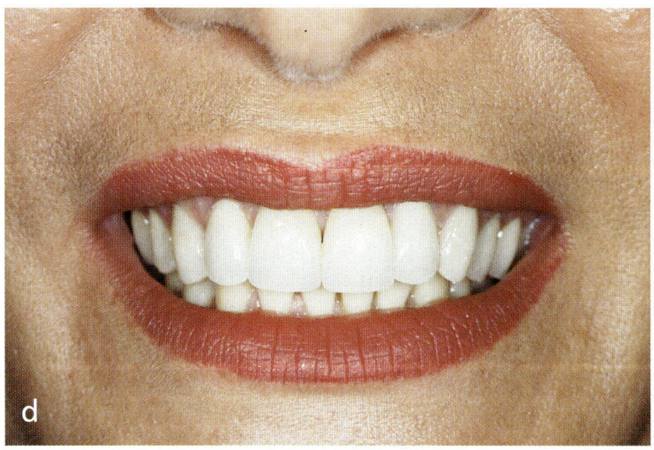

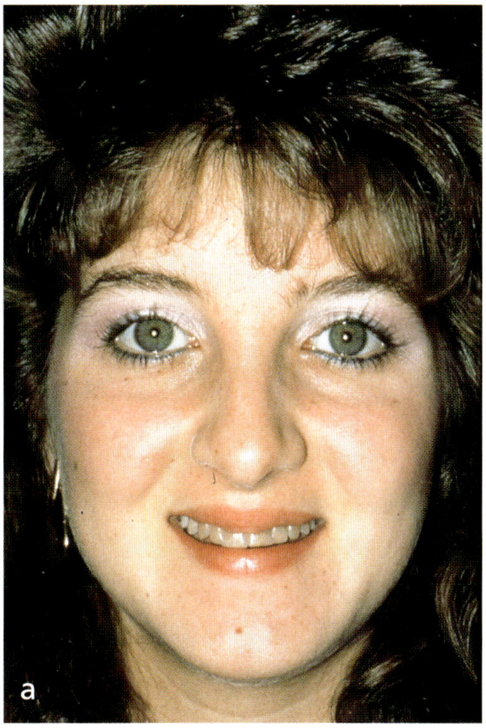

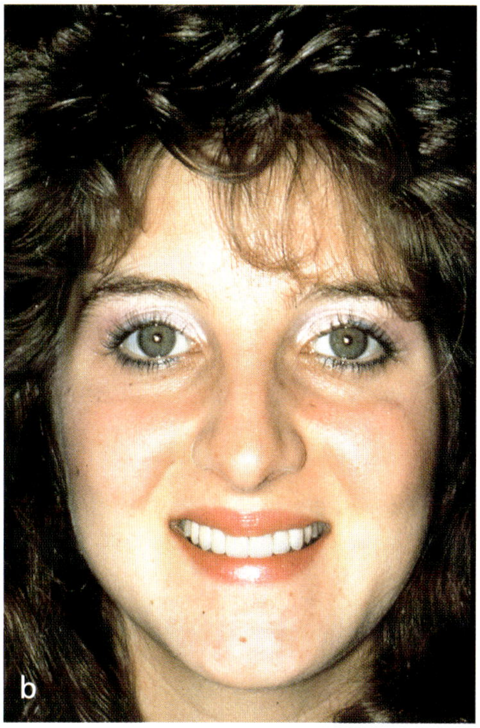

Figs 3-104a and 3-104b (a) A dentofacial restoration may not only emphasize the mouth or the lower facial third when the dominance factor fails to express its prevalence but may also moderate a too-strong disequilibrium. (b) Since the length, width, and color of the anterior segment have been emphasized, the disturbing dominance of the eyes has been moderated. (Courtesy Dr R. Nixon, Los Angeles, CA.)

Correspondence and contrast of character

The determination of the qualities of points, lines, and forms does not alone suggest, in the conception of a composition, the range of possible esthetic combinations. The elements in a composition will only appeal to our sensibility through the energetic qualities and the specific tensional relationships they develop in interaction with each other. These relationships are based on a correspondence of character and can be negated by the prevalence of a contrasting setup that does not respect specific conditions of arrangement.

It can be stated that the visual registration of a circle can be achieved in a continuity of movement impossible in the registration of a triangle, which must overcome three successive interruptions created by the sharpness of the angles. Moreover, these two forms, participating in different and even opposed geometric categories, display no similarity of charac-

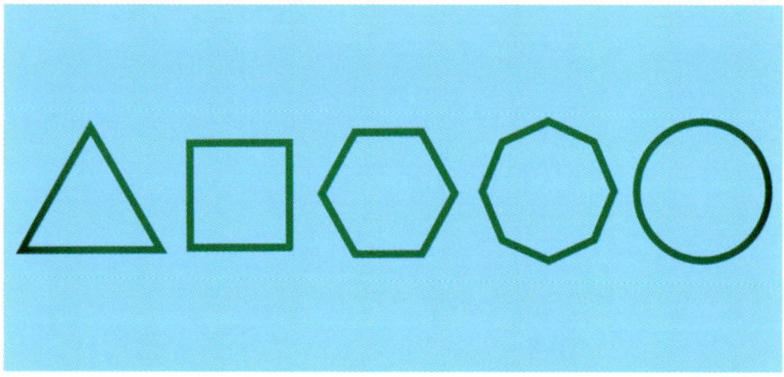

Fig 3-105 The triangle and circle are directly opposed in geometry and character. One could, however, imagine intermediate geometric forms that could create a smooth connection between them.

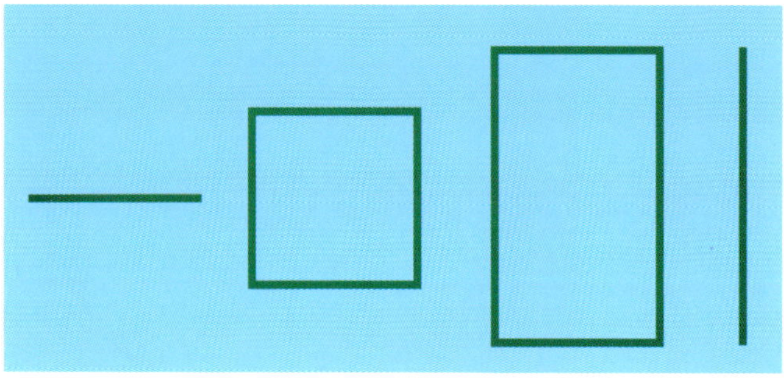

Fig 3-106 The horizontal and vertical lines are just as directly opposed. However, a comprehensive formal evolution of the first element may naturally result in the design of the second. These transformations are based on both geometric and psychological logic.

ter. A decagon, however, offers a smooth visual transition close to that presented by the circle, with which it therefore bears a very close identity of character. Yet one can easily imagine, between the circle, triangle, and decagon, intermediate geometric figures permitting the connection of structures that at first sight could be considered irreversibly opposed (Fig 3-105).

One could also consider that the cold and warm qualities expressed by a horizontal line and a vertical line are irreversibly opposed. However, a progressive formal evolution may lead to perfect correspondence of these lines when one of them is the dominating element in the form it produces. For example, in a horizontally elongated rectangle, the dominating element is the horizontal line. However, the rectangle also presents vertical lines that will find realization in the square shape, which in turn may be extended as a vertically elongated rectangle whose reduction will produce a vertical line (Fig 3-106). The transformation of a vertical line into a horizontal one, as well as the sequence of character evolutions leading to the transformation of a circle into a triangle, depends not only on geometric but also on psychological or physiological logic.

These relationships are purely schematic and do not correspond exactly to elements in the facial composition. Yet the tensions generated by the complex sequence of character correspondence participate in the variety of phenomena that trigger esthetic response. In the facial composition, this type of chain reaction has usually resisted realization. Yet elements of proportionate relationships are significant exceptions (Fig 3-107). For our purposes proportion is a

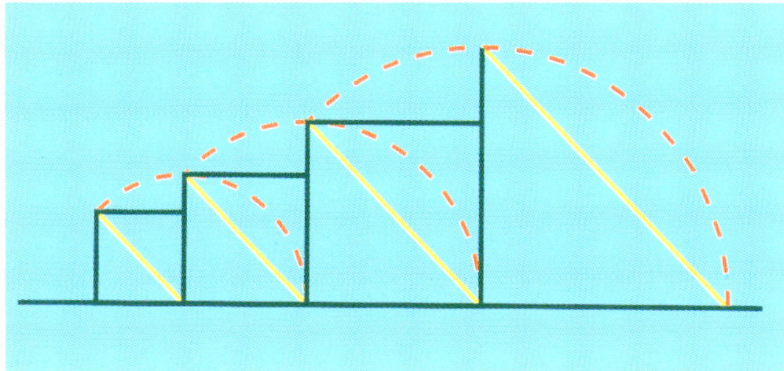

Fig 3-107 In the facial composition, these types of chain reactions have always resisted realization. However, a logical sequential progression, similar to that determined by the diagonal of a square and fixing the location of various entities of the facial composition, could perhaps offer opportunities of application in human compositions.

progressive sequence of ratios fixing specific relationships between different entities. So defined, proportion is no less important than correspondence and contrast of character, and therefore much attention will be dedicated to it in this chapter. The main reason correspondence and contrasts of character have not been investigated is in the irrepressible tendency to relate one element to another by formal similarity or by principles of symmetry.

Two elements, totally different but located close to each other, will always be visualized as a whole, probably simply by acquired habit, while elements displaying similarities of shape or color, even if located at opposite ends of the field of vision, will be mentally associated. This kind of association usually prevails over others in human perception—by which I do not mean to suggest that it lacks esthetic value. However, the combination of elements in character contrast is better suited to attracting our mind and spirit and appealing to our sensibilities.

Specific landmarks in the facial composition can constitute elements of real interest, provided they are readily identifiable. For example, a line drawn between the lateral protuberance of the forehead, the side of the zygomatic process, and the mandibular angle could, in a reduced dimension and a reversed position, foreshadow the design of the distal contour and angle of the central incisor. These lines present at the same time a correspondence of shape and a contrast of position (Fig 3-108).

These three different facial landmarks are easily identifiable and ideally projected from the incisal third to the cervical third of the central incisor. Practice has shown that particular attention should be paid to the correspondence between the line extending from the lateral protuberance of the forehead to the zygomatic process and the design of the distal angle of the central incisor. The design of this line is greatly influenced by the expansion, reduction, or location of the eye, which generates, by character correspondence, a more or less angular or rounded distal tooth angle. Whatever the level of the smile line, this part of tooth design will be perceptible (Figs 3-109 to 3-111).

The reproduction of a line running from the zygomatic process to the mandibular angle, marking the design of the distal curvature of the central incisor, or that of a line running from the angle to the interdental periodontal connection may create difficulties when recessions due to biological or acciden-

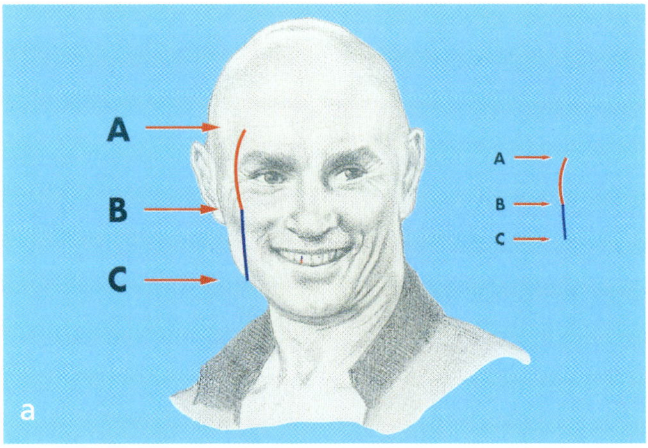

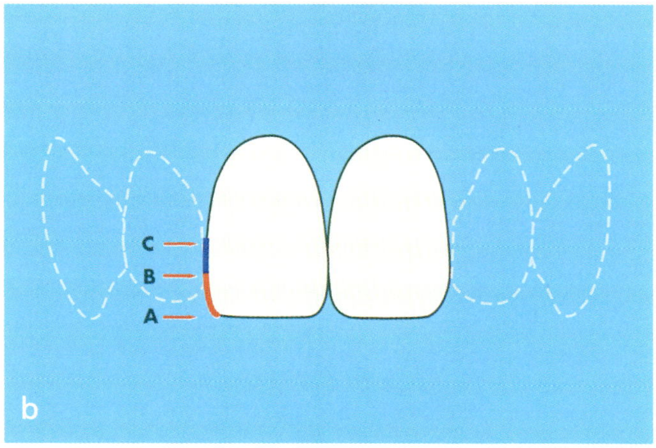

Figs 3-108a and 3-108b (a) A schematic representation of the lateral protuberance of the forehead, the side of the zygomatic process, and the mandibular angle, with a linear tracing between these entities surrounding the eyes. (b) The line *AB* surrounding the eyes traces the distal angle of the maxillary central incisor, while the line *BC* completes the tracing of its distal edge up to the level of the papilla.

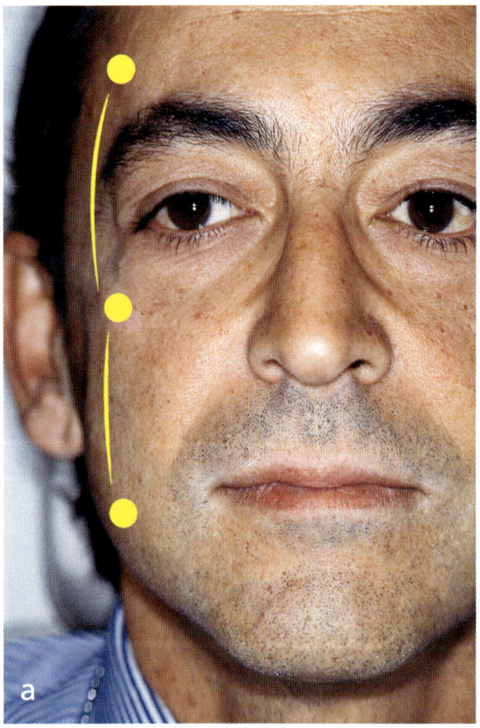

Figs 3-109a and 3-109b (a) It must be stressed that the design of the line *AB* may be more or less curved or straight according to the size and position of the eye and the location of the starting or finishing point. This element of evaluation must be translated into an angle design that will be more or less rounded or square. (b) Confrontation of facial landmarks and evaluative tracing with the natural design of the distal contour of the maxillary central incisor.

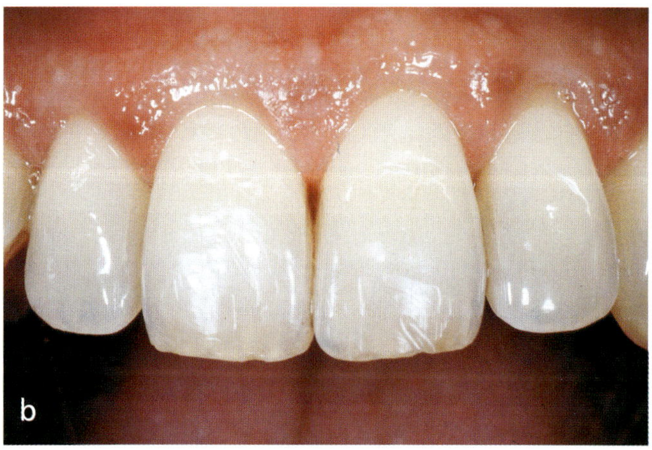

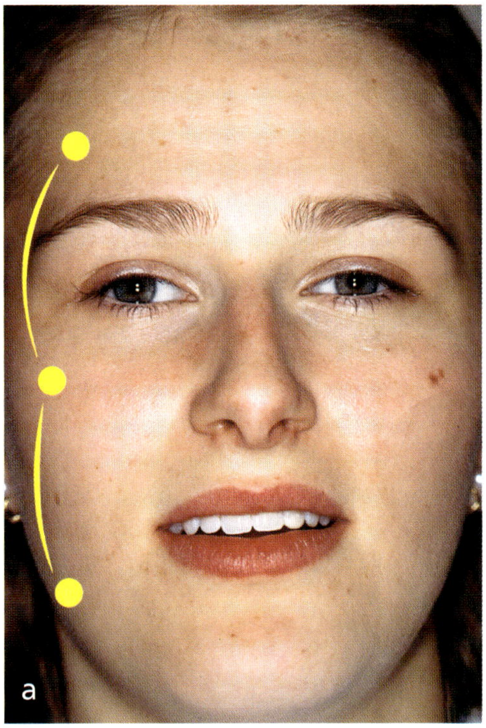

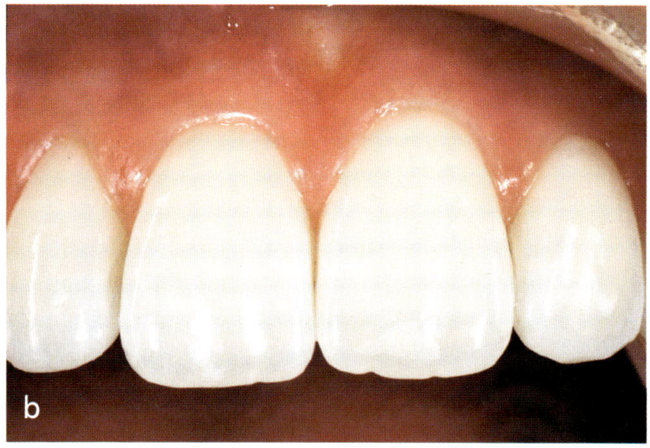

Figs 3-110a and 3-110b A facial composition displaying a more rounded distal angle, formed by the *AB* line traced around the eye, and a round distal curvature corresponding to a line drawn from the zygomatic process to the mandibular angle.

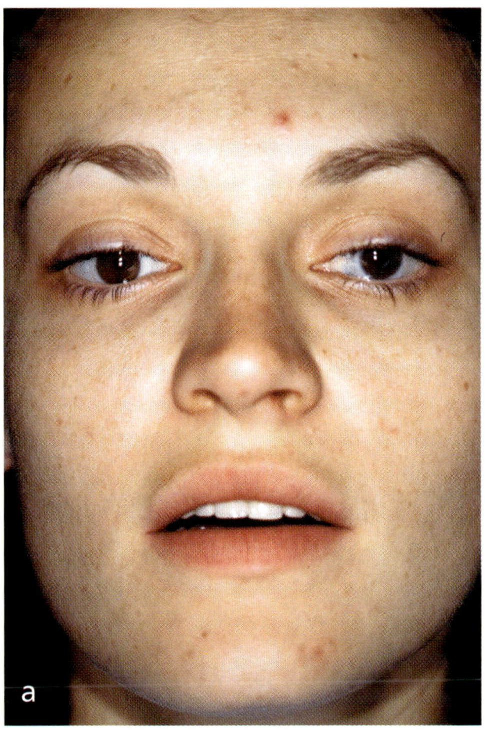

Figs 3-111a and 3-111b Restoration of the anterior segment with tooth design duplicating the linear tracing connecting facial landmarks. The rounded-square distal angle duplicates the practically straight line surrounding the eyes, while the distal edge duplicates the straight line between the zygomatic process and mandibular angle.

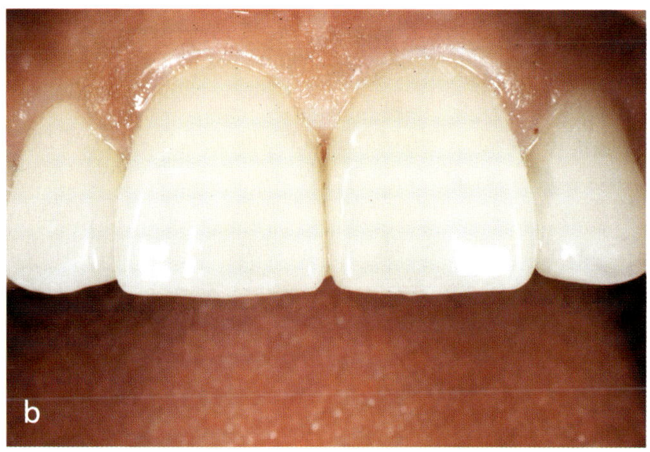

tal aging affect the gingival level. When tooth shape design can be established according to this rule of order, it can then be refined by the evaluation of personality traits. Pragmatically, one could say that tooth-design selection depends on a progressive evaluation: the elements of character significance define the nature of the angles while the elements of character correspondence modulate their contours.

Centers or "knots" of attention

Superficially, a composition appears to constitute a network of lines, shapes, and colors. Graphically, the importance of lines in a composition is predominant because no element really eludes the linear system, which either supports, separates, or serves as an abstract limitation of forms, space, and colors.

Observation demonstrates that lines, whether straight or curved, participate in a composition by way of association. While the combinations of lines can be reduced to a limited number of basic characteristic types, the variations that can be applied to these basic types are unlimited. Straight lines do not exist in nature and generate rigidity of expression in art. Their importance results from the human mental inclination·to codify things. This and our vision of nature lead us to recognize unlimited relations between straight and curved lines (Fig 3-112). These relations have esthetic effects arising from the congruence between what we discern and what is already written within us.

The esthetic value of a composition results from the sum of the tensions produced by its elements, and the impact of these associations is determined by irrational, esthetic logic.

Horizontal and vertical lines introduce opposed tensions. These two lines, symbols in the human experience of a vertical push on a horizontal plane, an attempt to liberate oneself from the effects of gravity to elevate oneself spiritually, morally, intellectually, or socially, generate a feeling of accomplishment. The perception of this resonance is conditioned by the maintenance of the significance of the basic constitutive elements. In this composition, made up of an association of two lines and leaving aside the effect of optical illusion, no one line really dominates.

The range of tensions that take place between lines may be illustrated by the plus and equal signs. The plus sign is made up of two straight lines crossing each other. This meeting reinforces their tensional strength, leading to a conflict and inducing a strong psychological effect. The equal sign is made up of two straight lines of identical tensional strength drawn in parallel. It generates a connotation of connection, of equality, between two parts and suggests one means of attaining cohesion in a composition.

These patterns also appear in the facial and dentofacial composition. For example, the plus sign may appear in the interincisal diastema, where it resembles a cross, while the equal sign may appear in the parallel lines made by the lower lip and the incisal line, which have, according to many authors, significant esthetic impact.

The plus and equal signs can be considered perfect illustrations of what has been called segregative and cohesive forces. The presence of these two forces, which in turn appeal, reject, and unify, is necessary to the esthetic quality of a composition (Fig 3-113).

In an esthetic composition, some elements may imprint their own image upon everything, entice eye

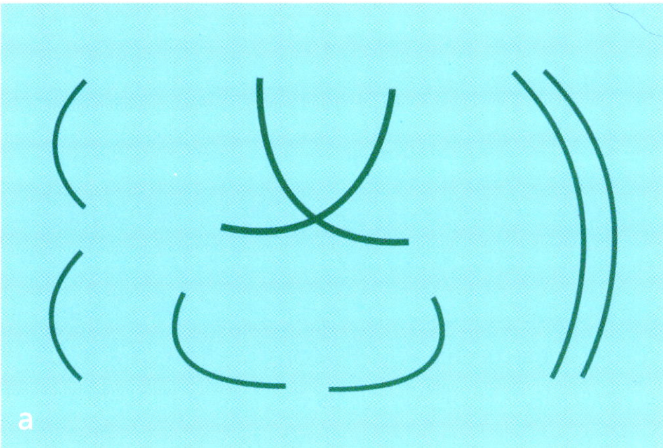

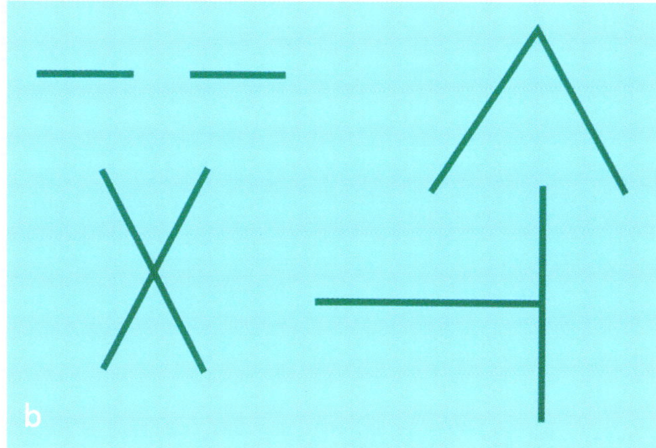

Figs 3-112a and 3-112b Compositions are constituted of a network of curved or straight lines whose combinations can be reduced to a limited number of basic types (a,b), yet in unlimited variations.

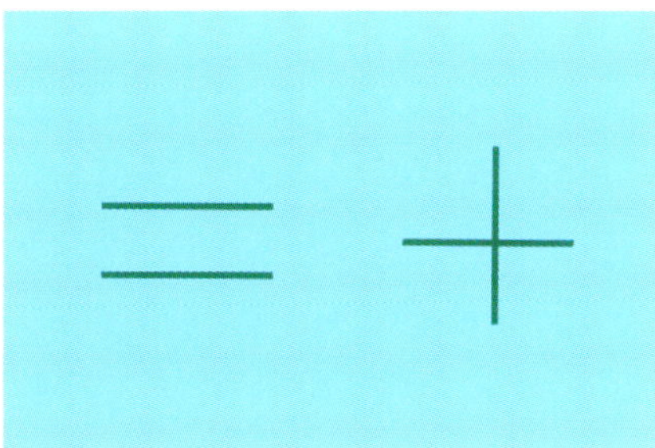

Fig 3-113 The graphic diversity of linear association is illustrated by two antagonist types: the equal and plus signs.

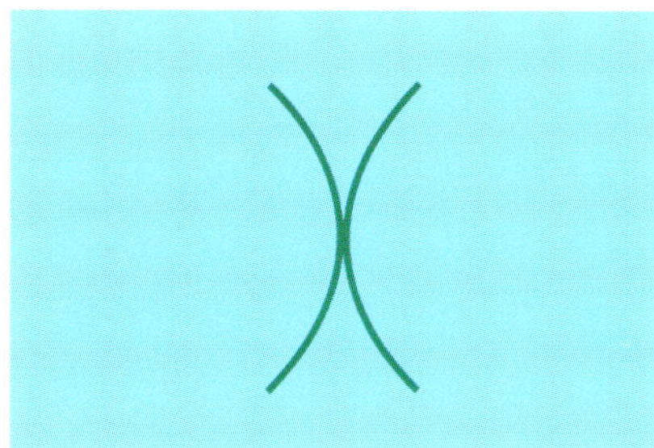

Fig 3-114 Nature very rarely displays the rigid types of association that respond to the human inclination for mathematical order; it tends rather to display associated designs susceptible to constituting elements of visual convergence or "knots of attention."

and soul, reduce the sonority of other elements, and engender an obvious tension that at first glance overwhelms our sensibility. These "knots of attention" are elements of visual convergence whose attractive potential depends upon the strength of their significance.

The dentofacial composition offers some perfectly identifiable knots of attention, to which one should attend in dentofacial rehabilitation while duplicating original tooth-lip relation. For example, the design of two curved lines of opposing curvature simulates a combination of the plus and equal signs; that is to say, it establishes a perfectly identifiable relationship between two elements while at the same time generating an intense visual impact (Fig 3-114).

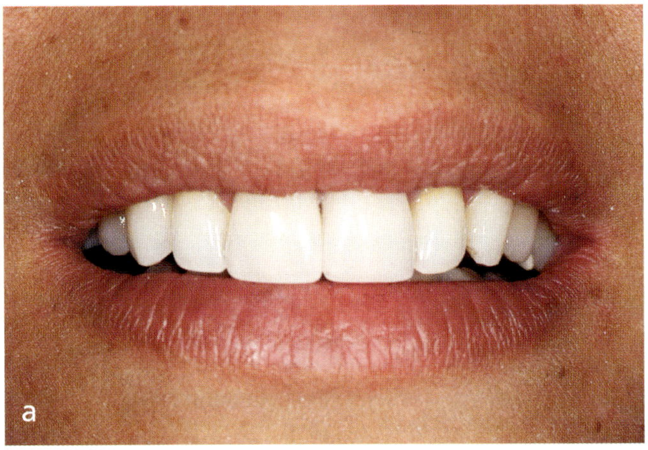
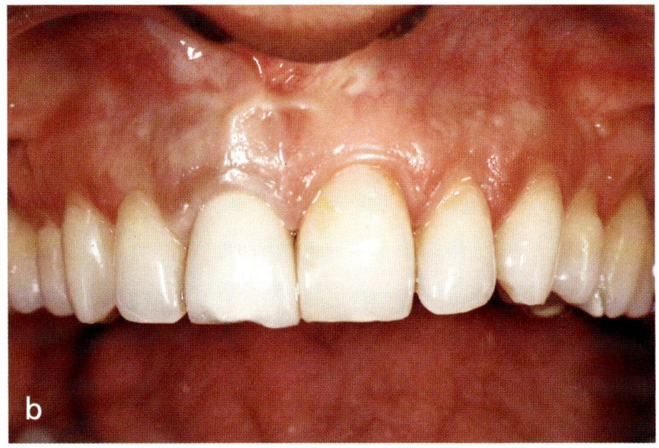
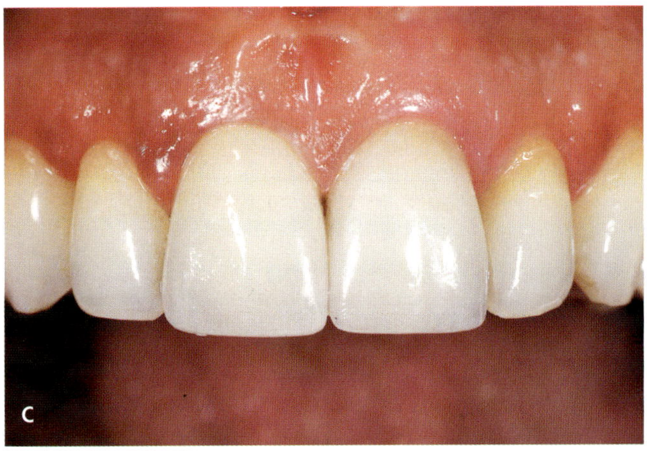

Figs 3-115a to 3-115c (a) Lower lip design has been described as presenting a decreasing width from lip center to lateral borders. (b) Initial clinical situation. (c) These characteristics are correlated with a regular dental alignment and an incisal line presenting a downward curvature that in this case required restoration.

In clinical reality these elements are realized by the specific relationships in the vertical plane between the maxillary incisal line and the lower lip. Tooth-lip relations are best examined in a position that can be described as dynamic, which means a mandibular rest position or one in which soft tissue is subjected to a slight pull from the corners of the mouth, simulating what has been described as the quarter of a smile. The lower lip design is usually described as presenting a progressively decreasing width from its central part of the corners of the mouth (Fig 3-115). Observation generally confirms this morphological design but reveals a variety of differences mainly affecting its upper border and thickness. These differences, concrete manifestations of the axiom "shapes create relations as relations create shapes," are not accidental but result from the stimulative action of the incisal border of the upper dental element contacting the lip in the dynamic of oral movements.

Though the morphological variations affecting the lower lip design seldom resist repetitive interrogations, a precise description of correlated tooth spatial

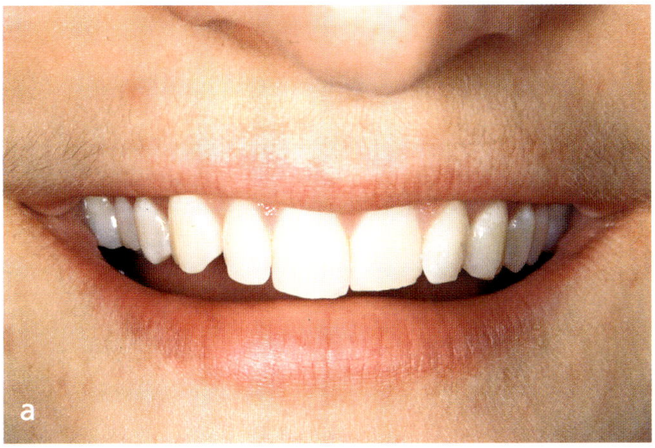

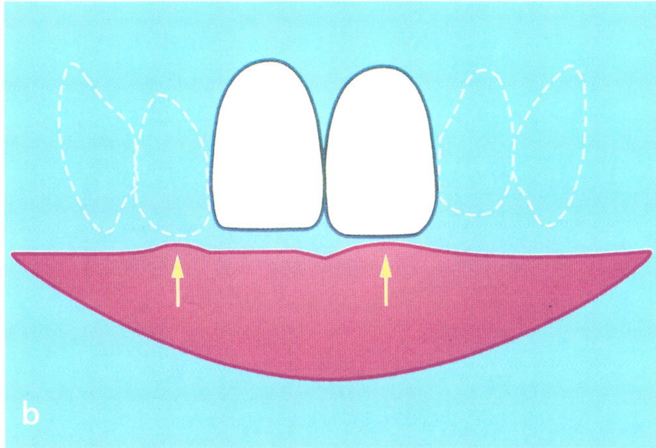

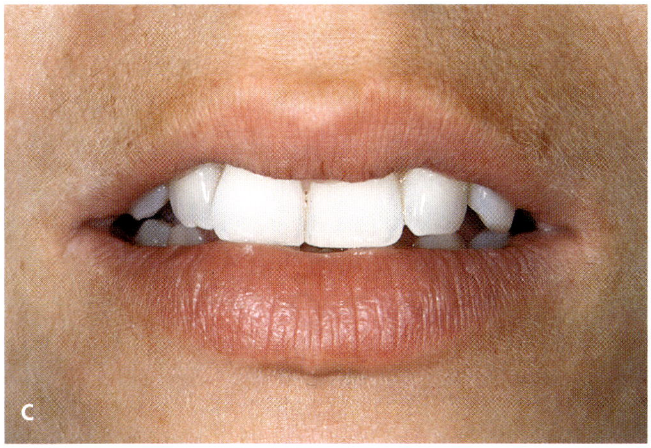

Figs 3-116a to 3-116c In reality, lower lip width and design undergo variations, while perfect tooth alignment remains theoretical. There are direct relationships between maxillary teeth and lower lip design dictated by the nature of the stimulative impact of the incisal edge on lip tissues during the dynamic of oral movements. (a, b) A tooth elongation generates a correlated increase of lip width that can be defined as a bump. (c) Two long and large central incisors correlated with significant lip thickness, which extends on the left side under the stimulative action of a lateral incisor in a more buccal location. But the absence of lip stimulation correlated with a right lateral incisor in a lingual position causes an important reduction of lip thickness.

location is more difficult to establish. A reading of natural tooth-lip particulars shows that major differences in lip width and lip thickness are correlated to specific anterior tooth spatial arrangements (Fig 3-116), while more delicate anatomic particularities, located in the center of the upper lip-line border, may be related to the characteristics of the interincisal space and even dictate the incisal design of maxillary central incisors.

A triangular depression in the upper lip-line border usually causes a similar but reversed interdental space design with closed and slightly rounded mesio-incisal angles, while a slight, smooth, and convex depression in this middle part is related to more rounded mesio-incisal angles (Fig 3-117). Nature shows that an extension of this central depression, ending bilaterally with well-marked convexities, is related to specific designs of the incisal edges (Fig 3-118). Conversely, an absence of interincisal space with square angulated mesial angles is usually related to a straight or slightly upward convexity of the lip in its center (Fig 3-119).

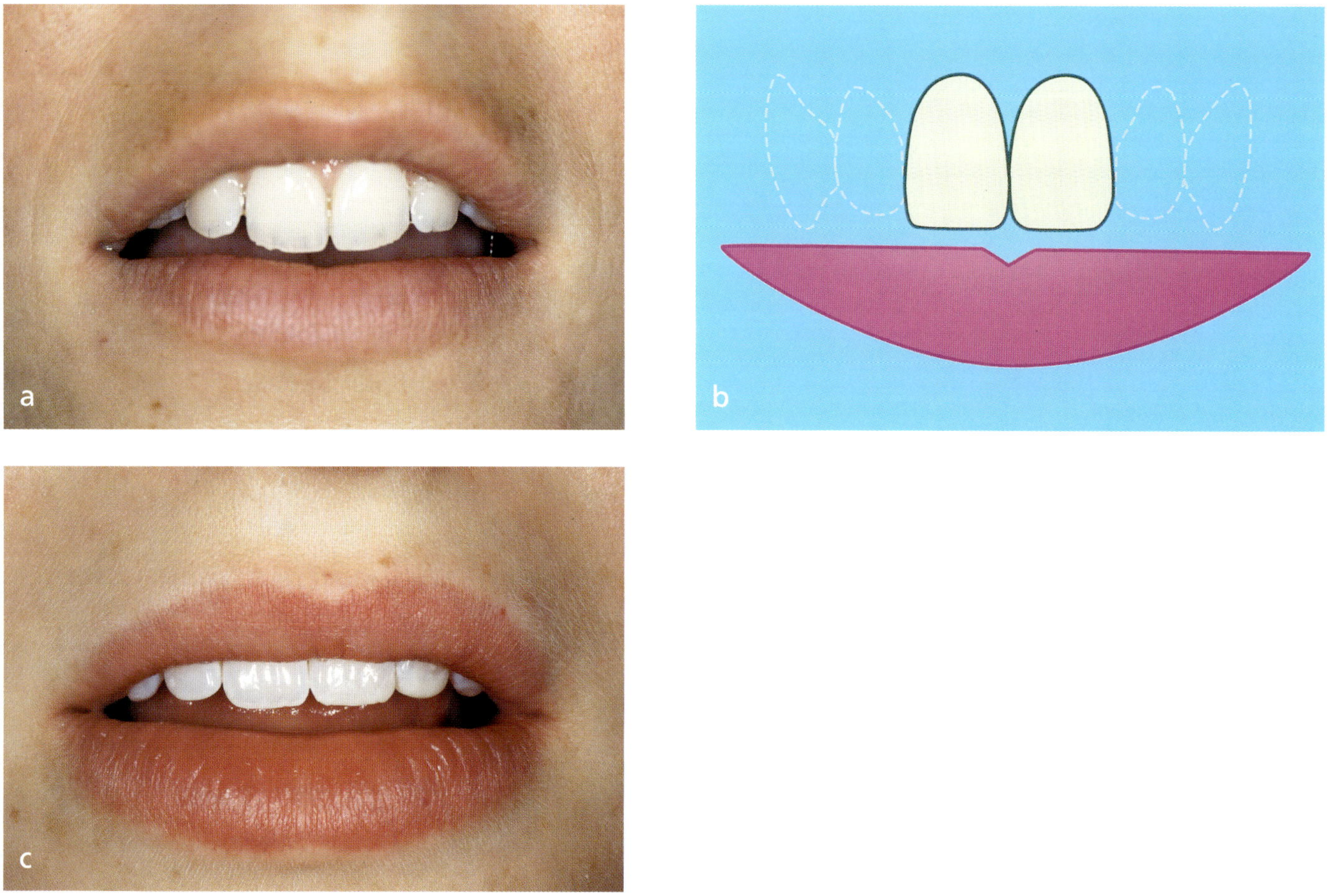

Figs 3-117a to 3-117c (a,b) A profound opening of the interincisal space with slightly rounded mesial angles of the maxillary central incisors is correlated with a triangular concavity in the center of the lower lip upper border line, (c) while a minor lateral extension of this lip depression is correlated with a proportional interincisal opening and rounder mesial angles.

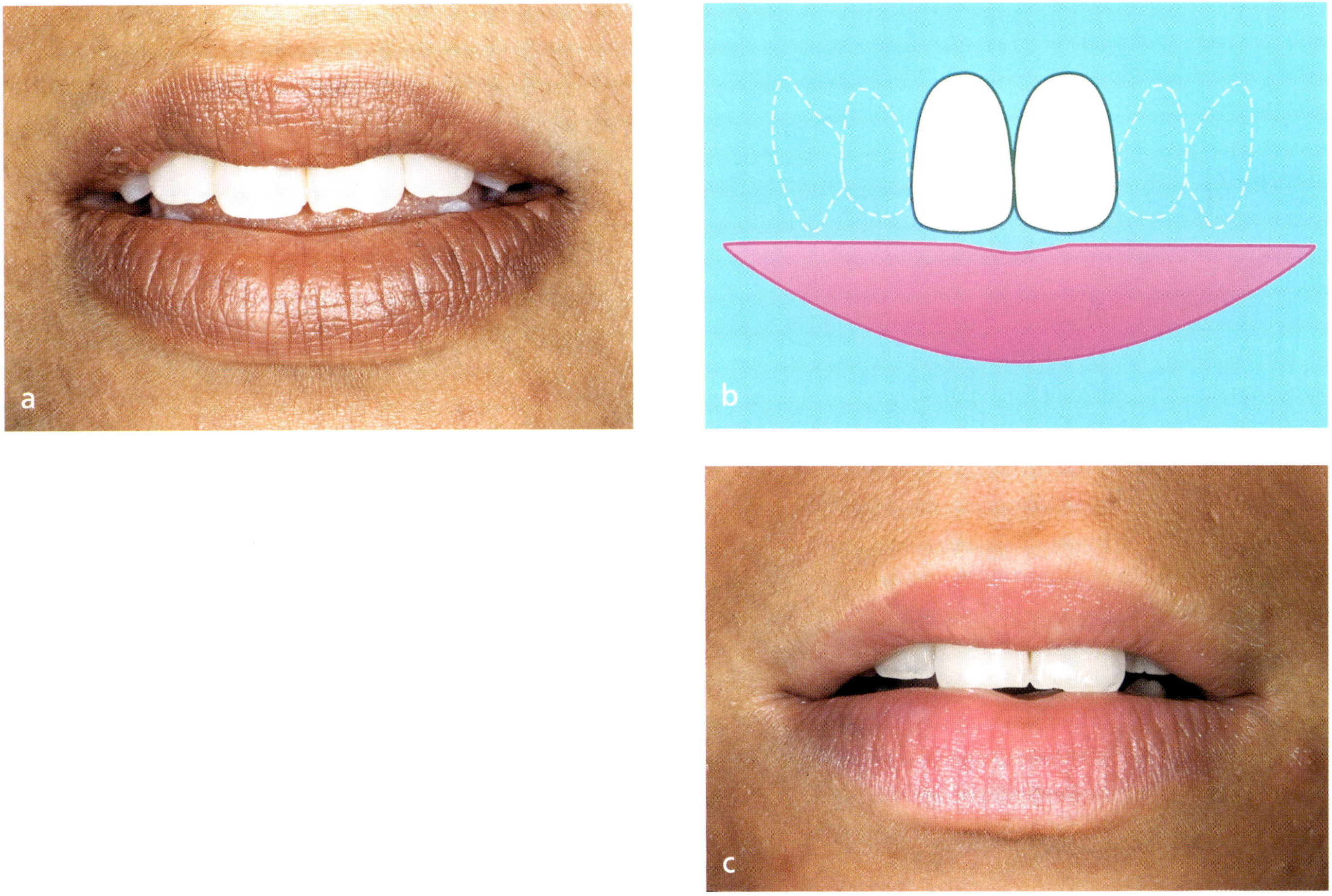

Figs 3-118a to 3-118c (a,b) A depressed central curvature in lower lip design ending with an increased lip thickness testifies to the roundness of the incisal edge and stresses the stimulative action of the tooth's incisal shape to antagonist lip tissue, (c) while a triangular depression surrounded by lower lip soft tissue "bumps" is correlated with a reverse incisal design. These observations confirm the accuracy of the basic esthetic principle: "shapes create relations as relations create shapes."

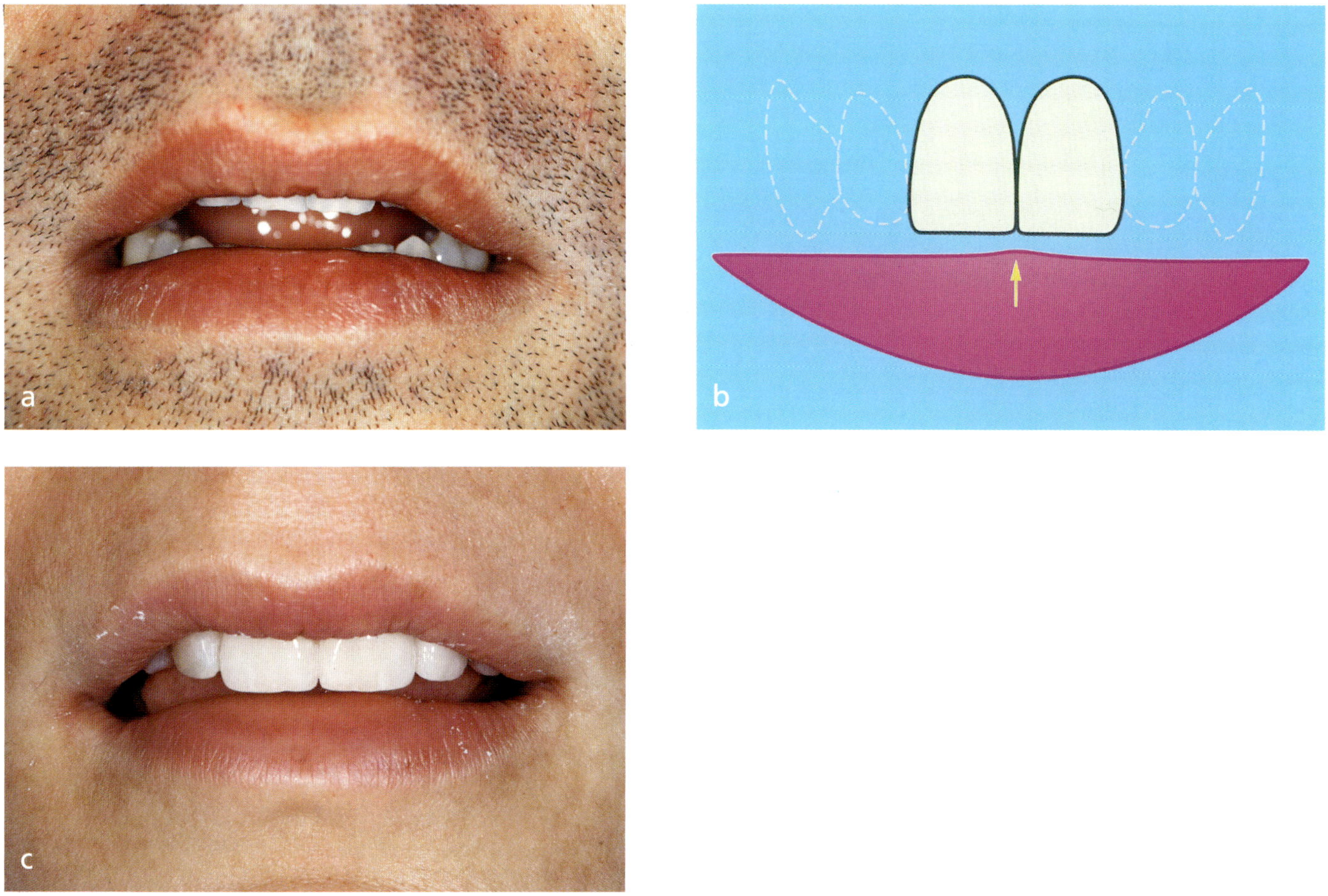

Figs 3-119a to 3-119c (a, b) A raised lower lip width with a straight upper border line are correlated with an extension of the maxillary central incisors' length, straight incisal edges, and square mesial angles. These are characteristics common to natural tooth-lip relationships. (c) These restorations must be reproduced in artificial restoration to attain proper esthetics.

We now need to find a clinical application of these elements to relational esthetic qualities (Figs 3-120 and 3-121) and observe some morphological characteristics that could enhance and provide credibility to our restorations.

When the particulars of the upper lip-line border conflict with the design of the interincisal space and perhaps reveal the nature of the maxillary central's mesio-incisal angles and incisal edges, the correct reading of the localized bumps or protuberances affecting lower lip width in its upper border may, depending on their position, serve as an indicator of the spatial location of the lateral incisors. Clinically, the strict alignment of the lateral incisors along a parabolic dental arch results from perceptive deficiencies and exists only in orthodontic samples and removable

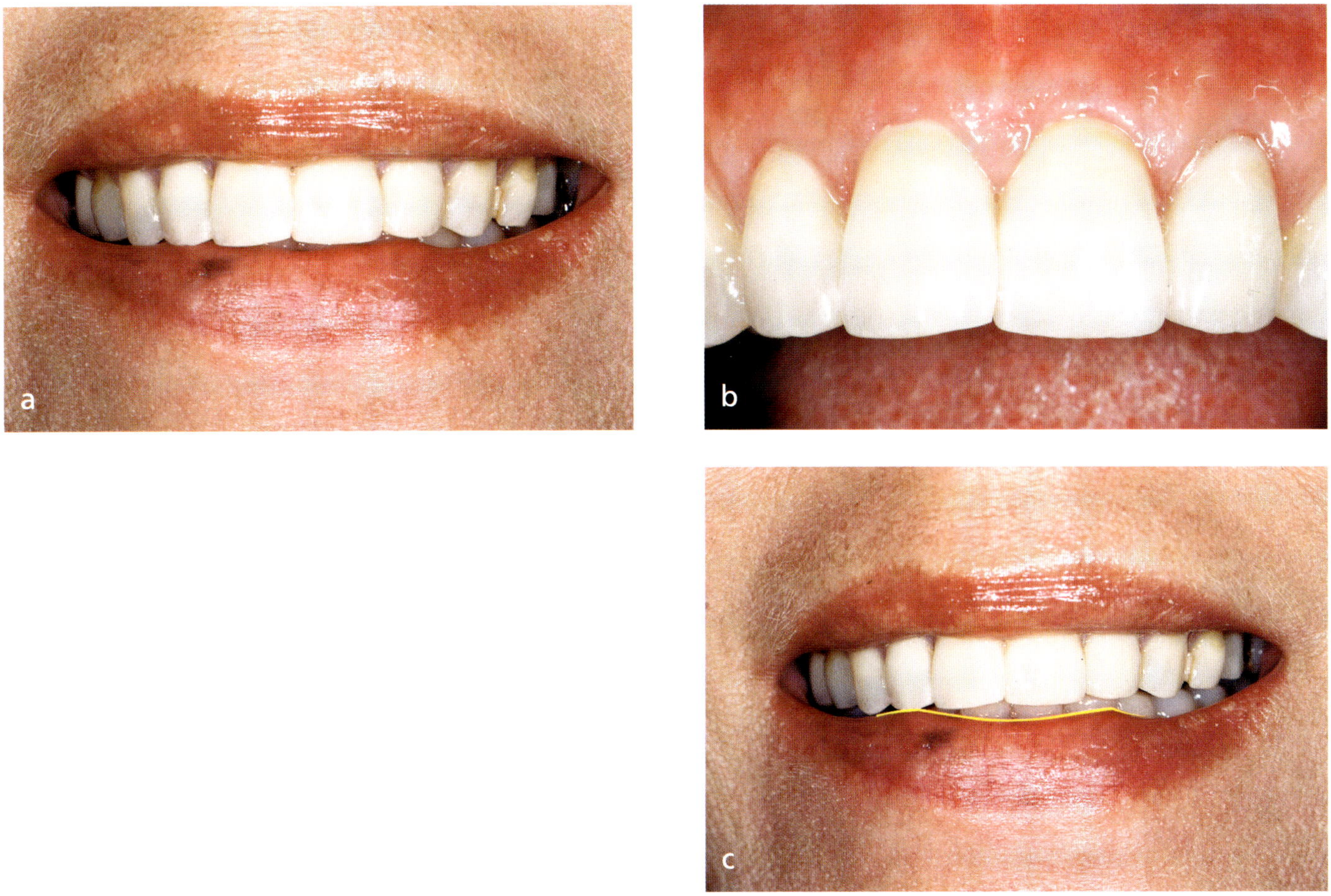

Figs 3-120a to 3-120c (a) In practice, only repetitive interrogations will reveal the real design of the upper border line of the lower lip and (b) progressively show that bilateral increases in lip thickness may also, according to their position, be correlated with variations in the spatial location of maxillary lateral incisors. The observation of the variations of lip width, the nature and location of the "bumps," should dictate the restoration of perfectly related dental elements. (c) Clearly, the retruded spatial location of the left and right lateral incisors is not perfectly correlated with lip design.

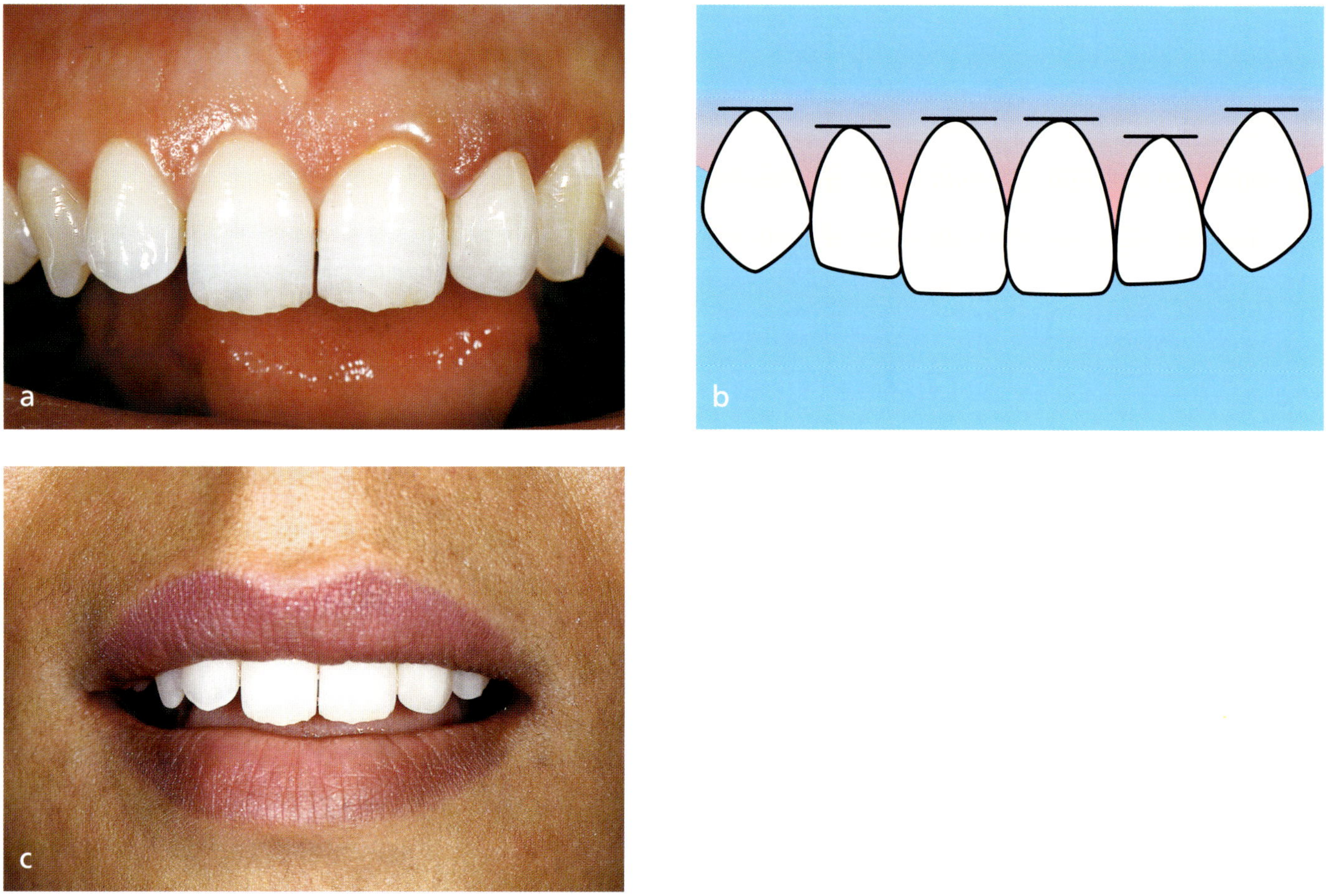

Figs 3-121a to 3-121c Tooth design and placement that have to be correlated with specific variations of lip design may very often challenge the imagination of the restorative dentist. Observation shows that the two natural maxillary central incisors, with rounded incisal edges and open interincisal spaces, are related to a slight and round depression of the upper lip-line border in its center, confirming our previous remarks. (a) We now have to explain the reasons that have dictated the restorations of the lateral incisors. (b) According to many authors, lip design presents a decreasing width from its center to its lateral borders, and the tooth-gingival level of the lateral incisors is lower than that of the central to realize the esthetic of the anterior segment. On the left side of a mouth that shows these characteristics, the lateral incisor is restored in the arch alignment. (c) Yet the restoration of the right lateral incisor will be more exacting and will be dictated, both in its design and location, by the level of tooth-gingival relations, which is higher than that of the centrals, and by the lateral "bump" seen on the right side of the lower lip, promoting the individuality and particular appeal of the dentofacial composition.

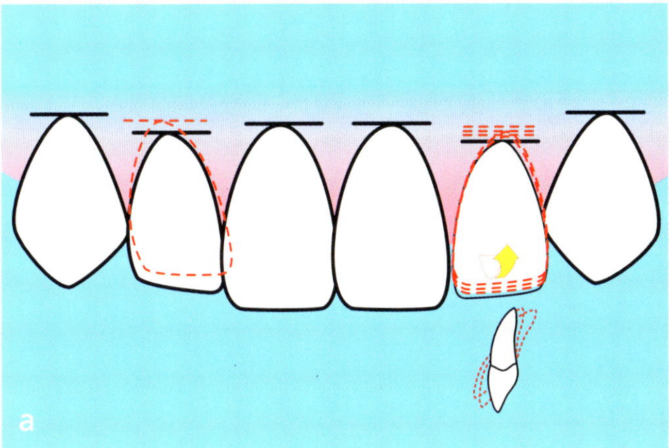

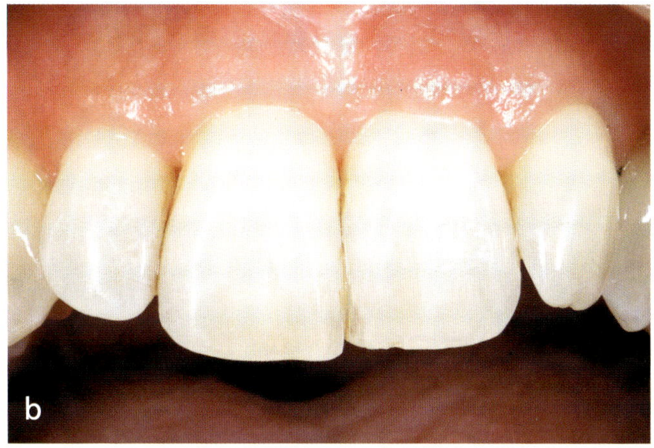

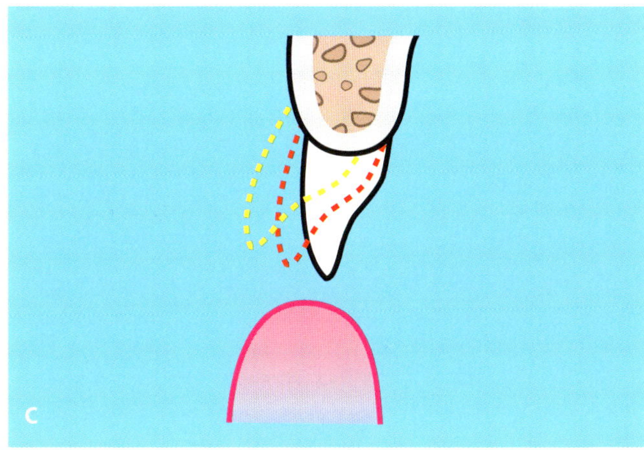

Figs 3-122a to 3-122c (a) A direct relationship exists between tooth-gingival level and tooth sagittal inclination. The higher the gingival level, the more buccal its inclination. (b) This rule is valid not only for the lateral incisors but also for the maxillary central incisors and leads to another consequential statement: (c) for a given tooth length and various tooth-gingival level locations, lip stimulation and lip thickness are identical.

complete-denture prostheses. Natural dentitions always show more or less marked malpositions affecting predominantly the lateral incisors as a consequence of arch form, tooth-gingival level, and tooth-lip relationships.

These three elements are inseparable and consequential. Basically, the spatial location of the lateral incisor is dictated by the space availability between canine and central incisor. This location has been described as ideal when tooth-gingival relationships are located lower than the tooth-gingival level around the central incisors. Yet clinical practice shows that variations in the location of the tooth-gingival level of lateral incisors are always related to the proportionate variations of tooth axial direction, either in the sagittal or in the frontal plane, as a result of reduced space availability (Fig 3-122). These variations of the lateral incisors' axial direction do not disqualify it esthetically. On the contrary, they usually break the monotony generated by a perfect tooth alignment, provided they establish adequate esthetic relationships with lower lip particulars.

From these observations it follows that the adequate positioning of the lateral incisor participates in and makes a significant impact on the characterization of the dentofacial composition. But it demands for its location a sensitive appreciation of parameters as diverse as lip design, gingival-level location, tooth-length normality, and space availability, as well as functional and phonetic requirements.

Tooth-lip relationships constitute elements of unconscious visual convergence or knots of attention corresponding to a logical esthetic design. In the facial composition the presence of these knots of attention determines points of support and rupture that will influence the sequence of facial reading which should travel from the most appealing elements to the others.

Rhythm and cohesion

Rhythm is a concept familiar to us all. In the succession of cold and warm seasons, of night and day, work and rest, heart pulsation, breathing, walking, rhythm is part of our existence. Rhythm is linked to most of our activities, physiological, mechanical, artistic, conscious or unconscious.

Rhythm can be defined as the recurrence of strong and weak periods at more or less regular intervals, moments of activity and moments of quiescence. These characteristics of ordered periodicity appeal to a collective sensibility; they are inherent in all the arts: music, dance, and poetry, as well as the plastic arts. The application to the plastic arts, characterized by static representation, of the rhythmic properties usually attributed to arts of duration like music and poetry perhaps needs some explanation.

The esthetic evaluation of any esthetic element or composition requires an active participation of the eye, which is invited to move along the object. This

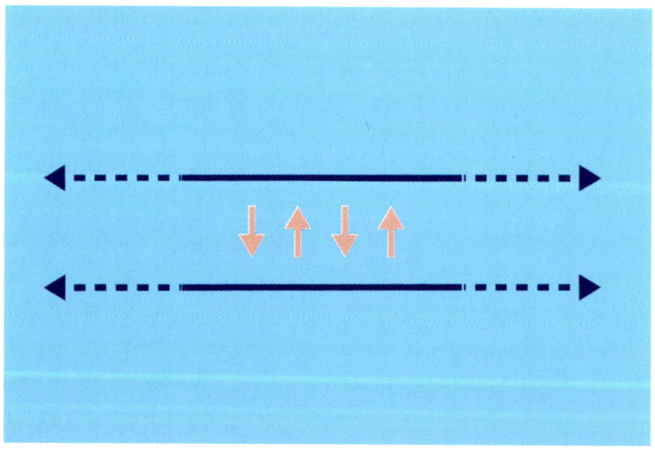

Fig 3-123 In the reading of two parallel lines, three tensional strengths can be perceived: the proper tension of these lines and the interconnective tensions they generate.

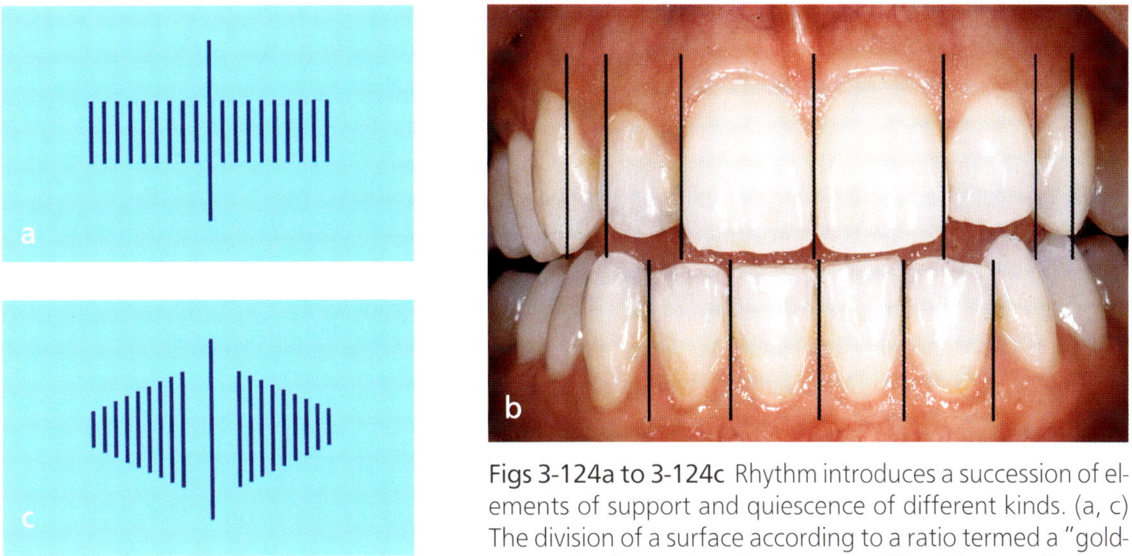

Figs 3-124a to 3-124c Rhythm introduces a succession of elements of support and quiescence of different kinds. (a, c) The division of a surface according to a ratio termed a "golden number" appeals to human sensibility. (b) A maxillary anterior segment duplicating this type of division generates the same impact, a feeling that nothing more takes place in the perception of its rhythmic qualities.

implies a phenomenon of duration and requires the same qualities of perception as the arts of duration.

In the reading of the two parallel lines of the equal sign, three tensional strengths can be perceived: the proper tensions of the two linear elements and the tension of their interaction (Fig 3-123). Two of these elements are basically static or in expectation of activation. Their meeting creates the conditions necessary for activation, a dynamic at the origin of their rhythm. Should we add to the composition another line parallel to the first two, the dynamism created by the interconnection between the two first lines will drive the eye to the third and introduce elements of duration, support, and rupture, ie, rhythm.

According to the painter A. Hölzel, rhythm requires three elements to really manifest itself. It has both qualitative and quantitative elements. Its qualitative elements work by accentuation and originate in the tensions displayed by lines, shapes, and colors; its quantitative elements work by zones of quiescence, retransmission, and duration.

Rhythm involves multiple combinations and variations whose appreciation is a characteristic of human sensibility. The division of a surface according to a ratio sometimes called a "golden number" represents one of these multiple combinations, whose qualitative and quantitative rhythmic elements have appealed over the centuries to the collective sensibility. Yet rhythm is not a more or less simple repetition of identical elements, but rather a composition of tensional relationships (Fig 3-124).

Any element placed on a plane surface generates new tensions as well as its own tensional strength, that will extend their action to the different parts of its plane. Consequently, the plane will be subjected to a new division of its surface into areas of increased or reduced quiescence. The presence of these multiple elements will generate dynamic or rhythmic areas of tension and relapse, areas of support and rupture, leading to a specific quality in the division of the plane surface that will appear agreeable, disagreeable, or even repulsive.

Whatever its perfection, each new dental composition introduced into the facial composition will create modifications in the facial rhythmic properties that may not necessarily be appreciated as esthetic improvement. These considerations suggest a reevaluation of the rhythm of each facial composition with the introduction of a new dental composition.

However, apart from its rhythmic qualities, the linear parallelism in a composition is an important factor of esthetic cohesion, connected or not to the lines of force generated by the shape of the plane, the basic element of esthetic construction defined above as the tension of the plane. In reality, the interconnective tensions resulting from linear parallelism generate not only the qualitative and quantitative variations at the origin of the rhythm but also the cohesive forces that control the unity of the composition. Rhythm is born from the tensions created between one element and another. In its absence, the cohesive qualities of the composition also disappear.

Relationships between the shapes and limits of the plane

The distance separating a form from the border of a plane serves a special and important esthetic function, as it may constitute an area of tension that interests both eye and spirit, a characteristic that was termed a "knot of attention." When a line lies free in a plane and approaches its border, it will be subjected at this end to an increased tension toward the border while the tension of the other end will weaken (Fig 3-125). At the moment the line makes contact with the border the tension suddenly ceases. The farther a line lies from the border of a plane, the weaker becomes the attraction of this border. Expressed differently, elements close to the limits of the plane increase the "dramatic" resonance of this particular relation, a term stressing the quality of the vibrations produced and thus the power of the esthetic appeal.

Once a line contacts the border, the tension of the other end suddenly increases but with a strength depending on its spatial position. The attraction of forces of gravity is always predominant. As a result, a downward tension generated by a line touching the upper border of a plane is felt with more strength than that generated by a line attached to the lower border of a plane. Upright tensions that underline the ambition of man to free himself from gravity are always overpowered by downward tensions (Fig 3-126).

The common preference for a smile anatomy that shows a lip position relative to tooth display described as "middle lip-line smile" results from the tensions created by the upper lip borders displaying the whole tooth and suggesting the presence of interdental pink gingival tissue in a position perceived as close to the

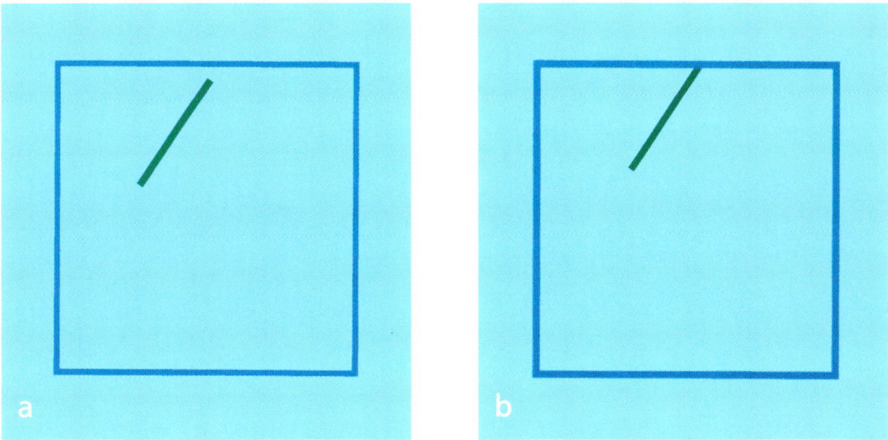

Figs 3-125a and 3-125b (a) A form approaching the border of a plane will be subjected to an intense tension that will be either strengthened or weakened the closer or the farther away it is from this border. (b) These tensions are suddenly released when the form comes in contact with the border of the plane. Tooth-gingival relationships displayed by lip-line level in smiling duplicate this type of situation, as do the relations between posterior segment and lateral negative space.

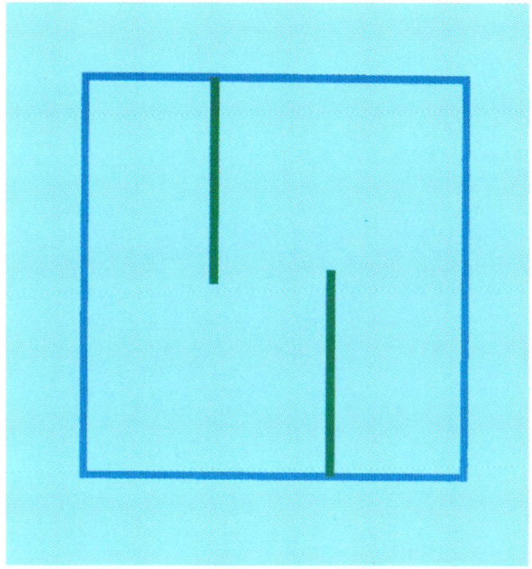

Fig 3-126 At their contact with the border of the plane, the forms are subjected to differentiated tensional strengths because forces of gravity always predominate in upward-directed tensions.

border of the lip frame. Should gingival display be increased, tensions will still be perceived until the moment the high lip line level exhibits a large amount of gingival tissue, breaking the tensional strength that takes place between the white of the tooth and the lip frame.

Tension dissipates when the mass of the anterior dental segment establishes a large contact with its lips frame, a situation experienced in low lip-line levels. Similarly, invasion of the lateral negative spaces, which has been advocated to increase visual attraction, only works when it maintains with the inner lip corner a distance that generates tension and esthetic attraction. When the integration of the dental composition into the geometric parameters of the facial composition appears natural, which is seldom difficult in practice, the voluntary creation of punctual elements of attraction or knots of attention necessary to improve the esthetic quality of a composition remains more aleatory. Yet it may greatly benefit from these simple elements of esthetic knowledge (Fig 3-127).

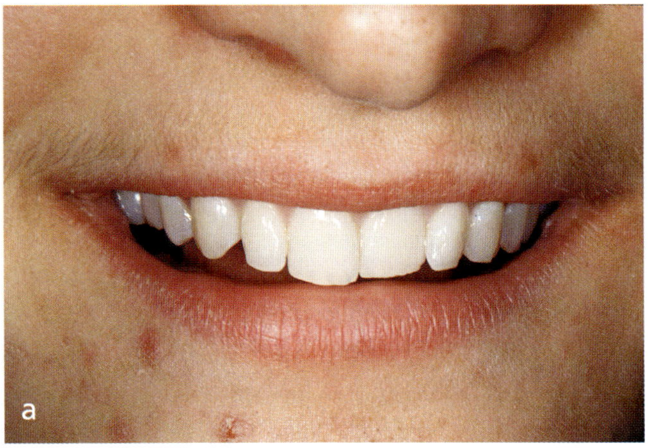

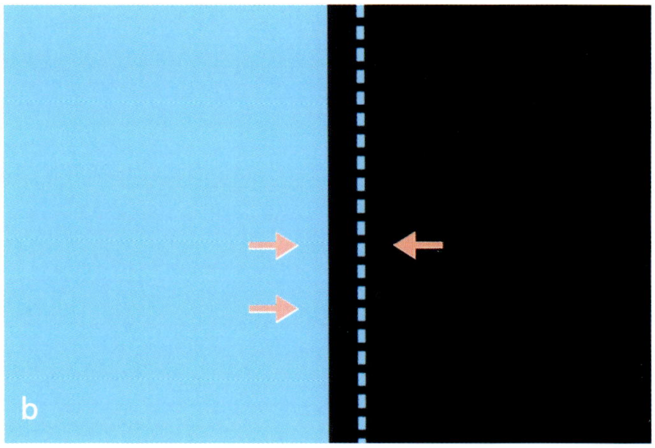

Figs 3-127a and 3-127b (a) The maxillary right central incisor barely contacts the lower lip in smiling: tension. The left posterior segment barely contacts the commissural angle: tension. Lip level barely displays interdental papilla: tension. Is the central interincisal line in the center of the smile or not? This feeling of a possible disequilibrium, the constant interrogations of eye and mind to restore the interincisal line in the center of the smile or (b) in the center of a plane, generates nothing else but . . . tension. A rather appealing smile for a chaotic tooth arrangement.

Proportion

Beauty has often been defined as harmony of proportion in numerical or geometric relationships. Many have claimed that the harmonious qualities developed by certain proportional relationships may originate in the talent or inspiration of the artist. In this particular field, however, talent alone is insufficient. Pleasing proportional relationships appealing to our visual and mental sensibilities can only be obtained by a conscious or unconscious application of laws. Where artists have ignored such laws they may well have produced harmonious relationships through a phenomenon of unconscious visual remembrance. Analysis has always shown similarities between the structures of attractive esthetic relationships and the most well-known or most frequently applied proportionate relationships. Consequently, we must reject the idea of a natural and spontaneous creation of harmonious relationships.

Philosophers have often considered language of mathematics as providing the only means of understanding nature, and generations of them have attempted to apply this language in the hope of reducing beauty to objective criteria. Proportion, a concept inherited from the Greeks, allows a quantification of norms applicable to every physical reality. The basic axiom of Pythagorean theory, *"Panta en arithmo"* (Everything is in the number), illustrated this concept and, with the expression of the "golden number," generated a mystique that has perpetuated its influence down to the present day. In the study of proportion, mathematical considerations cannot be ignored.

The belief that beauty should depend only upon numerical rules originates from a natural desire for simplification. However, the strict observations of laws and rules may not only limit creativity; it also leads to a failure to consider the individuality and cultural environment of the observer. Since the effect produced by proportion is physico-psychological, esthetic philosophers have advocated a more psychological approach. These concepts have moderated the claims of mathematical estheticians, who would have been limited to producing recipes if they really could create beauty by number.

In esthetics we are dealing with laws and rules that in their formulation and application require a marriage of science and emotion. Creator and observer represent the two poles of an identical phenomenon that embodies the transcription and the reception of an emotion. To the creator is left the choice of the best material means and proportions to attain the desired esthetic effect.

Definitions

In ordinary language the notion of proportion has been confused by association with different kinds of criteria. To clear this confusion, and in an attempt to provide clarification in a field that has and will constantly escape a definite solution, two types of definition can be proposed.

First, proportion can be defined as a quantitative relationship of size or dimension between two elements of the same nature. This type of proportional relationship embodies a simple arithmetic division. For example, a tooth proportion has been defined as the division of its clinical width by its length. Width-to-length ratio has been described as ideal when it reaches 75% to 80% for maxillary central incisors. It has been emphasized that below 65% teeth may appear too narrow, as could occur following periodontal surgery, and above 85% appear too short, as could occur following tooth wear.

The golden ratio has fixed at 1.618 the proportions of a rectangle of unanimous esthetic appeal. According to the experiments of the esthetician Fechner, these proportions received preferential rather than unanimous approval, which tends to show that the claim originating with Plato that other ratios not only could but also did exhibit a particular beauty, weakens the universality attributed to the golden number. This claim not only prevented condemning to ugliness all proportionate ratios diverging from the golden number but also suggested the vanity of expecting mathematical formulae to explain beauty.

Such a statement will certainly not meet with the approval of plastic surgeons who base their evaluation of human beauty on the application of the golden proportions. They observe that the relation between hip and waist only generates esthetic appeal when rated between 0.6 and 0.7. The same rule of order is claimed to be valid for facial proportions, supposedly ideal when approaching 1/3, 1/3, 1/3 for each facial segment according to a definition proposed by Leonardo da Vinci.

In reality, when applied to human elements, these proportional relationships can only be used in the definition of morphological normality, based on anatomy and the average proportions of the human body. Nothing but an anatomical normality determines the width-to-length ratio of dental elements, which does not satisfy the golden proportion.

Human beauty involves conformity to morphological normality. According to the arithmetic theory of the human body, normality can be defined by biometric measures. This approach has led to the definition of specific anthropometric norms expressing the dimensions of the limbs as fractions of the body's height. Greek standards, for example, determined that human proportions are ideal when the body's height is seven and one-half times the height of the head (the doriphore), while Roman standards extended this proportion to eight times its height (Lysippe, Apollo of Belvedere). These variations, stressing the importance of geographical and physiological factors, underline the relativity of beautiful proportions and promote a concept of multiple "canons of beauty."

However, these restrictions have never lessened the attraction of the arithmetic theory, which has generated multiple and various studies, one of which has demonstrated that the central incisor in its length and width should correspond to 1/16 of the length and width of the head. By facial width one has to understand the interzygomatic distance while facial height corresponds to the distance between the root of the hair and the lower part of the chin. These observations show that the notion of proportion is most usually understood as the confrontation of two numbers or two quantities of the same nature entertaining between each other simple quantitative relationships.

In the language of mathematics, the comparison of two numbers is called a ratio. It constitutes by subtraction an arithmetic ratio such as $8 - 3 = 5$ and by division a geometric ratio such as $10 : 2 = 5$. Mathematically nothing else exists but these two ratios, arithmetic and geometric, but the esthetic results have been variable. This does not mean that the idea of an association of organic beauty with a mathematical order must be dismissed as insignificant. In reality, a true system of proportions not only relies on ratios stating specific relationships between two elements but is also based on reciprocal and immutable connections between a main part, subordinate parts, and the smallest parts between them.

Mathematically, proportion emerges from the union of two equivalent ratios or, following Euclid, can be understood as the equivalence of ratios between two homogeneous elements. For example:

8 surpasses 5 as 6 surpasses 3 or

$$8 - 5 = 6 - 3.$$

This is an arithmetic proportion. But 15 contains 5 as 18 contains 6 or

$$\frac{15}{5} = \frac{18}{6}$$

produces a geometric proportion. This type of proportionate relationship is characterized by four terms, two mean terms and two extremes. It is called discontinuous.

When the middle terms are equal, the proportion is reduced to three terms whose sequence will generate a progression. For example:

$$12 - 10 = 10 - 8$$

generates a continuous arithmetic progression and

$$\frac{48}{12} = \frac{12}{3}$$

generates a continuous geometric progression.

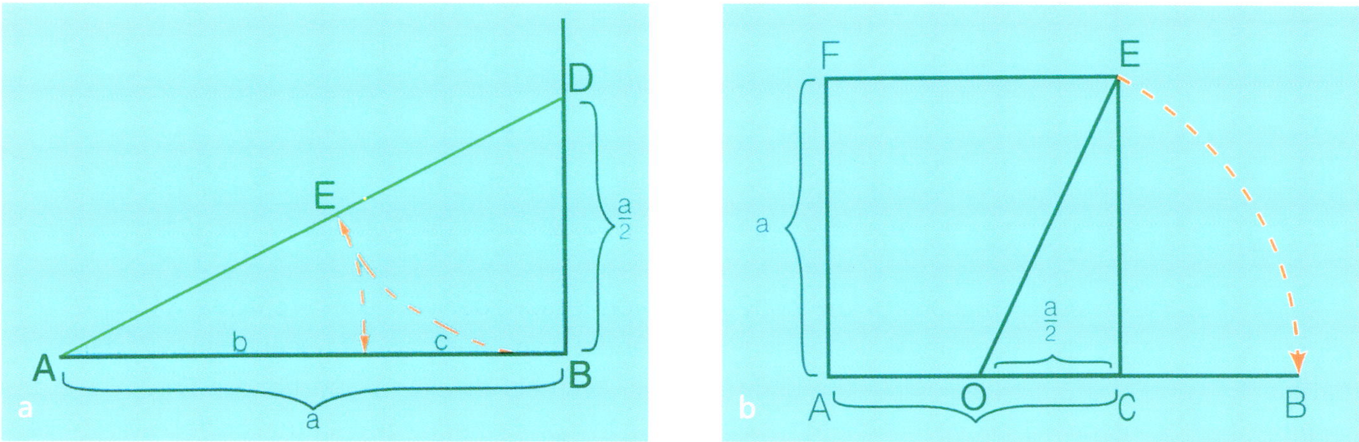

Figs 3-128a and 3-128b (a) A tracing of a golden segmentation using right angle and compass, with the tracing of a line *AD* perpendicular to a line half its length, followed by the tracing of an arc of length a/2 with the compass in *D*, crossing the diagonal *E* drawn from *A* to *D*. With its point in *A* the compass traces an arc from *E*, crossing *A* at a point dividing *A* in two segments *b* and *c* in golden relationships. (b) For a specific linear length *AC*, an extrusion of this line, a golden progression, can be obtained using a square shape of identical dimension, bringing down on the extension of the tracing *AC* a diagonal line drawn from half the width of *AC*.

In the simple equality of ratios must be included a notion of equivalence, or analogy of ratio, fixing the specific relationships existing between different entities. This type of relationship is such that, taken individually, each part will reveal, by simple quantification, the measure of the whole as well as that of its subordinates. In other words, proportion is constituted of a series of terms or a progression in which each term is related to that which precedes it or to that which follows in such a way that it determines its relationship to the whole.

This introduces into the nature of the proportion a qualitative element or a common denominator that unifies the elements of a whole to generate esthetic appeal. Proportion then realizes its full potential and can defined as follows:

The division of a surface into parts contrasted in shape and dimension, yet related to each other.

Next, one has to confront the mathematical expression and the graphic realization of a progression without assuming that the golden number may be involved at each manifestation of a continuous progression. Other examples of continuous geometric progressions, like the series of Fibonacci, do exist and find interesting applications in the visual arts, where the esthetic result depends predominantly on the quality of the division of a defined geometric space. The continuous geometric progression presents a regular but complex movement, a rhythm and a capacity to reorganize itself with its own elements.

Every segmentation of a line, every shape built according to this rhythm of division, is correlated in a

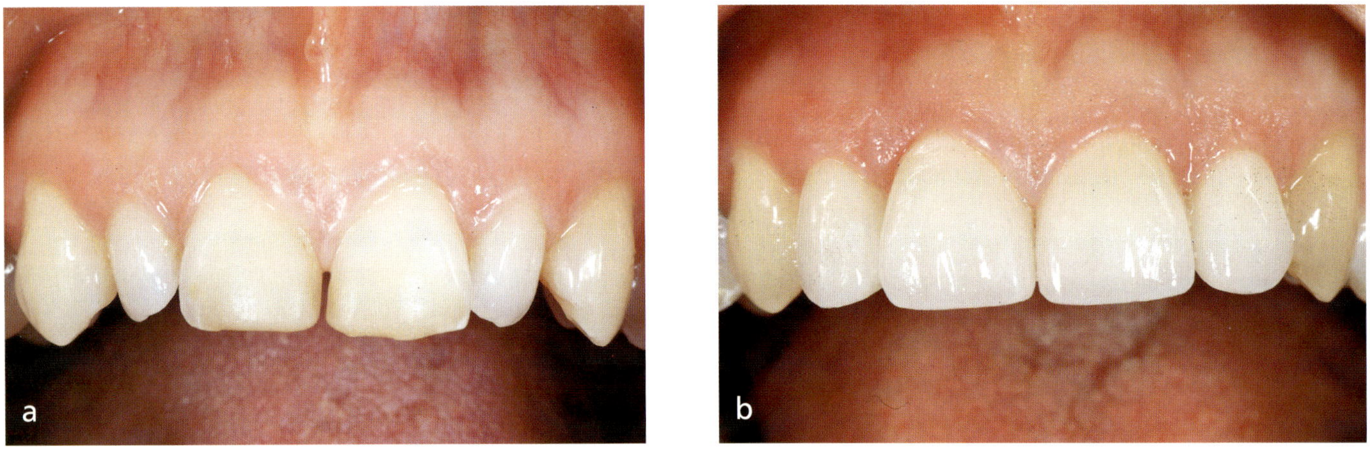

Figs 3-129a and 3-129b The restoration of perceptible golden relationships in an anterior dental segment that did not display these qualities in the original dental elements.

similarity of form and surface. Indeed, the ratio of the continuous geometric projection results from the partition of a segment of a line in mean and extreme terms. This operation permits the segmentation of a given linear length into two unequal segments in such a way that the relation between the smallest and the largest is equal to the relation between the largest and the sum of the two. Consequently, the addition of two terms gives the value of the third one.

In focusing on the golden segmentation of a linear tracing (Fig 3-128), we should remember that it responds to the arrangement of the anterior dental segment as described by Lewis (Fig 3-129) and could also be applicable to the linear relationships ruling the width of the eyes and interocular distance (Fig 3-130). But other structures present a segmentation arising from the golden number, in particular the pentagon and decagon that, generating the subsequent tracing of rectangles closely related to this golden number, have permitted its schematic application to the various elements of facial composition. The significance of this correlation has not only been appreciated by orthognathic and plastic surgeons but has also contributed to the definition of the constraining guidelines used to attain the facial integration of dental compositions.

The appeal to human sensibility of the esthetic and rhythmic qualities of continuous geometric progressions has long been accepted; in surgical practice, however, the conscious application of the golden number becomes pure speculation. Our working capabilities are limited to operating in an arithmetic discontinuity which, unfortunately, offers few elements of perfect proportion, and for decades or even longer we have anticipated in vain ready-made schemes of continuous geometric progressions.

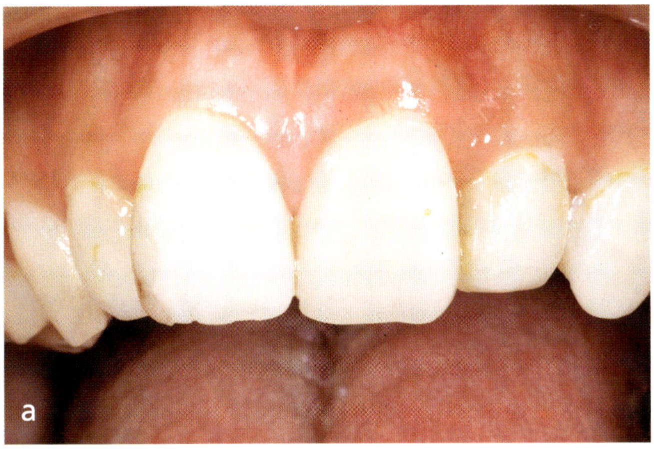

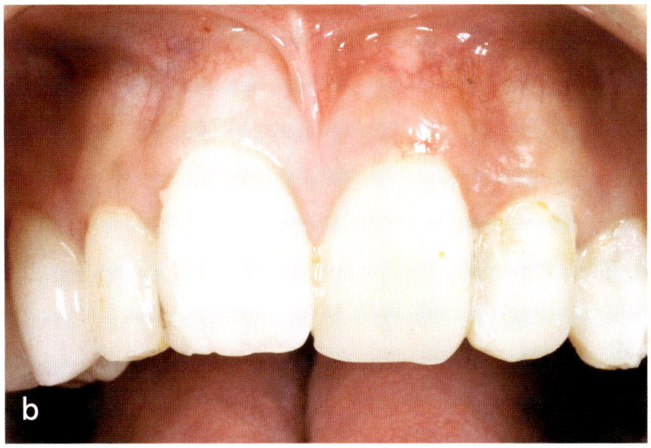

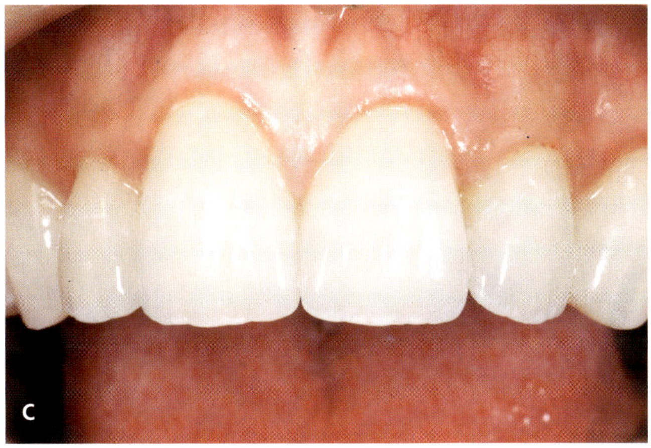

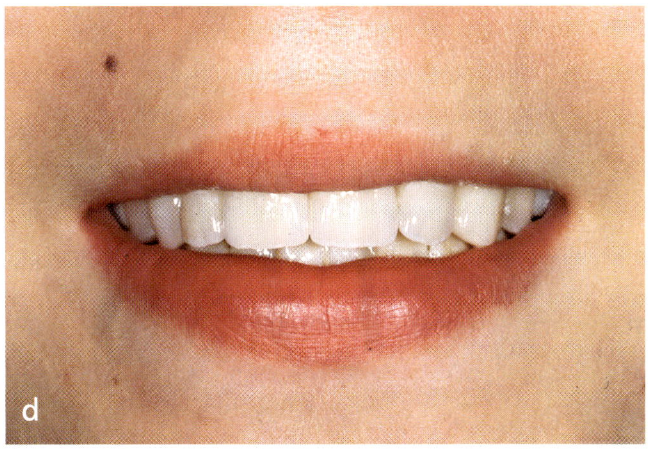

Figs 3-130a to 3-130d An attempt at the restoration of golden relationships in an anterior segment (a) by means of a modification of the right canine and lateral incisor's axial direction and optical illusions. These modifications can be appreciated (b) during the esthetic setup and (c) following cementation. (d) A lower lip line in smiling, showing correct shaping of maxillary central incisors relative to the lower lip but insufficient modifications of the axial direction of the maxillary right canine to meet the requirements of a golden progression. To attain a real level of esthetic qualification, these elements should be correlated with facial parameters, displaying identical proportionate relationships.

Selected Readings

Alain. Propos sur l'esthétique. Paris: Presses Universitaires de France, 1959:14–16.

Angsburger RH. Occlusal plane relation to facial type. J Prosthet Dent 1953;6:755–770.

Arnheim R. Visual Thinking. Berkeley:Univ of California Press, 1971:xii–345.

Arnheim R. Art and Visual Perception, a Psychology of the Creative Eye. London: Faber and Faber, 1956.

Arnheim R. Forms and the consumer. College Art J 1959; 19:2–9.

Art and Language, 1966–75. Oxford: Museum of Modern Art, 1975.

Ash MM. Wheeler's Dental Anatomy, Physiology and Occlusion. Philadelphia: Saunders, 1984.

Barthelemy J. Traité d'Esthétique. Paris: Ed. de l'Ecole, 1964:496.

Bayer R. Traité d'esthétique. Paris: A. Colin, 1956:304.

Berenson B. Seeing and Knowing. London: Chapman and Hall, 1956.

Berger R. La Mutation des Signes. Paris: Denoel, 1972:4

Brisman AS. A comparison of dentists' and patients' concepts. J Am Dent Assoc 1980;100:345–352.

Chiche GJ, Pinault A. Esthetics of Fixed Anterior Prosthodontics. Chicago: Quintessence, 1994.

Cley MM. Le nombre d'or. Paris: PUF, 1973.

Copper DF. Interrelationships between the visual arts, science and technology. Leonardo 1980;13(1):29–33.

de Sausmarez M. Design: La dynamique des formes. Paris: Dessain et Tolra, 1973.

Duthuit G. Le feu des signes. Genève: Saira, 1962.

Eissman H. Visual perception and tooth contour. In: Dental Porcelain: The State of the Art. Los Angeles: Univ of Southern California School of Dentistry, 1977:297.

Frush JP, Fisher RD. Introduction to dentogenetic restorations. J Prosthet Dent 1955;5:586.

Frush JP, Fisher RD. How dentogenetic restorations interpret the sex factor. J Prosthet Dent 1956;6:160–172.

Frush JP. Fischer RD. Dentogenetics: Its practical applications. J Prosthet Dent 1959;9:915–921.

Frush JP. Fischer RD. The dynastic interpretation of the dentogenetic concept. J Prosthet Dent 1958;8:588.

George W. Présence de l'esthétique de Hegel. Paris: Arted, 1967.

Ghylka M. Essai sur le rythme. Paris: Gallimard, 1952.

Goldstein RE. Change Your Smile. Chicago: Quintessence, 1984.

Goldstein RE. Esthetics in Dentistry. Philadelphia: Lippincott, 1976.

Golub J. Entire smile pivotal to teeth design. Clin Dent 1988;33.

Gombrich EH. Norms and Forms: Studios in the Art of the Renaissance. London: Phaidon, 1966:vii–167.

Graber LW, Luckner WG. Dental esthetic self-evaluation and satisfaction. Am J Orthod 1980;77:163–173.

Gredon S. Space, Time and Architecture. The Growth of a New Transition. Cambridge, MA: Harvard Univ Press, 1965.

Green B. The Doctrine of Pure Aesthetic. College Art J 1959-60; 19 (Winter): 122–133.

Greenberg JR. Shaping anterior teeth for natural esthetics. Esthet Dent Update 1992;3:81.

Guillaume P. La Psychologie de la Forme. Paris: Fammarion, 1984.

Hegel G. Wilhelm Friedrich. Esthétique, Textes choisis par Claude Khodoss, ed 3. Paris: PUF, 1962: intro–16.

Hogrebe W, Naredi-Rainer P, Klein J, Stüben J, Hasenfuss J. Geschichte der Ästhetik und der Kunsttheorie. Zeitschrift für Ästhetik und allgemeine Kunstwissenschaft. Vol 23 (1978);130–283.

Hughes GA. Facial types and tooth arrangement. J Prosthet Dent 1951;1:82–95.

Huyghe R. Dialogue avec le Visible. Paris: Flammarion, 1995.

Kandinsky W. Ecrits Complets. Paris: Denoel-Gonthier, 1970.

Kandinsky W. On the Spiritual in Art. Guggenheim Foundation. New York: Solomon, 1946.

Kandinsky W. Point, Ligne, Surface: Contribution à l'Analyse des Éléments Picturaux. Paris: ed. de Beaune, 1963.

Kant E. Le jugement Esthétique. Paris: PUF, 1966.

Klee P. Die Ordnung der Dinge. Teufen: A. Niggli, 1975.

Kuhn R. Komposition und Rhythmus: Beiträge zu Neubegründung einer historischen Kompositionslehre. Berlin: W. De Gruyter, 1980.

Lalo C. Les sentiments esthétiques. Paris: F. Alcan, 1910.

Lalo C. Notions d'esthétique, ed 5. Paris: Presses universitaires de France, 1969.

Landow G. The Aesthetic and Critical Theories of John Ruskin. Princeton, NJ: Princeton Univ Press, 1971:xii–462.

Lejoyeux J. Les 9 clefs du visage. Paris: Solar, 1991.

Levin EL. Dental esthetics and the golden proportion. J Prosthet Dent 1978;40:244–252.

Lombardi RE. The principles of visual perception and their clinical application to denture esthetics. J Prosthet Dent 1973;29:358–382.

Lucio-Meyers J-J. Visual aesthetics. London: Lund Humphries, 1973.

Mavroskoufis F, Ritchie GM. The face form as a guide for the selection of maxillary central incisors. J Prosthet Dent 1980;43:501–505.

Moles AA, Rohmer E. Psychologie de l'Espace. Tournai: Casterman, 1972: i–16.

Muriro T. Form and Style in the Arts: An Introduction to Aesthetic Morphology. Cleveland: Case Western Reserve Univ Press, 1970: xvii–468.

Norberg-Schulz C. Existence, Space and Architecture. London: Studio Vista, 1971.

Pound E. Applying harmony in selecting and arranging teeth. Dent Clin North Am 1962;241–258.

Ratel P. Naissance de l'odontographie: Prothèse dentaire. 1998;139: 23–29.

Ricketts RM. The biologic significance of the divine proportion and Fibonacci series. Am J Orthod 1982;81:351–370.

Sanginola RA. Prothèse compléte: Choix des dents artificielles. Encycl Med-Chir. Paris; Stomatologie, 12-1997, 233 25 F-10.

Schüling H. Theorien der malensischen Linear Perspektive. Giessen: Universitätsbibliothek, 1973:xii–28.

Sourian Etienne. Clefs pour l'esthétique. Paris: Seghers, 1970:i–16.

Torroya E. Logik der Form. München: GDW Callwey, 1961.

Tritten G. Education par la forme et par la couleur. (Erziehung durch Form und Farbe). La Tour de Peilz: Ed. Delta, 1968.

Tweed CH. The diagnostic facial triangle in the control of treatment objectives. Am J Orthod 1969;55:651–657.

Weyl H. Symmetry. Princeton, NJ: Princeton Univ Press, 1952:iii–168.

Woelfels JB. Dental Anatomy: Its Relevance to Dentistry, ed 4. Philadelphia: Lea and Fabiger, 1990.

CHAPTER

4 Functional Integration

"However pleasing a restoration may be, it may well represent a perfect example of functional illusion and reveal itself as intrusive to the gnathic system" (Robert Lee). Good relations between esthetics and function involve the philosophical acceptance that shapes will be subconsciously felt as ideal and beautiful if they are felt as responding to the requirements of function.

If we understand the function of natural elements it becomes easy to reproduce them in a verisimilar artificial form because function generates form. Unfortunately, the functional explanation has never explained specifically which functions generate which forms. We are left with the feeling that morphology alone must guide us in the restoration of the beauty of things in their form and function.

But feelings are just feelings and can hardly resist the convincing power of theories. What has always prevailed in the field of occlusion is the elaboration of functional theories producing ever-reproducible dentate pseudoforms that fail to meet the primary requirement of esthetic dentistry: respect for morphological reality.

Nothing is more disturbing to clear understanding than the repetitive influence of theories generating absurd forms; nothing is more disturbing to understanding than the controversies resulting from the multitude of occlusal concepts; and nothing is more disturbing than the statement that no concept or system has proven superior to another and that no concept can be harmoniously associated with another or to the existing reality.

In the restorative approach, the road to good occlusion and esthetic excellence involves respect for tooth morphology and the respectful application of a variety of parameters that investigations of the functional mechanisms of the stomatognathic system have discovered.

Aside from sound scientific knowledge, the most important element in the outcome of prosthodontic procedures remains the sensibility of clinicians. They alone can appreciate individual physiological or morphological variations. Only they can compensate for the limitations of professional instrumentation, which, whatever its degree of sophistication, remains purely mechanical and repetitive and too often clouds clinical judgment. Sensibility is not a gift from heaven but results from constant training and repeated observation. It is the most important instrument of the esthetic dentist.

But sensibility must nonetheless be supported by scientific knowledge, which today requires that a certain number of parameters be considered to ascertain the integration of restorative elements into the mechanisms of the stomatognathic system and their long-term stability.

Architecture

The nature of the gnathic structure is genetically established. The study of the osseous trabeculation of the stomatognathic system and that of the whole human body shows us that these structures are shaped by function. This means that the percussive function of teeth is in full coordination with their structure. This structure appears to be sinuous or undulating. Undulating structures in electromagnetic waves are considered the fundamental elements of energetic transmission; energy develops its power by undulation. In fact, the structure of every living organism is in harmony with undulating structure, and the elements of the oral architecture do not escape this phenomenon.

Dental arches present sinuous buccal and lingual contours. The morphological progression of the cuspidal arrangement presents sinuous dentitions. The sagittal and frontal lines of occlusion also share these sinuous characteristics.

Long dental axis root canal designs are sinuous, as is the whole occluso-articulated complex, including the condyle pathways. These elements are fully adapted to the impact of the percussive clashes and vibrations they generate. They oppose a resistance arising from their elasticity and rupture of pressure.

Contrary to the notions of Cartesian spirits who always connect two points with a straight line, human architectural reality establishes connections between these same points with a sinuous undulation. Therefore it must be stressed that the esthetic reading of linear elements that was described in the previous chapter was simplified to fulfill didactic and analytical objectives.

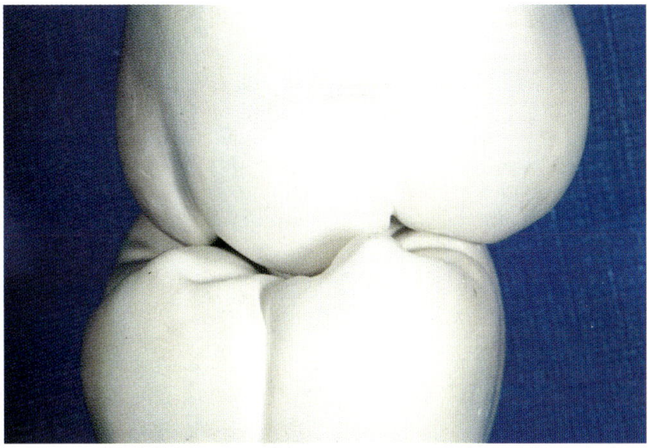

Fig 4-1 Cusp to fossa, cusp to ridge, or tripodization, the nature of interocclusal contacts has no importance as long as they are simultaneous, reduced in size, and multiple, with resultant forces directed along the long axis of the root to ensure stability. These characteristics are best achieved with well-designed cusps and fossae such as in the tooth morphology proposed by A. Tanaka, CDT, Chicago.

Respect for the morphological and architectural characteristics of oral design is the true answer to the restoration of the beauty of living things in their form and function. However, it behooves us to state that the restorative elements commonly used to integrate the stomatognathic complex do not always exhibit this respect and achieve their purpose only approximately. We have settled for this because we have been fooled by the incredible adaptive capacity of the system, which always delays an inevitable future breakdown.

Coordinated Interocclusal Relationships

In a good occlusion all the teeth in the mouth make simultaneous contact. However, and even if this statement results only from a feeling, contacts should be lighter on the anterior than on the posterior segments. The tripodization of posterior contacts promoted by the gnathological concept, though most valuable from a mechanical point of view, is rarely seen in nature where cusp-to-ridge relationships usually prevail over cusp-to-fossa relationships.

Though the preference for one system or another has no importance, the aim of occlusal stability forces us to attend to direct occlusal forces along the long axis of the root. The key to occlusal stability is intercuspal precision. Precision means contacts should be simultaneous and contact areas should be reduced as much as possible to minimize occlusal loading strength (Fig 4-1).

Mechanically, three interocclusal contacts ideally located on the arch may achieve this stability. In practice, the cuspidated nature of helicoid antagonist closing surfaces, differences in the distance from the rotational center of the mandible, and tooth axial position interfere with simultaneous contacts. To reach this objective and to limit the impact of minor undetected interocclusal failures or interferences, the largest possible distribution of occlusal contacts (usually 16 to 22, numbered on each quadrant) is advisable.

The maximum contacting position of the mandibular teeth to the maxillary teeth has been called centric occlusion (CO) or intercuspal position (IP). Centric occlusion (CO) represents the end point of natural functional movements. Studies have demonstrated that in CO the condyles are three-dimensionally displaced from all the three walls of the border pathways, suggesting that CO generates an unloaded joint position.

The way to the end point of functional movements may be strewn with encumbrances and a variety of deflective contacts. Once free from any type of interference, this end point coincides with a mandibular rotational position denominated centric relation or CR. This means that centric relation position may be repeated at any rotational location of the mandible and can be defined as a craniomandibular relationship in which the condyles are in the most anterior-superior region of the fossa. CR is not a rest position since intense electromyographic activity may be observed in this position.

CR is a physiologically functional and indefinitely repeatable position. This explains its interest and the importance of its registration. It has been stressed that its clinical registration should result from a repetitive, unstrained, nonmanipulated mandible closure. MacNeill has concluded that centric registration is best achieved with the mandible in function. During this recording procedure, muscular activity apparently places the condyle-disc assembly in the most anterosuperior position of the fossa, a fact of evident clinical interest.

Consensus has made of CR the best location for the intercuspation of teeth. In other words, craniomandibular tooth relationships can be considered ideal when CR = IP. This gives a clear indication for selecting a procedure of CR registration that at the same time ascertains ideal interocclusal relationships and the location of the condyle-disc assembly. Formerly this has been impossible during the whole restorative process for lack of an easy clinical means of evaluation. Now, however, two distinct procedures for CR registration can be used: intraoral and extraoral. The usual intraoral registration techniques are done at a fixed occlusal height that cannot be modified. Extraoral registrations of the terminal hinge location allow an immediate determination of CR at all possible variations of the occlusal height by simple rotational opening or closing of the articulator.

Yet the ideal clinical registration procedure remains to be determined, since the total negation of the patient's adverse muscular activity during registration is impossible, and the absence of manual interference is not credible. In today's state of knowledge, one has to stress that the objective of the clinical registration of CR and its prosthetic applications is not an occlusal relationship coordinated with a specific location of the condyles, but the achievement of occlusal stability.

Controlled Tooth Closure

It clearly appears that these elements of the occlusal schema—optimum distribution, location and size of interocclusal contacts in centric relation, and simultaneous coordination of interocclusal relationships—

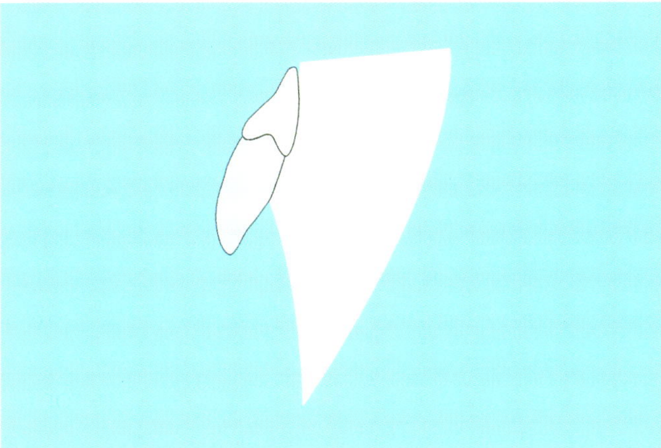

Fig 4-2 The range of action of mandibular movements is limited by the anatomical characteristics of the temporomandibular joints. It scribes a three-dimensional tracing delimiting an area defined as "the envelope of mandibular motion," represented here in its sagittal development.

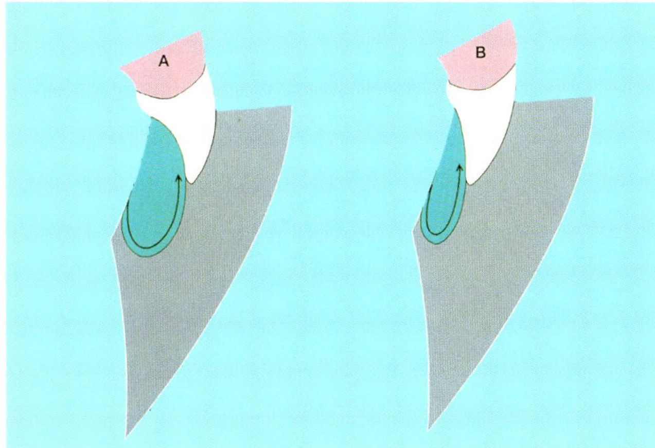

Fig 4-3 The nature of functional movements is dictated not only by condylar pathways but primarily by antagonist tooth morphology and tooth position, generating for each individual a different three-dimensional tracing (a,b) delimiting an area defined as the "envelope of function," represented here in its sagittal development.

have to be considered important contributors to long-term occlusal stability. Yet clinical observation shows that these common characteristics are far from leading to identical results. To reach the objective of occlusal stability it remains for the restorative dentist to master the application of these schematic similarities in light of multiple individual differences and the dynamic of mandibular movements.

Mandibular movements can be described as simultaneous rotations and translations around three axes, transverse, sagittal, and vertical. The range of action of these movements is limited by the anatomical particulars of the temporomandibular articulation and associated muscles and ligaments, encompassed by a spatial area that has been described as "the envelope of mandibular motion"(Fig 4-2). The registration of these movements is required for the development of articulators or mechanical devices aimed at simulating them.

Born from mechanically inclined imaginations to serve a concept, articulators have become symbols of intellectual perversion. They have succeeded in brainwashing generations of professionals convinced that they will reach new levels of accomplishment by the mere possession and sometimes the use of the newest or most sophisticated models. Yet in the complex stomatognathic system, mandibular movements are not the same as function. Function takes place at the moment teeth enter into action. Consequently, the nature of functional movements is not only dictated by condylar pathways but also by anterior antagonist tooth morphology and position, all of which takes place in an area called an "envelope of function" (Fig 4-3).

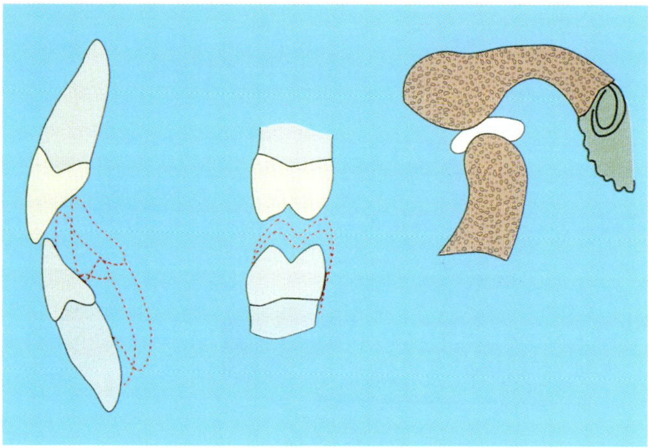

Fig 4-4 Function takes place at the very moment teeth enter into action. Long-term stability of anterior teeth is evidence of the atraumatic mandibular approach to CO along the anterior pathway, whatever the head posture, and attests to the presence of self-protective neuromuscular mechanisms.

The envelope of function, limited to the area of the teeth, is naturally included within the spatial area containing the full range of mandibular movements, or the "envelope of mandibular motion." In clinical applications the importance of mandibular movements has been fading since we have realized the importance of the mechanisms dictating tooth closure and disclosure patterns. Research has shown that teeth, along with condylar pathway characteristics and neuromuscular activity, are the primary factors in tooth closure patterns.

Indeed, only the presence of neuromuscular mechanisms can explain the repetitive and "atraumatic" mandibular approach to centric occlusion, whatever the head postural position. Even if the mechanisms involved are not completely understood, we know that this approach is influenced by proprio feedback information controlled by the central nervous system (CNS), which in turn dictates appropriate muscular closure (Fig 4-4).

The hypothesis that the CNS could develop new engrams for occlusion when anterior relationships are submitted to restorative modifications affecting tooth morphology or tooth position has received clinical confirmation. This means that the primary concern in the restorative process remains the restoration of morphological normality, with respect for specific conditions that permit autoprotective neuromuscular mechanisms to develop their action.

The objective of the restorative process, once simultaneity and multiple occlusal contacts have been achieved, is to gain control of the dynamic of tooth closure and disclosure patterns, since the majority of problems of occlusion originate from improper or nonfunctional tooth closure.

Any closure of teeth producing visible or invisible stress, damage, or overload to the teeth, joint, muscle, bone, periodontium, or nervous system has been defined as traumatic occlusion. The dental literature is replete with descriptions of the various interfer-

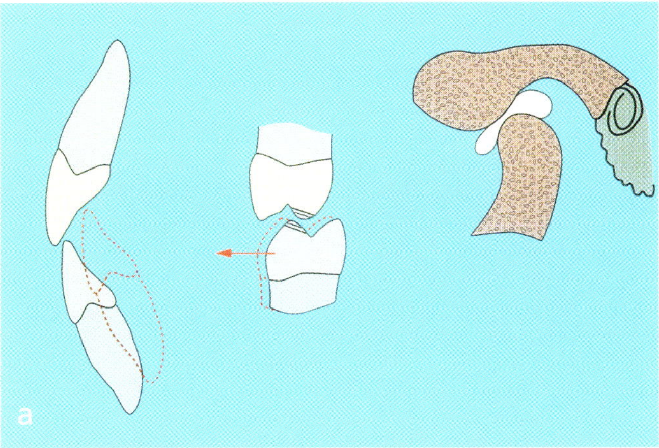

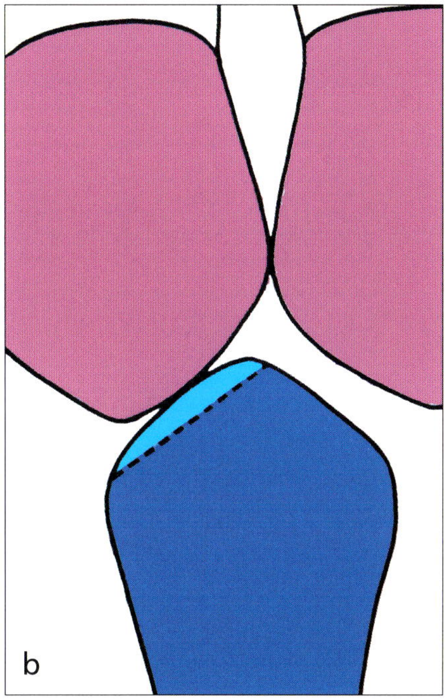

Figs 4-5a and 4-5b The free pathway to CO may be disturbed by two types of interferences or centric interferences. (a) The first type generates a slide from centric either laterally or in protrusion. (b) Centric interferences must be eliminated by selective grinding.

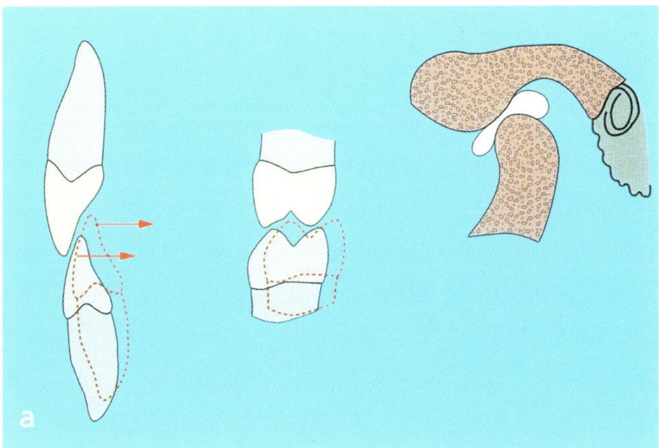

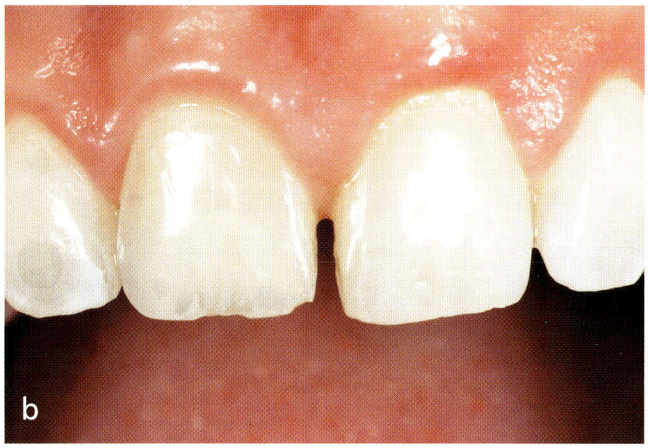

Figs 4-6a and 4-6b (a) The second type of centric interferences has been defined as incisive or protrusive-retrusive. (b) This is more difficult to eliminate because an approach with selective grinding could only increase the already-existing tissue damage, affecting the incisal-lingual aspect of maxillary incisors.

ences that may impair centric relations from the moment of first contact between antagonist anterior teeth. Those interferences that take place within the envelope of mandibular function are defined as centric interferences. They are of two kinds: *(1)* centric relation (anterior or lateral slides, fulcrum), and *(2)* incisive (protrusive-retrusive).

All authors agree that these interferences are responsible for the delivery of excessive lateral forces to the teeth, a prime triggering factor in the initiation of bruxism and a predisposing factor in temporomandibular joint dysfunctions and so must be eliminated (Figs 4-5 and 4-6). This will open the way to free functional closure which must be understood as an atraumatic tooth closure engagement and disengagement whose development remains under neuromuscular control whatever the process in play, mastication or swallowing.

This freedom of movement can hardly be attributed to articulators whose protrusive and lateral disengagements invariably strike against the obstacle of the teeth in the absence of neuromuscular control. No real freedom of movement can be experienced with articulators until destructive forces have erased the particulars of tooth anatomy. This is most confusing and invites us to consider the nature and importance of complementary parameters to ascertain long-term occlusal stability.

Reduced Muscular Activity

Occlusal forces can be uniformly distributed along the arch and precisely directed along the tooth axis. Tooth closure patterns can be free from interferences and under neuromuscular control. It remains for us to investigate the impact resulting from the variations of dental architecture when submitted to the dynamic of mandibular movements.

The studies of Kelly have claimed that 80% of the population present a Class I interocclusal relationship. In this type of relationship the maxillary and mandibular anterior teeth overlap both vertically and horizontally. Variations of this type of relationship in the vertical and horizontal planes and in tooth inclination are unlimited (Fig 4-7). More pronounced variations in the inclination and spatial position of the teeth may affect the remaining 20% of occlusal types, defined as malocclusion, which include Class II angle relationship, horizontal overjet, open bite, edge-to-edge, and Class III relationships, in decreasing order of occurrence. Concomitantly, it is interesting to note that the incisal pathway, which depends upon tooth position, tooth inclination, and tooth morphology, also deviates from the standard in 20% of cases.

The eccentric disengagements of these different architectural dental arrangements, or so-called lateral eccentric occlusions, have been classified according to tooth contact conditions as self-protected articulation or tooth guidance, group function, and balanced articulation. Currently the belief that all these eccentric occlusal schemes are designed to distribute occlusal forces evenly finds no scientific support. Research has shown a progressive increase of muscular activity from eccentric tooth articulation to group function to balanced articulation. This progressive increase, related to an increase of tooth contacting surfaces in eccentric occlusion, can appear in the development of tooth wear resulting from bruxism. Bruxism generates a force 6 times that of normal function and longer lasting. This illustrates the

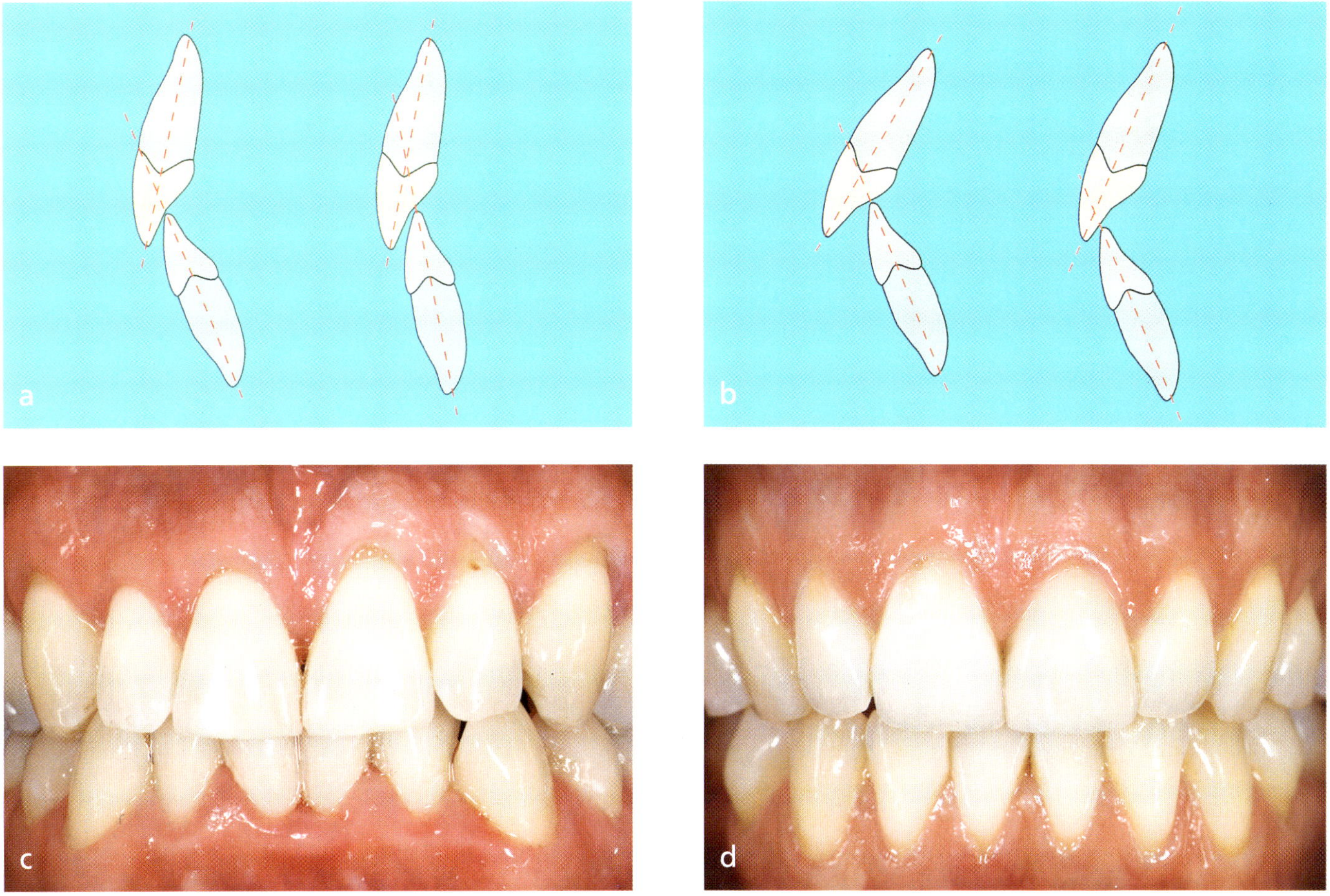

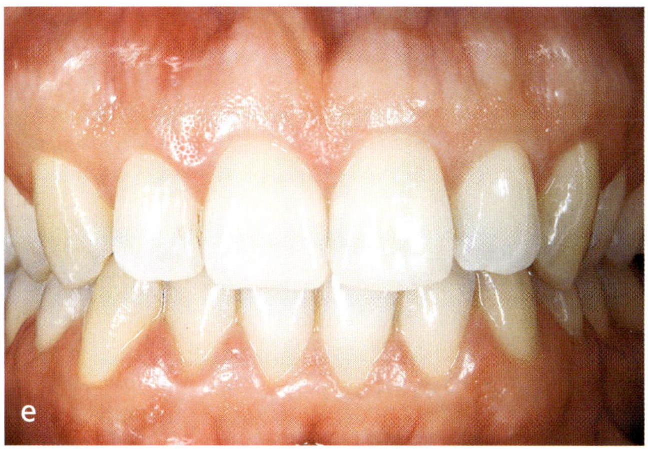

Figs 4-7a to 4-7e (a,b) Eighty percent of the population presents a Class I relationship, but variations in anterior axial inclinations, interocclusal relationships, and incisal pathways are unlimited. Yet they do not have identical effects. Samples of various interocclusal designs in individuals between 40 and 50 years of age show (c) moderate manifestations of wear on maxillary left incisors with gingival recession on a lateral incisor, pathologies that could be correlated with the loose interocclusal relationships affecting the canines; (d) reduced vertical overbite with an advanced abrasion of the mandibular anterior segment and signs of wear predominantly on the maxillary canines and central incisors; and (e) good anterior relationships and morphological integrity and all the characteristics of occlusal stability.

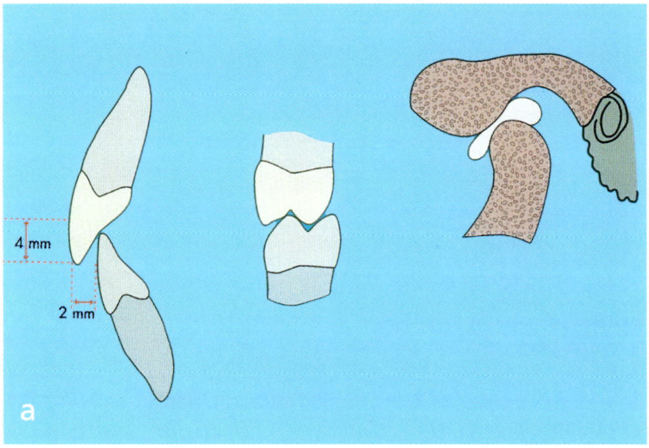

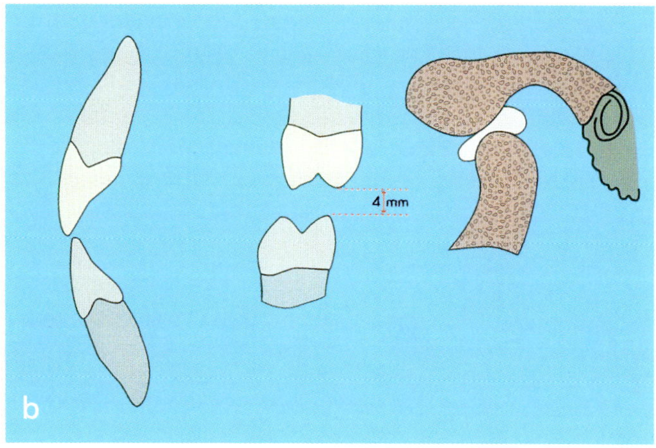

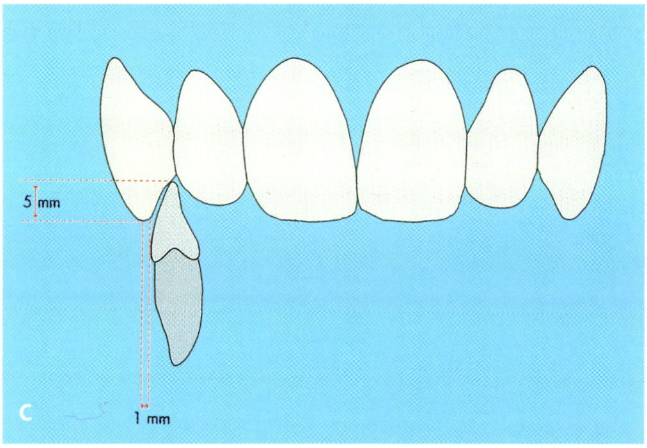

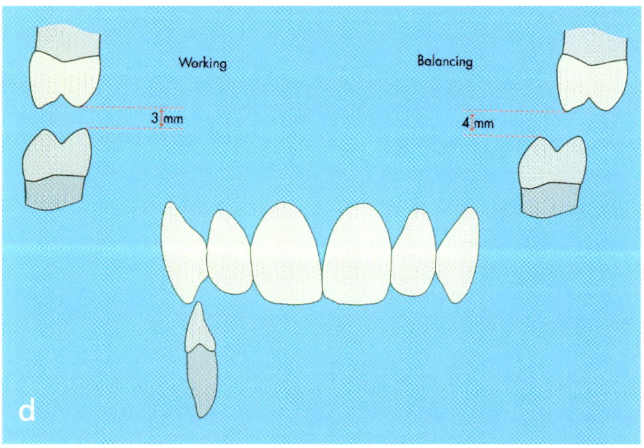

Figs 4-8a to 4-8d Long-lasting dentitions exhibit not only tooth guidance in eccentric occlusal relationships but similarities in tooth morphology and in vertical and horizontal overbite. (a) Scheme of ideal relationships between maxillary and mandibular incisors in centric and (b) eccentric protrusive occlusion. (c) Scheme of ideal relationships between maxillary and mandibular canines in centric and (d) eccentric lateral occlusion.

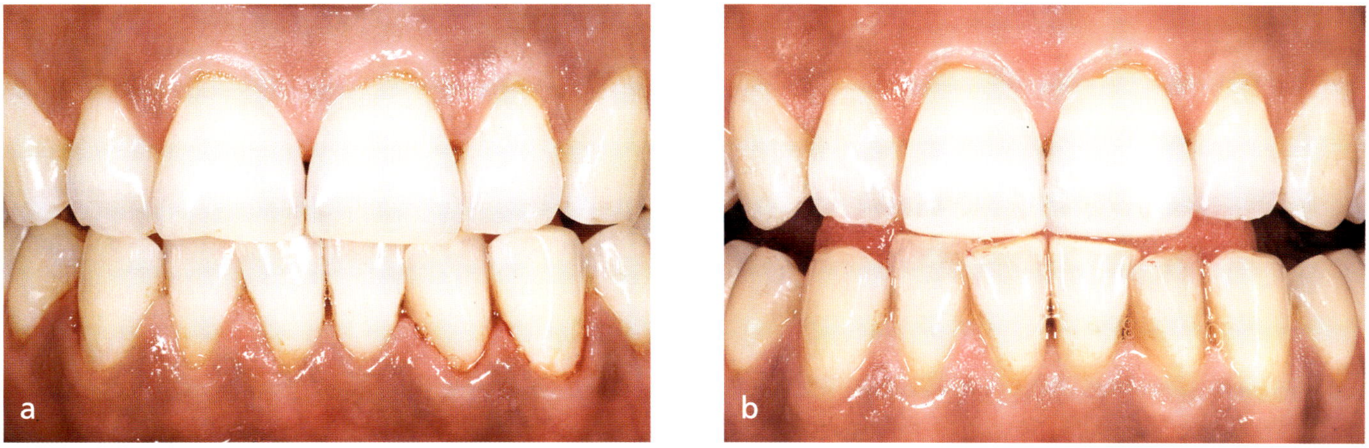

Figs 4-9a and 4-9b The morphological characteristics of a tooth are a key element in ideal interocclusal relationships in both centric and eccentric occlusions. A 1.5-mm maxillary incisor length increase to modify the angle of the incisal pathway has succeeded in obtaining the expected posterior interocclusal clearance in protrusive eccentric occlusion.

unphysiological and traumatic nature of the phenomenon.

Reduced muscular activity is one of the parameters that may help identify occlusal stability. Eccentric tooth articulation, or tooth guidance, represents the only scheme of occlusal architecture that permits us to reach this objective. Tooth guidance (self-protected occlusion or anterior guidance) involves the contribution of self-protecting neuromuscular mechanisms. It involves two parameters: incisal guidance (protrusive-retrusive movement) and canine guidance (mediotrusive lateral movement).

Clinical observation shows us that long-lasting, untreated, and atraumatic dentitions not only exhibit this type of eccentric occlusal relationship but (whatever the age) present similarities in tooth morphological design and interocclusal relationships (Figs 4-8 and 4-9; Table 4-1).

Table 4-1 Average morphological designs and interocclusal relationships

Occlusal relationship	Average clearance
Maxillary central incisors	12 mm
Maxillary canine	12 mm
Mandibular incisor	10 mm
Incisal horizontal overbite	2–3 mm
Canine	1 mm
Incisal vertical overbite	3–4 mm
Canine vertical overbite	5–6 mm
Posterior clearance in	
eccentric protrusive occlusion	2–4 mm
lateral occlusion	
working side	2–3 mm
nonworking side	3–4 mm

These types of morphological designs and anterior relationships prevent any possibility of posterior eccentric interference and allow for the most verticalized mandibular tooth closure to load in CR posterior teeth with the most reduced possible strength. It must be stressed that few dentitions are so arranged as to satisfy these conditions. Variations are unlimited, pure canine or incisal guidance is not the rule, and corrective measures are usually unavoidable.

Verticalization of the occlusion can be defined as the therapeutic approach to duplicating these conditions. The decision to verticalize occlusion rests on the dentist's experience and can only be reached in the light of dentofacial esthetic evaluation. These two elements, function and esthetics, are indissociable.

Guidelines to Occlusal Stability

Correct, stable, long-lasting natural or restored occlusions are always identical and respond to identical functional principles. In the organization of the occlusal plane, interocclusal contacts are multiple, reduced in size, and simultaneous; the inclination of the tooth closure pathway is dictated by maxillary and mandibular tooth position, tooth inclination, and antagonist tooth morphological design, as well as the condylar pathway; the engagement of the mandibular anterior incisor along the lingual surface of the maxillary incisor or incisal guidance and the engagement of the mandibular canine along the lingual surface of the maxillary canine or canine guidance, is under neuromuscular control; tooth closure engagement or disengagement responds to similar neuromuscular mechanisms; and neuromuscular mechanisms implicate proprioceptive receptors that constantly feed the brain with information relative to the position of the mandible. This dictates appropriate and atraumatic tooth closure patterns. This is a reflex mechanism, repetitive in the onset and development of its action. These mechanisms, which are self-protective, are among those that prevent anterior overload during function until posterior teeth provide large occlusal support when tooth closure is completed. Centric interferences that could disturb free tooth closure engagement must be eliminated. During all the stages of tooth closure, engagement, or disengagement, with the exception of complete tooth closure, posterior disocclusion is the rule.

The following observations can be made:

The interocclusal void that takes place during all the phases of tooth closure, engagement, or disengagement or during mandibular movements can also be observed in rest position; this rest position, which constitutes the starting point of all mandibular movements, remains impossible for the articulator.

Deviations from these standards, disharmonies in the static of occlusion, or disrhythmia in the dynamic of function influence mandibular closing patterns and bring stress into the stomatognathic system.

It is left to clinicians to recognize among the variety of occlusal schemes the potential sources of instability. They must adopt sound and appropriate treatment modalities for the control of occlusal stability, including corrective measures; when these corrections are impossible to apply, they must adopt maintenance measures.

Malocclusion and Maintenance

Few dentitions present the ideal conditions that guarantee long-term occlusal stability. The objectives of occlusal maintenance therapy are to prevent the destructive action of parafunctional forces and to prevent or control any migratory movement in all cases where corrective therapies, for one reason or another, cannot be applied.

Occlusal maintenance will have to be adapted to existing clinical conditions. They should be applied as early as possible to make up for interocclusal deficiencies involving all types of occlusal relationships, from so-called normocclusions to Class II, open bite, and edge-to-edge relationships (Fig 4-10).

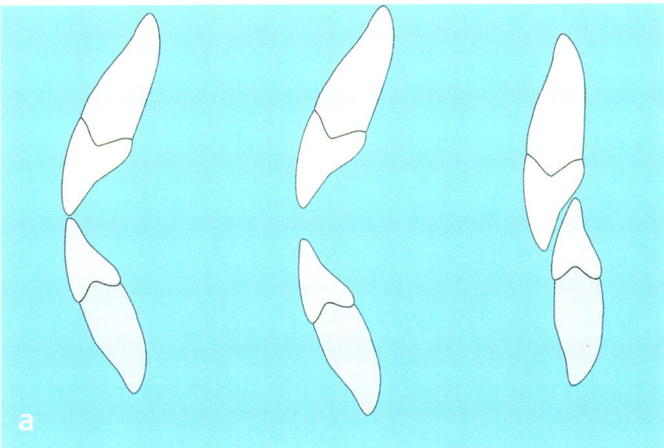

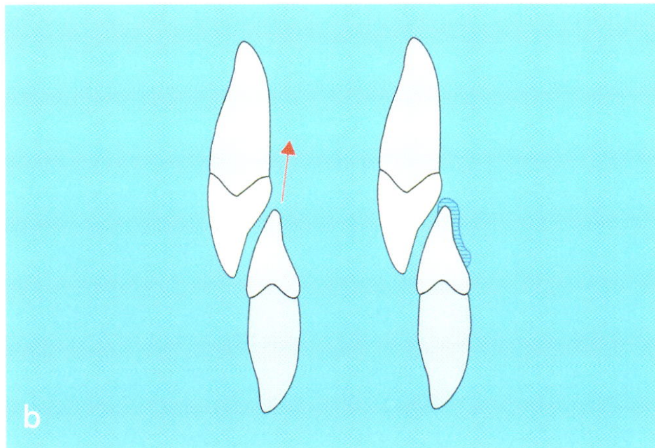

Figs 4-10a and 4-10b Over the years, migratory movements or morphological alterations can affect dentitions showing deficiencies in interocclusal relationships like edge-to-edge relations, open bite, and excesses in horizontal and vertical overbites. When these conditions are present, maintenance measures must be systematically applied.

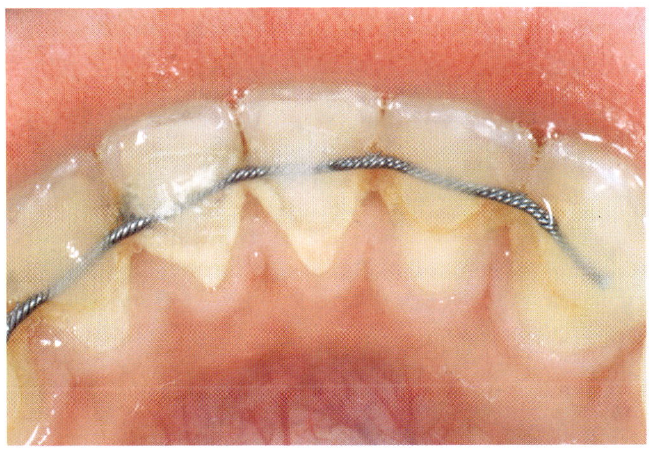

Fig 4-11 Prevention of migratory movements with any type of appliance, fixed or removable, has to be adapted to each particular clinical situation and integrated in the panoply of therapeutic measures dedicated to oral maintenance.

Most of the criteria of occlusal stability and good function involve the anterior segment of the dentition. They consequently involve esthetic considerations. In dealing with these, the clinician should realize that esthetic dentofacial excellence is not linked to a Class I relationship and that malocclusions are not synonymous with dentofacial ugliness.

Few adult patients will give up dentofacial esthetic satisfaction or occlusal excellence. Most are reluctant to accept major orthodontic treatment. Therefore, we can offer these patients no palliative treatment other than occlusal maintenance (Fig 4-11).

Prevention of migration

It has been stated that the percussive function of teeth develops from the contact of antagonist dental elements. In the absence of such contacts this repetitive and atraumatic functional stimulation may fail, but will be compensated by the palliative action of the tongue or lip to maintain the spatial stability of the dental elements. Yet this palliative soft tissue stimulation does not automatically develop its action in the absence of interocclusal contact.

It can be observed that in a poor alignment of the mandibular anterior segment, tooth eruption systematically affects the most lingually positioned element. In a Class II occlusion with the progression of age, the eruption of the whole mandibular anterior

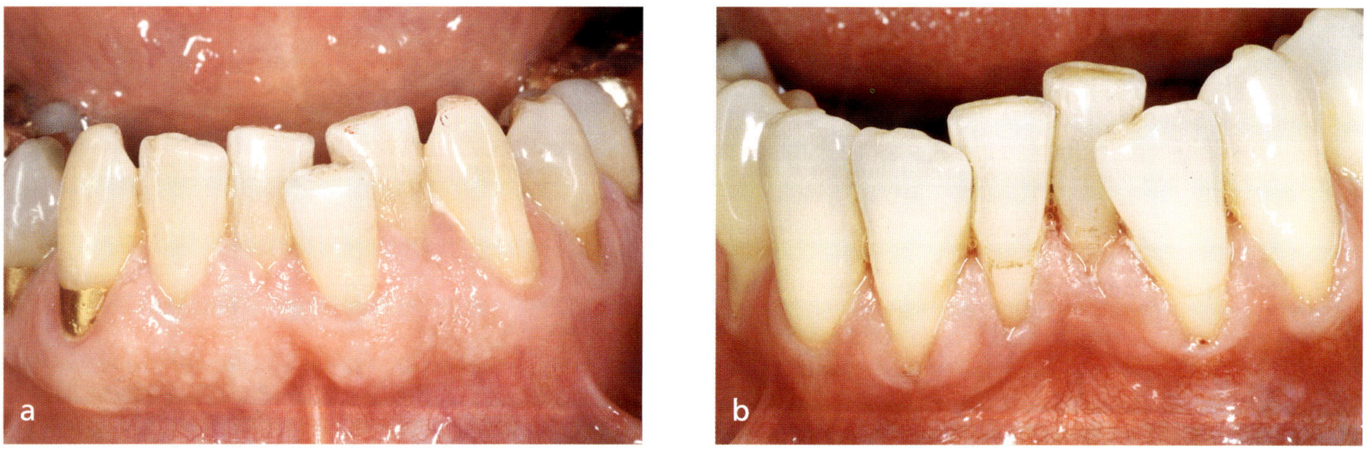

Figs 4-12a and 4-12b (a,b) Preventive maintenance measures should not neglect a category of patients affected by sudden increase of mandibular incisor crowding generated by a reduction of mandibular arch width, which usually takes place between 50 and 60 years of age. In such a situation, intracoronal or extracoronal retention, fixed or removable, from canine to canine is the rule.

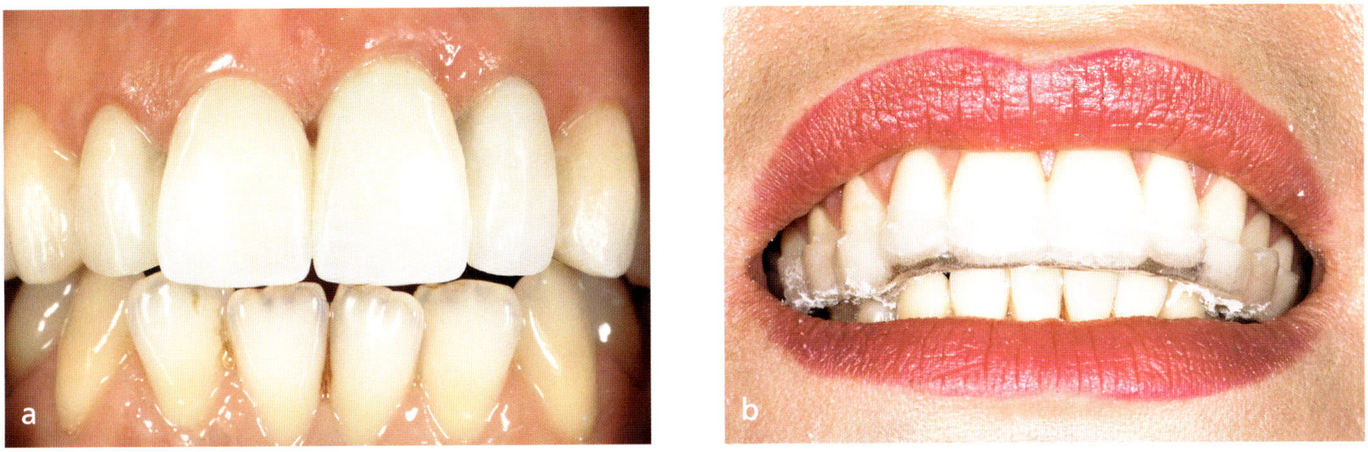

Figs 4-13a and 4-13b These preventive measures also implicate individuals showing deficiencies in interocclusal relationships and are foreseen for the maintenance of both natural and restored dentitions. (a) This particular case presents an occlusal scheme with an anterior open bite malocclusion. (b) Twelve individual porcelain veneers are maintained with a removable acrylic bite guard.

segment is not unusual. Migratory movements may take place each time normal tooth function cannot be accomplished in a repetitive manner (Fig 4-12).

These types of events cannot be expected in youth, but the insidious progression of these migrations, impairing dentofacial esthetics, calls for the early institution of preventive measures, depending on the nature of the malocclusion. We are speaking here of simple therapeutic means including morphological tooth modifications, all types of splints, and retention from bonded orthodontic retainers to the usual acrylic bite guard or night guard (Figs 4-11 and 4-13).

Occlusal stress control

Bite guards seem to be ideal therapeutic devices for diluting the effects of clenching. Clenching is usually characterized by gingival recession, cervicular erosion, overgrowth of the osseous buccal plate, and muscle spasm. Depending on the circumstances, it can also achieve a temporary occlusal stabilization. To fulfill the objectives of reduced muscular activity, bite guards should also be designed to simulate a verticalization of occlusion.

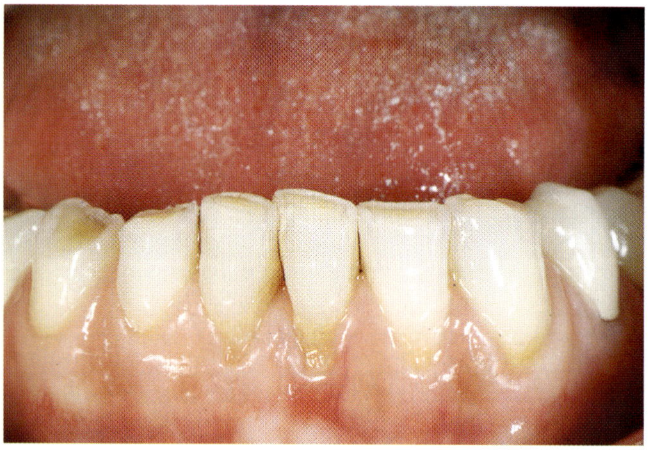

Fig 4-14 Various manifestations of tooth-wear disease, from dentin involvement to dentinal crevices and breaks of the enamel walls through loss of structural integrity.

Eccentric Interferences and Avoidance Patterns

In general dental practice, the dentist's occlusal knowledge and ability to diagnose is subject to variables, while working habits are focused on fulfilling punctually the patient's needs. Therefore the restoration of the physical damage resulting from dental diseases has always been effected without much analysis of etiologic factors. Dental disease may be defined as a permanent alteration or loss of function affecting teeth, periodontal tissues, and associated structures.

The loss of anatomical tooth structure from causes other than carious lesions can be considered a disease and labeled *occlusal disease*. It has been demonstrated that occlusal disease results from adverse forces and that the structural, or abrasius, alterations it causes may affect either the incisal or occlusal surface of the tooth. Sometimes the neck of the tooth on its buccal cervical side both in the anterior and in the posterior segments manifests a curved indentation, a pathologic situation called *erosion*.

This last type of structural alteration, erosion, brings about the best financial yield for the restorative dentist and has been the most common area for experimentation using updated materials. Eroded areas are most of the time associated with a localized gingival recession and buccal exostosis, whereas increase in masseter muscle development is not unusual after years of repeated occlusal clenching.

This suggests that the most simple acrylic appliance, such as a bite guard, can in many cases perfectly control the progression of eroded surfaces and associated structural losses by reducing the impact of adverse forces exceeding the resistance of the gnathic system. Long-term clinical practice has demonstrated the efficiency of this preventive measure but has not ended speculation on the etiology of erosions, in which psychological and physiological factors seem to predominate.

Occlusion, physiology, and psychology have also been proposed as predisposing factors of bruxism, but investigation of the causes of abrasion are rather limited because of its incidence in the population. As an occlusal disease, tooth wear is totally disregarded. This lack of interest in a problem that pervades the fields of restorative dentistry, periodontics, and occlusion results from the fact that occlusal wear is currently considered physiological. Why should incisal or occlusal wear be fixed when the whole system seems to work; when the patient remains free from pain; and when etiology, development stages, and treatment modalities have not been found? Why, when, and how interfere in the progression of the disease that will anyway be left finally to the therapeutic competence of the prosthodontist?

But why not interfere before both esthetics and function are completely compromised? Why not interfere when comprehensive treatment modalities can be applied at any stage of the progression of the disease ? The progressive alteration of incisal and occlusal surfaces, or abrasion, has recently been codified and this should help in the early detection and recognition of the disease.

Like any other part of the body, the tooth suffers the impact of biological aging that alters either its morphology or its color, which tends to saturate. The newly erupted anterior dentition presents along its incisal edges an undulating design that is called *mamelons*. In response to the imperatives of biological aging, the mamelons gradually disappear and give place to the natural shaping of the incisal edge. This phase of adaptation of enamel design can be considered a nondisease stage.

The stage I abrasion is limited to the enamel. Its early recognition is extremely important as it represents a functional emergency because of the rapid progression of this disease. Without preventive measures, wear will reach the dentin, which is less resistant than enamel. Further destruction will lead first to dentinal crevices between enamel layering, then to more breaks of these enamel walls, then to reduced tooth length, and finally to full occlusal destruction. This apocalyptic occlusal progression, labeled stage V on the index, depends only on time and resistance to the impact of parafunctional movements (Fig 4-14).

It remains to determine the factors that can cause the parafunctional movements that lead to tooth-wear disease. One must analyze and explain its spatial progression. In fact, the various occlusal designs that apparently relate to occlusal stability as described in the preceding pages may also lead to the development of tooth-wear patterns (Fig 4-15).

A punctual posterior interocclusal contact registered prior to the usual initial incisal or canine contact during the process of tooth closure could trigger avoidance patterns. In other words, a punctual occlusal contact might take place within the envelope of mandibular motion and outside the area of the envelope of function during tooth closure. This posterior interference, felt as a foreign body by the cerebral cortex, generates, as a neuromuscular reaction of avoidance, a pivoting movement and projection of the mandible. Such avoidance patterns constitute a self-protective response generated in the absence of the usual proprioceptive mechanisms dictating the sequential development of anterior tooth closure following initial contact.

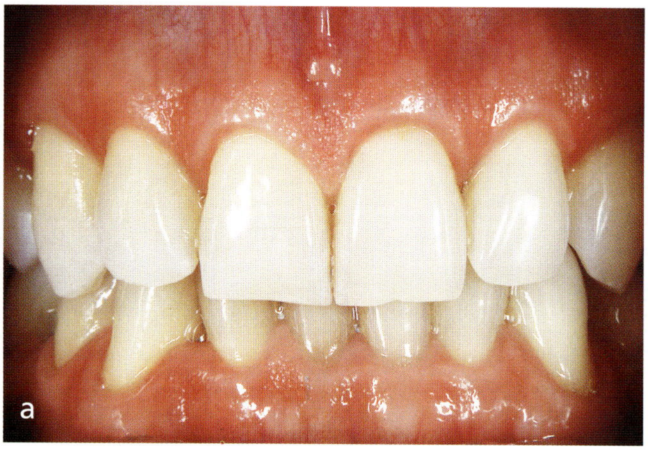

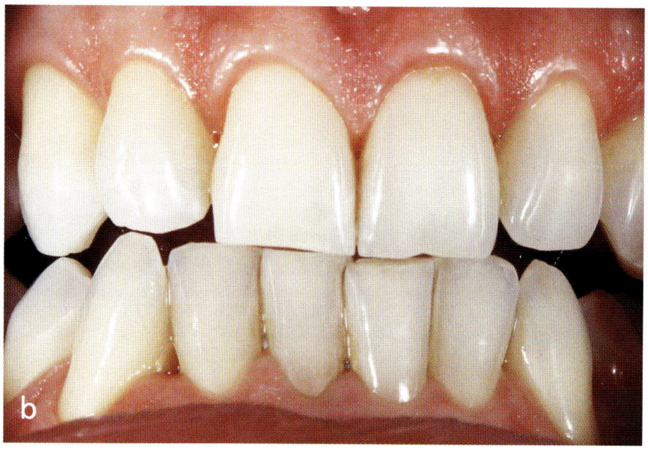

Figs 4-15a and 4-15b Correct anterior relationships both in the vertical and horizontal planes for incisors and canines with early manifestations of wear despite sufficient posterior interocclusal void in eccentric protrusive occlusion.

This hypothesis of a neuromuscular mechanical answer to an interference is supported by scientific research (Figs 4-16 and 4-17). It has been demonstrated that in the presence of an occlusal obstacle in the molar area, the horizontal fibers of the temporal muscle—and to a lesser degree the lower fibers of the inferior head of the lateral pterygoid muscle—are solicited, which in a combined action guide the mandible around the obstacle. The result of the contraction of these muscles initiated by the triggering effect of the occlusal obstacle is a mandibular tracing corresponding to the clinical location of the abraded tooth surfaces of the anterior segment. The hypothesis that the location of the occlusal obstacle can appear either on the working or balancing occlusal surface has led to the definition of two types of interference: *(1)* the eccentric working interference, and *(2)* the eccentric balancing interference.

While the etiology and the mechanism of avoidance patterns deserve further investigation, it remains for us to consider the impact and developmental stages of avoidance movements and the

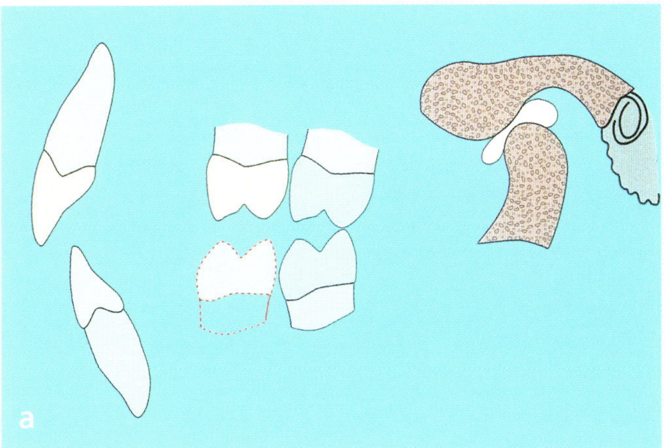

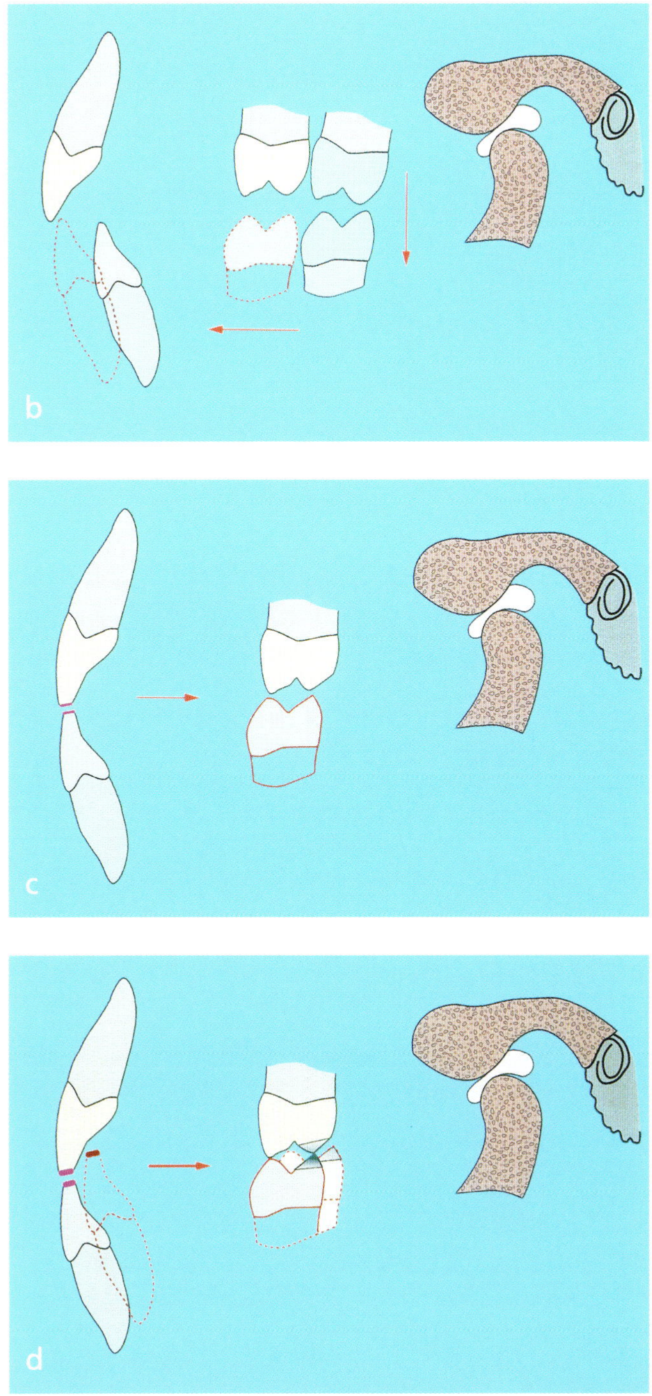

Figs 4-16a to 4-16d (a) Schematic representation of the development of avoidance patterns when an eccentric precontact takes place in an unusual mandibular position, (b) generating a neuromuscular reflex action leading the mandible to avoid this prematurity with a pivoting and protrusive movement. (c) As the mandibular incisors slide back and forth against maxillary incisors, both progressively lose substance, (d) which reduces posterior clearance until elements of the posterior segment participate in this degradation process. This process, which apparently takes place during periods of sleep, escapes conscious control.

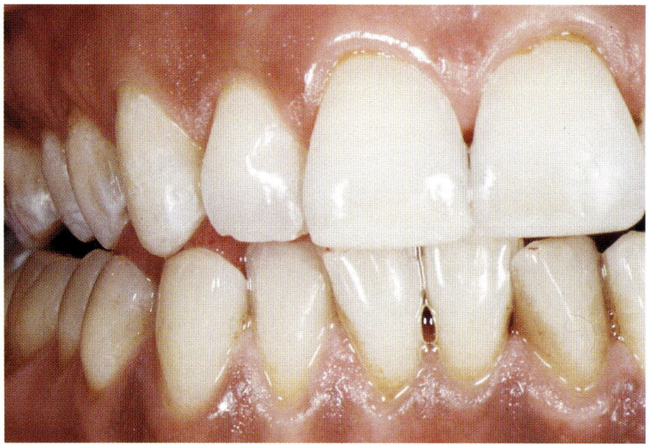

Fig 4-17 The location of eccentric interferences usually escapes clinical observation. In this particular case, the possibility of a posterior precontact (cusp tip erupting from the occlusal plane) preceding canine contact in a lateral eccentric occlusion can be envisaged.

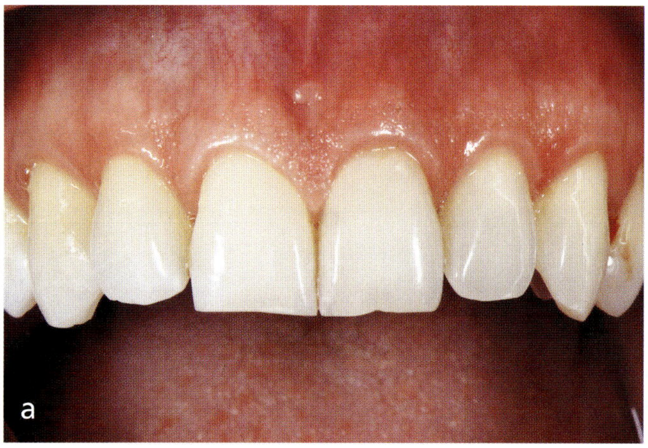

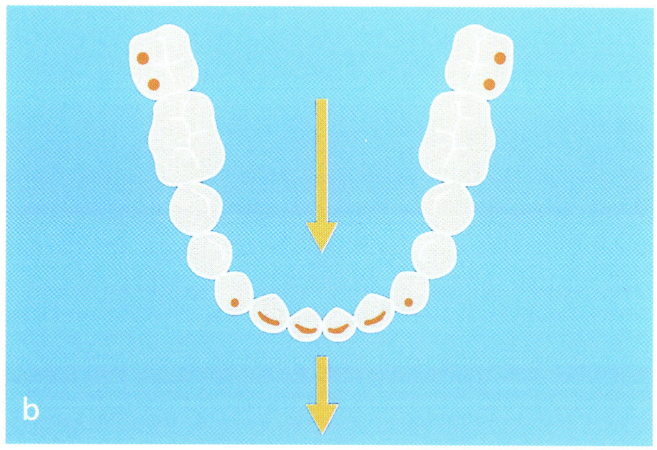

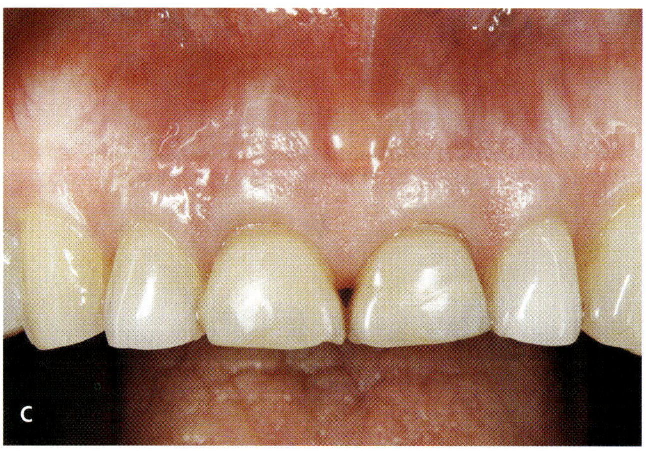

Figs 4-18a to 4-18c Bilateral simultaneous eccentric interferences will project the mandible straight forward, imposing first the overload of this back-and-forth movement generating the abrasion of the maxillary central incisors and mandibular incisors (a,b). Wear will then progressively extend from the central to the lateral incisors and canines (c). It is imperative to adopt adequate therapeutic measures in the initial phase of tooth-wear disease to stop its progression and its unattractive manifestations. These will consist of increasing the incisal pathway to prevent possible posterior interferences.

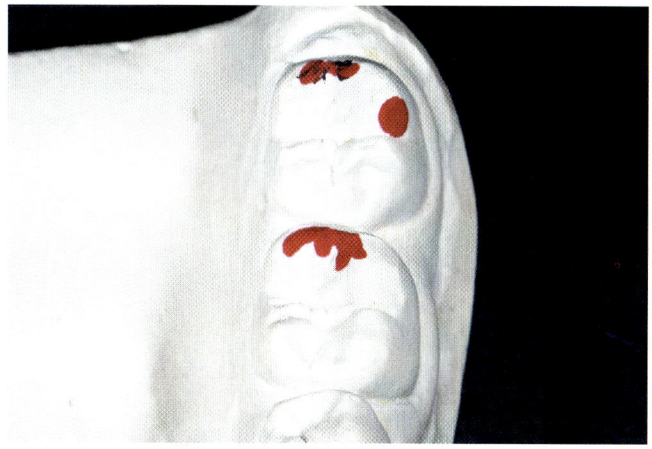

Fig 4-19 Wear faceting affects the mesial incline of the distal marginal ridge of both mandibular molars and starts eroding the elements of the posterior segment. This follows the abrasion of maxillary and mandibular incisors. Note the elements of abrasion visible on the buccal or working aspect of both molars, resulting from the loss of canine tooth substance.

means to protect the dentition from the progression of destructive abrasion. Bilateral simultaneous and posterior eccentric interferences generate avoidance patterns projecting the mandible against the maxillary central incisors, which are obliged to support the overload of the initial protrusive-retrusive movement, and respond by tooth abrasion (Fig 4-18). When the abrasion of the incisal edges reaches the level of the lateral incisors, the abrading effects of these parafunctional movements are supported by the four anterior teeth until these effects extend to the canine area (Fig 4-19).

Whatever the minor differences in this scenario effected by variations in tooth length, tooth position, and arch forms, nothing will prevent the extension of occlusal surface deterioration except appropriate therapeutic measures. In an advanced case, the following clinical observations may be made: anterior tooth morphology has been erased, anterior relationships have been modified, incisal and canine pathway angulation has decreased, and posterior disocclusion has either been reduced or vanished.

In this case the way to posterior faceting and abrasion is wide open. The destructive action of protrusive-retrusive avoidance patterns in erasing anterior tooth morphology progressively establishes in eccentric protrusive occlusion posterior interocclusal contacts.

Faceting of the mesial incline of the distal marginal ridge of the first molar can then be observed as well as that of the antagonist tooth surface incline when the whole anterior segment has been erased as the result of protrusive-retrusive avoidance patterns (Fig 4-19). Concomitantly, the gradual canine morphological erasure in changing the verticality of lateral tooth closure patterns contributes to the overload of the premolars, creating in eccentric mandibular positions group function occlusions leading to a progressive extension of the wear with the development of balanced occlusion and complete occlusal destruction. Great similarities exist in the scenarios that originate from unilateral eccentric interferences. The triggering effect generated by these unilateral eccentric interferences produce avoidance patterns de-

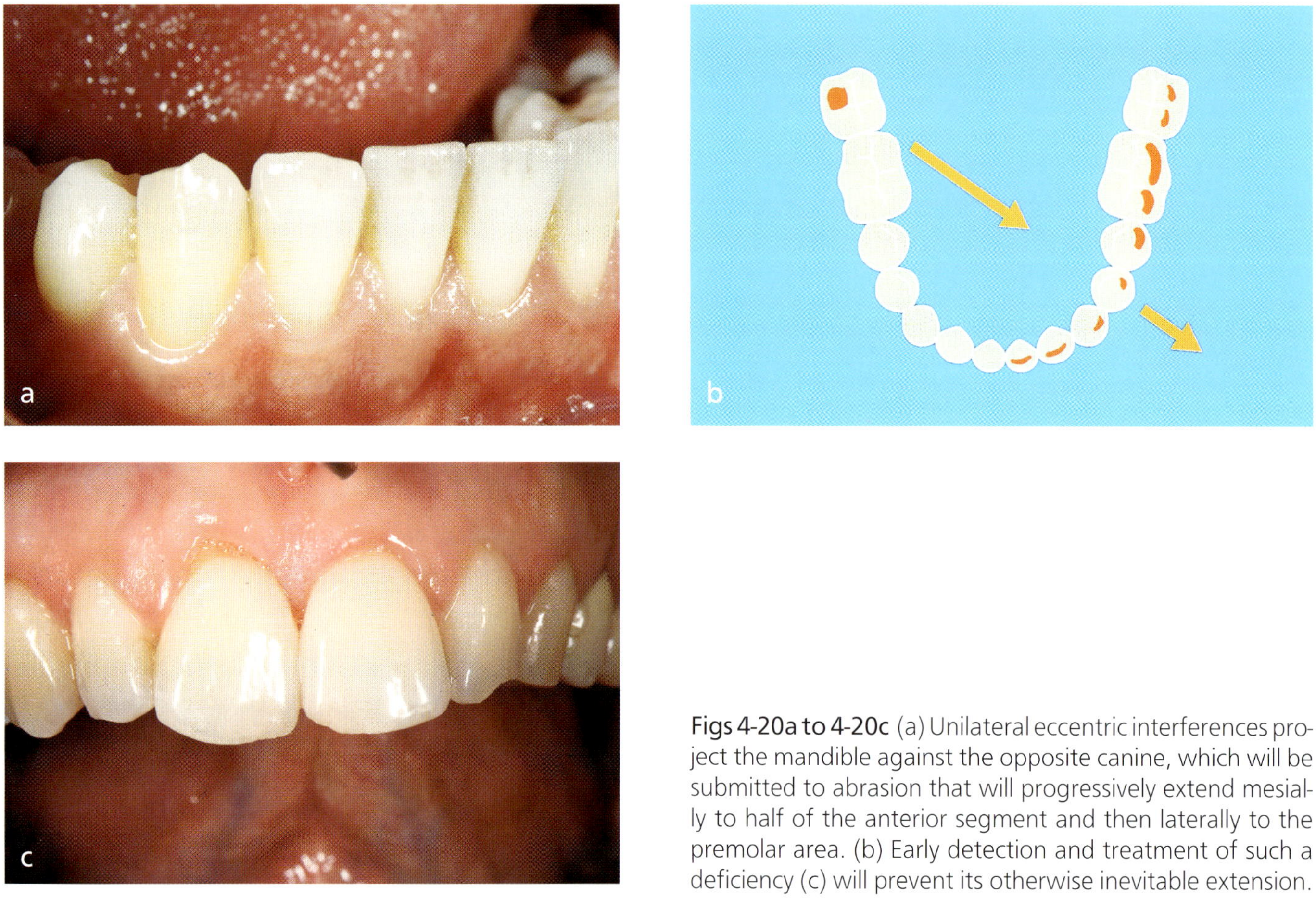

Figs 4-20a to 4-20c (a) Unilateral eccentric interferences project the mandible against the opposite canine, which will be submitted to abrasion that will progressively extend mesially to half of the anterior segment and then laterally to the premolar area. (b) Early detection and treatment of such a deficiency (c) will prevent its otherwise inevitable extension.

veloping their action against the opposite canine as the result of neuromuscular protective mechanisms.

This laterotrusive-retrusive back-and-forth movement will erase upper canine morphology in such a way that the mesial cusp incline will be progressively flattened and the cusp tip will move distally while the mandibular canine, submitted to identical loading, will exhibit a concomitant abrasion of opposite surfaces (Fig 4-20).

The laterotrusive tooth closure patterns linked to canine morphology and interocclusal relationships flatten tooth structure and will progressively abrade lateral and central incisors. And when the abrasion of the inner inclines of the buccal cusps of the maxillary premolars and that of the opposing outer inclines of the mandibular buccal cusps have been realized, group function in eccentric occlusion is instituted and contralateral disocclusion suddenly vanishes. At one moment or another, balancing contacts start apply-

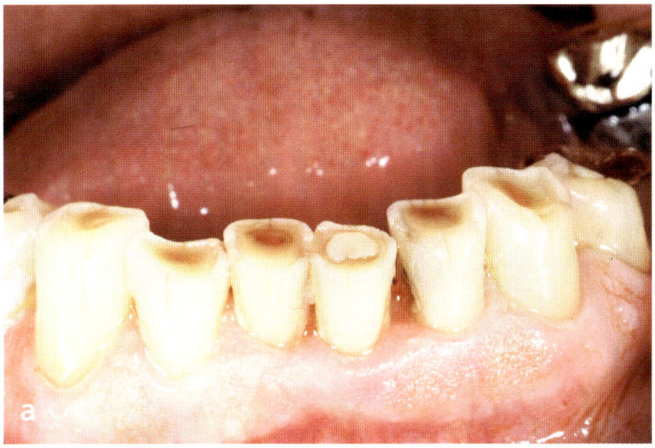

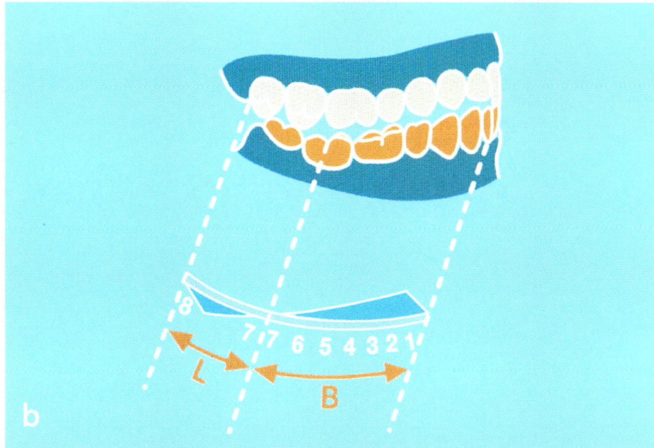

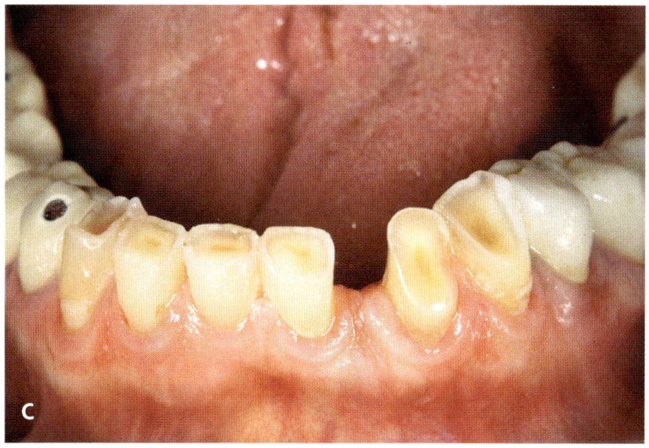

Figs 4-21a to 4-21c The complete destruction of the occlusal surface results in a helicoid shape. It usually leaves the distal buccal cusp of the mandibular second molar intact while the mesial cusp, first molar, and premolars present a completely erased design and a reversed frontal inclination. L = lingual inclination, B = buccal inclination.

ing severe and destructive lateral overload, opening the way to complete occlusal surface destruction.

Complete occlusal destruction can be observed in places where the combination of all of these progressive faceting and wear patterns affecting the occlusal architectural design create together a helicoid shape, characterized by a generalized, reversed Wilson curve that still presents a normal inclination at the level of the distal buccal cusp of the second molar, which has been maintained and will be maintained intact. This final helicoid shape of the occlusal plane may represent a physiological attempt to provide resistance to the overload created by parafunctional forces (Fig 4-21).

At this point, to meet the requirements of dentofacial esthetics, to satisfy the expectation of atraumatic functional tooth closure patterns, an extensive restorative treatment must be begun.

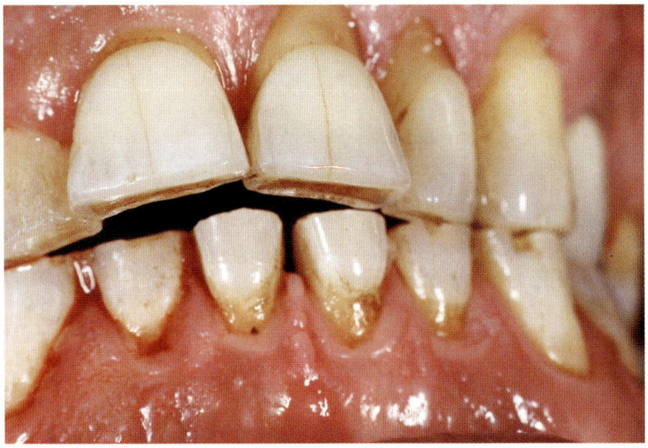

Fig 4-22 What explanation can be given for maxillary and mandibular incisor wear in an open bite interocclusal relationship, aside from that of the destructive impact of a mandibular projection?

Tooth Wear Control

Clinical observations have stressed that nontraumatic, stable, and long-lasting occlusions present identical occlusal parameters whether static or dynamic. The objectives of the restorative process, of the therapeutic approach to prevent tooth wear progression, will consist in integrating in the occlusal architecture all of the parameters necessary to ascertain occlusal stability.

The stage index development has shown that tooth-wear progression predominantly affects tooth morphology and tooth occlusal surfaces. This clearly suggests that the restoration of abraded dental elements should be exclusively extracoronal, either onlay type or full-coverage crown.

It has been established that the impact of avoidance patterns impinges, in the initial phase, upon central incisors or canines and progressively erases all the teeth of the anterior segment. This suggests that the treatment of tooth-wear disease will involve esthetic considerations requiring technical competence and esthetic knowledge and limit the choice of extracoronal restorations to tooth-colored material.

Avoidance patterns have been described as self-protective mandibular movements triggered by undetected working or balancing eccentric interferences (Fig 4-22). These interferences have been made possible in occlusal schemes presenting insufficient verticalization of the anterior segment, which generates reduced posterior interocclusal clearance in eccentric mandibular positions.

It has been observed that in nontraumatic occlusions the distance between cusp tips of the maxillary and mandibular posterior segments in eccentric occlusal positions should average 2 to 3 mm in protrusive position, 2 to 3 mm (balancing side), and 2 mm (working side) in laterotrusive positions. But one may also observe apparently ideal occlusal schemes that surprisingly exhibit symptoms of abnormal function (see Fig 4-15).

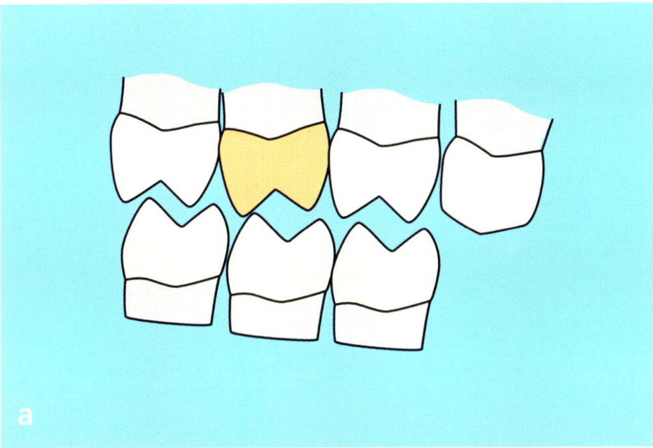

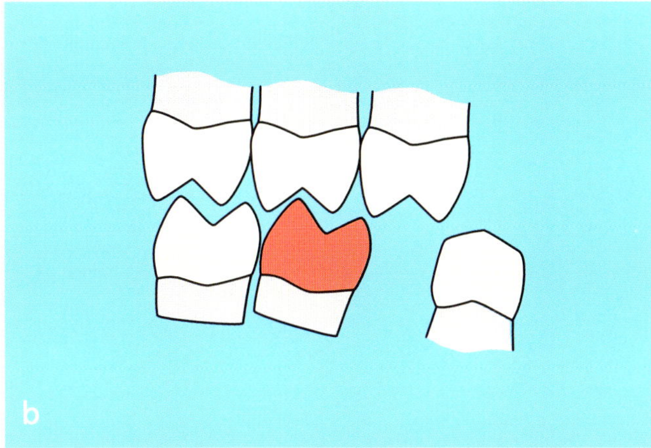

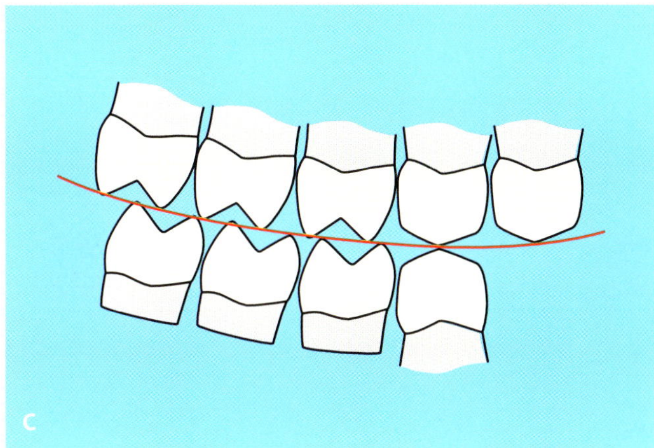

Figs 4-23a to 4-23c Every cusp design erupting from the level of the occlusal plane—for example, (a) second maxillary molar and (b) second mandibular molar—must be considered a potential site of undesirable precontact during tooth closure patterns. (c) A too-pronounced curve of Spee and posterior interocclusal relationships that appear totally locked from the frontal view introduce the same potential, even if the amount of anterior guidance seems to be sufficient.

Clinical examination of natural dentitions present ideal occlusal schemes and yet symptoms of functional deficiencies will regularly identify identical elements that seem to participate in the initiation of avoidance patterns, such as a mesial inclination of a mandibular molar with a distal cusp erupting into the interocclusal space; a mesial or distal tilting of a maxillary molar with corresponding cusp eruption into the interocclusal space; a generalized increase of axial tooth inclination toward the center, affecting the frontal maxillary front-back progression; a localized or generalized increase of mandibular frontal axial inclination; a poorly carved extracoronal restoration; and migratory tooth movement following antagonist extraction or contact-points deficiency (Figs 4-23 and 4-24).

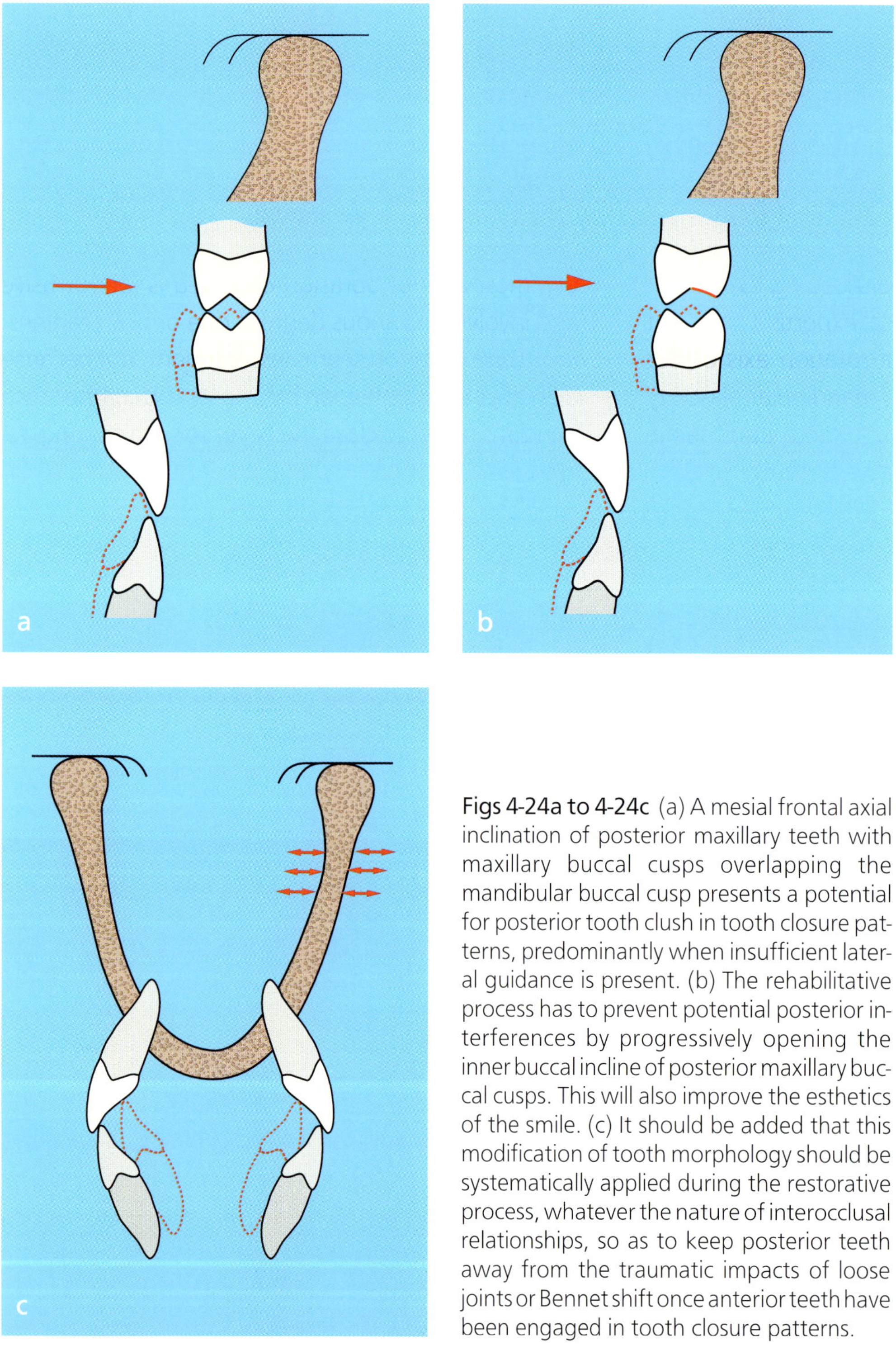

Figs 4-24a to 4-24c (a) A mesial frontal axial inclination of posterior maxillary teeth with maxillary buccal cusps overlapping the mandibular buccal cusp presents a potential for posterior tooth clush in tooth closure patterns, predominantly when insufficient lateral guidance is present. (b) The rehabilitative process has to prevent potential posterior interferences by progressively opening the inner buccal incline of posterior maxillary buccal cusps. This will also improve the esthetics of the smile. (c) It should be added that this modification of tooth morphology should be systematically applied during the restorative process, whatever the nature of interocclusal relationships, so as to keep posterior teeth away from the traumatic impacts of loose joints or Bennet shift once anterior teeth have been engaged in tooth closure patterns.

The presence or the combination of one or two of these parameters in the occlusal scheme and the development of their effects in the sagittal or frontal plane may modify the design of the area of functional movements and promote an uncontrolled collusion with specific mandibular movements without a real possibility of clinical pantographic control. Indeed, in investigating the initiating factors leading to anterior wear, common sense and clinical expertise point out that the impact of the vertical rotation axis of the condyle remains unknown, the mandibular elasticity may well produce some harmful effects, and the nature of the condylar side shift, stated as having no impact on canine location and morphology, could well produce its effects in the posterior area, once canine-canine engagement has been realized under the action of neuromuscular mechanisms (Fig 4-24).

These statements directly address orthodontists who very often present finished cases with insufficient anterior guidance, with the mesial cusp of the maxillary molars erupting from the sagittal plane of occlusion as the result of improper head gear manipulation, with a too-important axial frontal inclination, that is to say, a great vertical overlap of buccal cusps of premolars and molars opening the way to posterior tooth clash during tooth closure patterns.

These statements also address prosthodontists who, facing insufficient parameters in anterior guidance, may use these elements to compensate this deficiency by means of a modification of the inclination of the sagittal plane of occlusion, an alignment of the buccal and lingual cusps of the posterior segment along this plane, a reduction of the curve of Spee, and a progressive opening in the frontal plane of the buccal cusp of maxillary posterior elements. This setup of posterior parameters will help prevent posterior interference in mandibular closure. It is left to the sensitive dentist to appreciate all these contradictory elements in improving esthetics and function.

The observation of tooth-wear progression will determine a need for therapeutic interference at three different levels of tooth wear. Clinically, the most common type of abrasion observed is laterotrusive and involves in various degrees one or both canines. Protrusive abrasion seems less frequent, not because it escapes early detection but most probably because clinicians prefer to close their eyes to such starting defects because invasive treatment modalities will be difficult for patients to accept. Yet protrusive or laterotrusive early stages of abrasion should be considered functional emergencies requiring immediate therapeutic measures. If this opportunity of limited treatment, which either involves the restoration of one single tooth or its antagonist, is missed, tooth wear will ineluctably progress (Fig 4-25).

The second key opportunity for intervention takes place when tooth wear has affected the whole anterior segment, leaving intact posterior tooth morphology, thus limiting therapeutic measures to the prosthetic restoration of the anterior segment (Fig 4-26). But when the posterior segments start exhibiting the deleterious effects of tooth attrition, when eccentric interocclusal relationships are ruled by group function, and when vertical dimension has collapsed, only total rehabilitation is indicated, including an increase of the vertical dimension of occlusion (Fig 4-27).

Treatment modalities to control or prevent tooth wear progression will consist in introducing all the parameters generating an increase of verticalization in the anterior segment. This means more vertical incisal

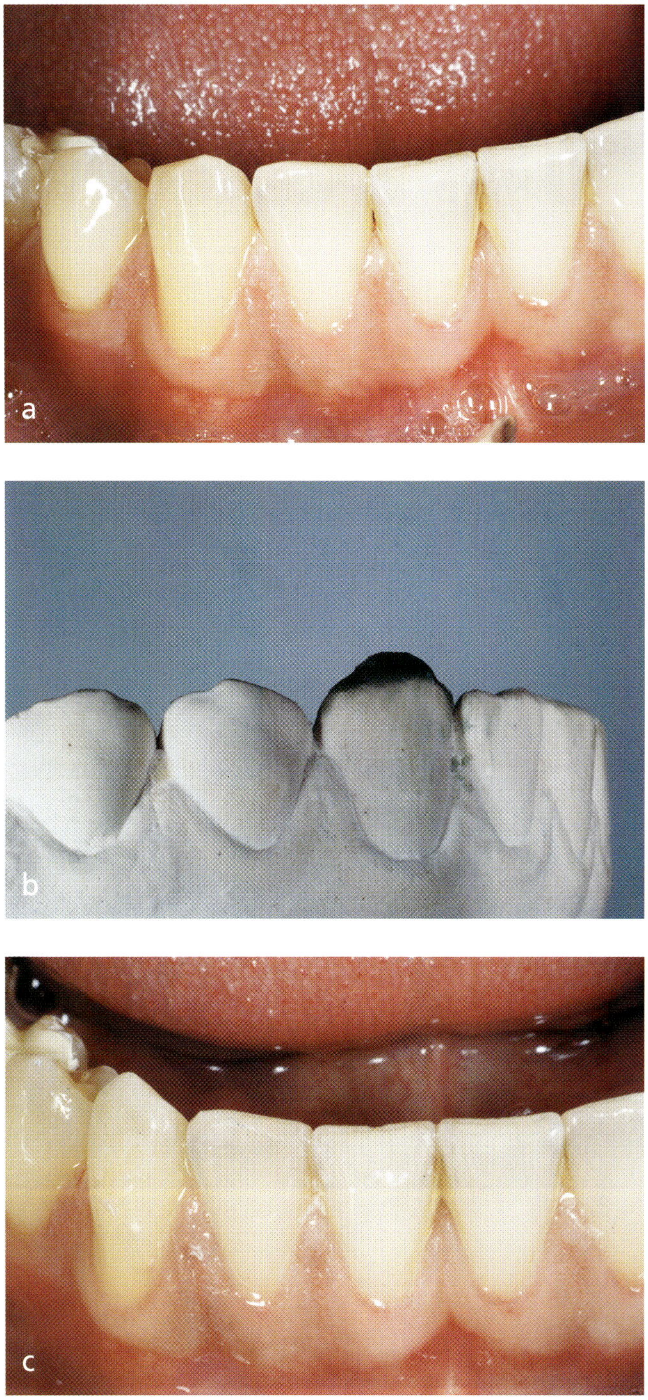

Figs 4-25a to 4-25c (a) Initial phase of tooth wear affecting the mandibular canine. (b) Treatment modalities include an increase of canine tooth length and vertical interocclusal relationships that can be translated to an increase of canine guidance steepness (c) by means of a porcelain veneer bonded on the lingual-incisal aspect of the canine.

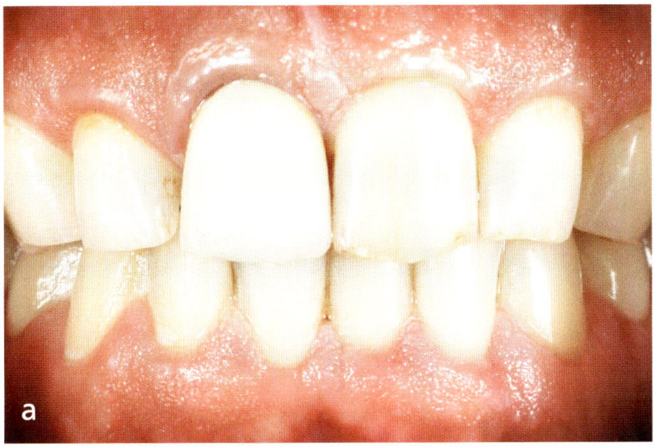
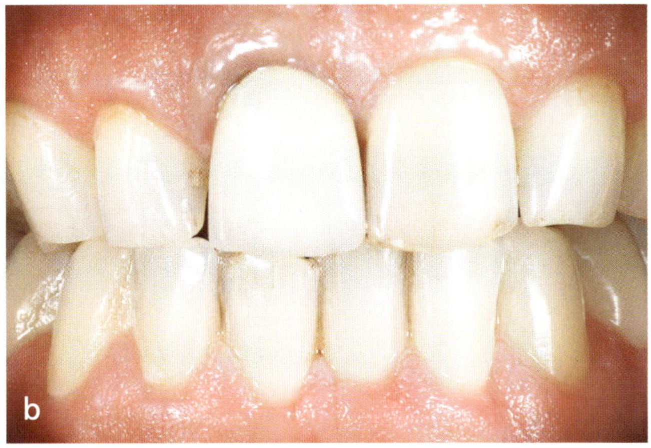
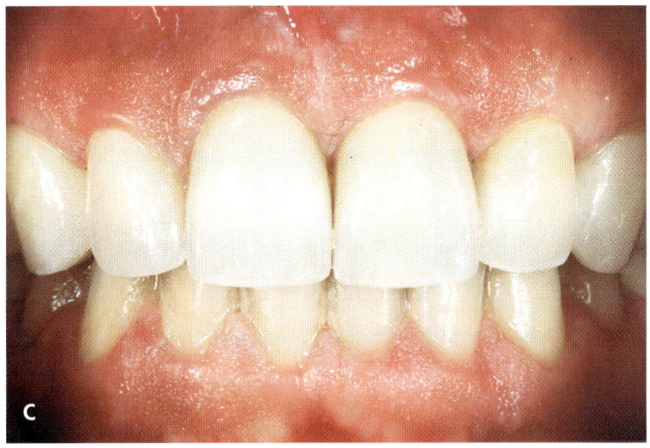
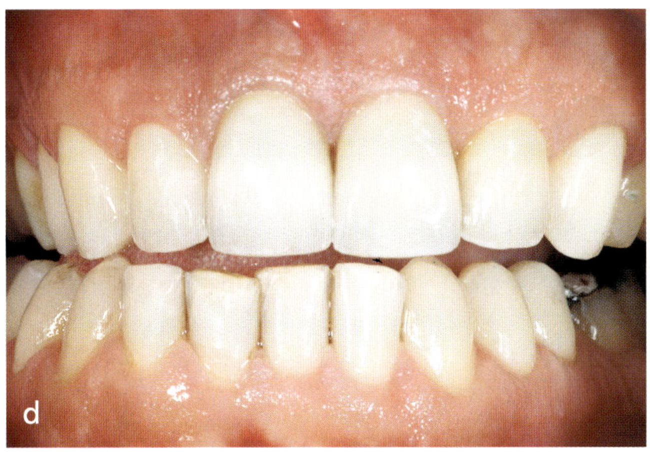

Figs 4-26a to 4-26d The abrasion of the whole anterior segment leaving intact the morphology of posterior teeth represents the last opportunity to limit the restoration to the six maxillary anterior teeth. The therapeutic approach to the mandibular segment, which depends upon tooth visibility in rest position, will be limited to tooth recontouring. (a) Anterior relationships in centric occlusion. (b) Anterior relationships in right eccentric occlusion. (c) Increase of interocclusal anterior relationships. (d) Right eccentric occlusion with steeper guidance preventing posterior tooth clush in tooth closure patterns. To satisfy esthetic requirements the mandibular teeth have been recontoured.

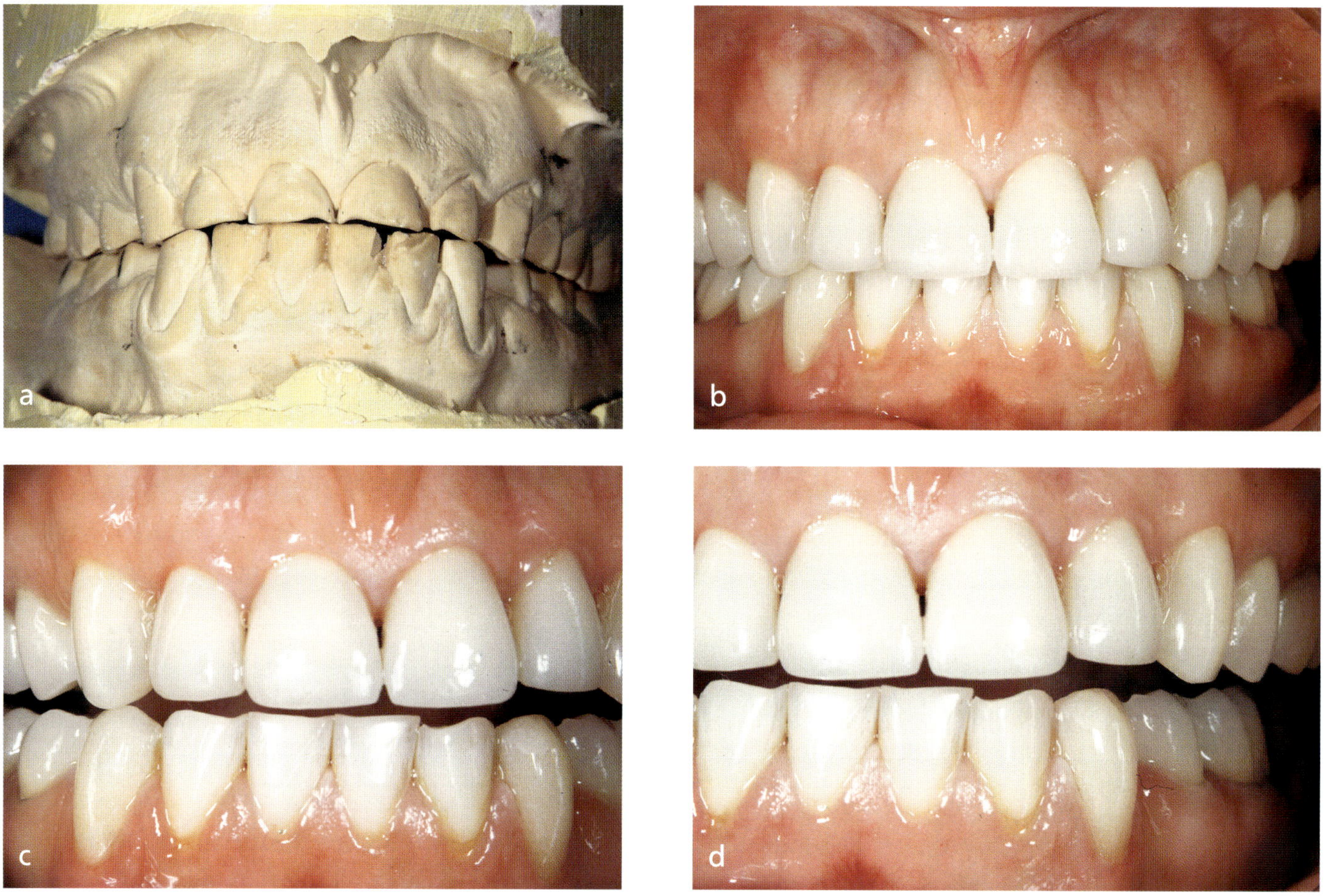

Figs 4-27a to 4-27d (a) Fully abraded dentition of a 30-year-old woman. (b) Restoration of anterior relationships, leaving intact the mandibular anterior segment with the exception of the canines. Right lateral eccentric occlusion with (c) an interocclusal void in the working side and (d) the balancing side, preventing posterior tooth clush in tooth closure patterns.

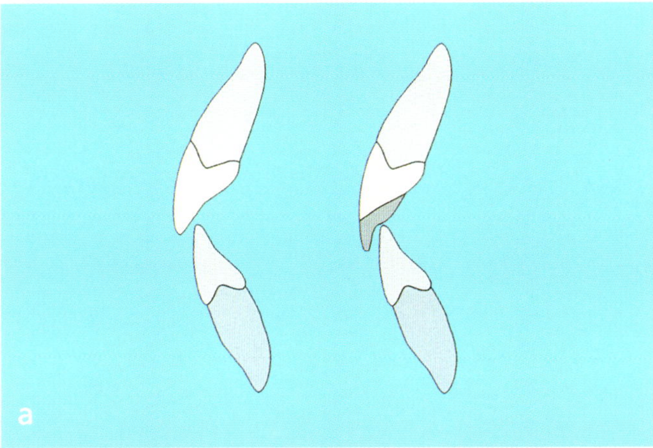

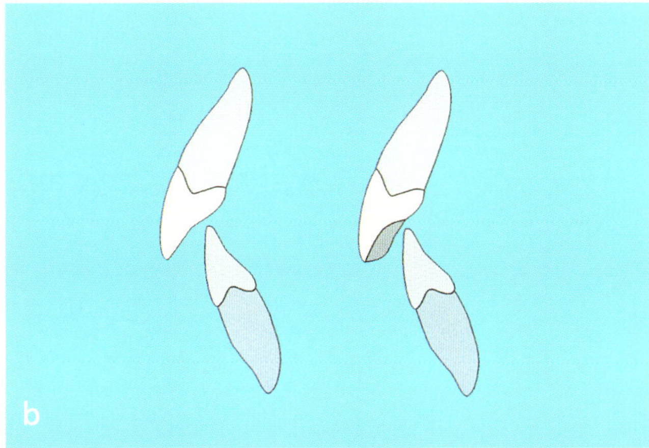

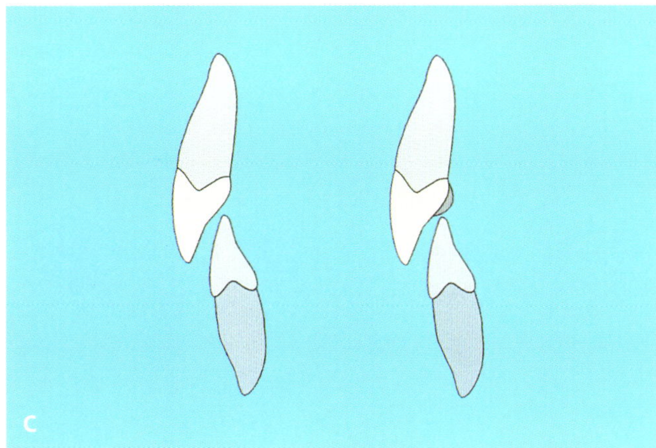

Figs 4-28a to 4-28c The restoration of ideal anterior relationships implies an adaptation of the lingual aspect of maxillary anterior teeth to the mandibular incisors' spatial location, previously evaluated to conform to esthetic criteria. (a) When reduced anterior relationships are present, the increase of tooth length provides the means of increasing guidance steepness. (b) One should not refrain from increasing maxillary tooth width or redesigning lingual morphology to restore ideal anterior relationships. (c) Occlusal stability also involves a maxillary lingual design aimed at preventing mandibular tooth eruption when ideal occlusal relationships are not present.

and canine pathways to increase interocclusal posterior clearance in eccentric occlusions so that posterior teeth cannot contact during tooth closure engagement and disengagement and other mandibular movements. Clinically, this is best achieved by a comprehensive augmentation of the vertical anterior overlap together with a modulated morphological modification affecting the lingual contour of maxillary dental elements (Fig 4-28). This approach will allow the central nervous system to develop new engrams for controlled tooth closure engagement or disengagement.

An examination of the existing interocclusal relationships, a live try-in of eccentric occlusal positions, and extension of the posterior clearance will determine the nature of the necessary morphological modifications, while esthetic dentofacial considerations, including occlusal line direction, tooth length, and tooth-lip relationships will determine the location and nature of these other modifications.

Whenever possible, teeth should be prepared on their lingual aspect with a buccal extension, an approach dictated by psychological and esthetic considerations and resistance requirements. This type of preparation will help to support the patient's feeling that abraded tooth surfaces are really restored and not further destroyed to satisfy the clinician's inclination for specific occlusal relationships.

It is imperative to control that the restored anterior interocclusal relationships permit an atraumatic tooth closure engagement and disengagement, that is to say, one free from any centric interferences, fortunately easily detectable and always identical: laterotrusive for the canines and mainly protrusive-retrusive for the incisors. Since these are pure centric interferences, corrective measures consist simply of grinding off interfering restored surfaces, keeping in mind that the likelihood of encountering these interferences, greatest following the insertion of restoration, is proportionate to the degree of incisal or canine guidance.

Vertical Dimension

The dental literature has never expressed a clear clinical concept of the vertical dimension of occlusion. This dimension is determined by the measurement of the distance between two arbitrarily selected points, one on the maxilla, the other on the mandible.

But practically, this dimension, or facial height, consists of two elements: *(1)* the shortest facial height involving the contact of teeth in centric occlusion or the vertical dimension of occlusion (VDO), and *(2)* a more subjective facial height without tooth contact and the mandible in rest position or the vertical dimension of rest (VDR).

The rest position of the mandible is established by neuromuscular posturing. This position can also be defined two ways: clinical rest position and EMG rest position, which is a point of muscle elongation generating minimal EMG activity. These two entities are characterized by significant differences in facial height: 5 mm to 12 mm beyond the VDO for the EMG rest position and 1 mm to 3 mm beyond the VDO for the clinical rest position.

It has been stated that the VDR position is far from static, as variations during the day and the influence of posture or tension have been observed. Clinically, it is important to understand the nature of the possible relationships between the clinical rest position and the vertical dimension of occlusion. It is currently believed that interocclusal space may be obliterated as the result of the introduction of an increased crown height. This seems possible after a single occlusal contact occurs but is obviously totally erroneous when an increase of VDO is consistent with function.

It has been demonstrated that clinical rest position varies with changes in the VDO. An elevation of the VDO is correlated with an increase in resting facial height. We know that facial height is neither static nor limited by muscle resting length. Observation has shown immediate adaptation in the resting length of masticatory muscles when the vertical dimension has been increased. This immediate adaptation results from a neuromuscular response, whereas the physiological acceptance of increases in muscle resting length is evidenced by structural reordering that takes place after 21 days.

This can be considered the key clinical parameter for the successful long-term increase of vertical dimension that is required for most periodontal prosthetic patients. These patients have suffered the collapse of occlusion following tooth wear or the loss of posterior teeth, which generates an augmentation of forces applied to the anterior segment of the dentition that suddenly has to provide full support for the occlusion.

For all those cases demonstrating various degrees of bite collapse, gaining vertical dimension is unavoidable not only to provide sufficient room for the insertion of well-contoured posterior and anterior restorations but also to restore at the same time the original design of perioral structures. Establishment or reestablishment of harmony in the vertical dimension of occlusion must be approached subjectively with esthetic sensibility and objectively with full appreciation of the clinical reality.

But esthetic sensibility will have to develop within the limits of physiological, morphological, and occlusal parameters in restoring stomatognathic function and improving dentofacial and facial esthetics. The complexity of these elements requires some attention.

Physiological limitations

As facial height increases, EMG masticatory muscle activity diminishes to a minimal point. Beyond this point of muscle elongation, or EMG physiological rest position, reflex muscle contracture takes place as a protective mechanism. This restriction in the augmentation of facial height should receive consideration in orthognathic surgery when important increases of facial height may be necessary to correct dramatic facial deficiencies. Similar extensive augmentation of facial height in the restorative process is neither imaginable nor possible by reason of limitations that could affect tooth morphology.

Morphological limitations

The augmentation of the vertical dimension of occlusion multiplies its impact the farther away it is from the rotational axis of the mandible and may require elongation of the dental elements of the anterior segment that surpasses the realistic normality.

In this particular field, however, criteria of excessive tooth length based on the average norm need to be replaced with criteria allowing for greater esthetic tolerance. Such tolerance will depend on the amount of tooth display in smiling, which depends in turn on the vertical placement of the incisal edge of the central incisors relative to the lip-line level in rest position.

In facial height augmentation, these two parameters can hardly be dissociated; their evaluation should be coordinated with the restoration of dentofacial parameters such as the remodeling of lip design and the effacement of the nasolabial ridge and the labial and mental grooves.

All elements determined arbitrarily by the clinician's esthetic sensibility must be reevaluated on the articulator to ascertain if they can meet with the restrictions imposed by interocclusal requirements.

Interocclusal restrictions

An arbitrary and progressive opening of the articulator to simulate increase of facial height will invariably create undesirable tip-to-tip interocclusal relationships in the posterior area that may embarrass the most talented technician. Thanks to the increase of vertical dimension, sagittal Class I occlusion becomes a Class II malocclusion and interdentated relationships can only be restored by distorting dental morphological normality. But there is a level of tolerance in tooth morphological distortion. A tooth should look like a tooth to function like a tooth, which most often implies moderation in VDO increase.

It remains to correlate these elements of esthetic and functional knowledge in sensitive clinical applications.

Bibliography

Amsterdam M, Abrams L. Periodontal prosthesis. In: Goldman HM, Cohen DW (eds). Periodontal Therapy, ed 4. St. Louis: Mosby, 1968.

Amsterdam M. Periodontal prosthesis: Twenty-five years in retrospect. Alpha Omegan 1974;67:8–52.

Assal J. Basculement mandibulaire provoqué par une surélévation des dents postérieurs: étude anatomique et électromyographique. Rêv mens suisse odonto-stomatol 1988;98(5):459–464.

Assal J. Modification de la position de la mandibule chez l'adulte suite à une surélévtion des dents postérieurs. Rêv mens suisse odonto-stomatol 1986;96:1022–1035.

Carlsson GE, Ingervall B, Kocak G. Effect of increasing vertical dimension on the masticatory system in subjects with natural teeth. J Prosthet Dent 1979;41:284–289.

Celenza FV, Litvak H. Occlusal management in conformative dentistry. J Prosthet Dent 1976;36:164–170.

Celenza FV. The centric positions: Replacement and character. J Prosthet Dent 1973;30:591–598.

Celenza FV. The condylar position: In sickness and in health. Int J Periodont Rest Dent 1984;4:63–86.

Courtade GL. Occlusal rehabilitation. Dent Clin North Am 1963;Nov:577–679.

D'Amico A. The canine teeth: Normal functional relation to the natural teeth of man. J South Calif State Dent Assoc 1958;26.

Dawson PE. Evaluation, Diagnosis and Treatment of Occlusal Problems. St. Louis: Mosby, 1974.

Hellsing G. Functional adaptation to changes in vertical dimension. J Prosthet Dent 1984;52:867–870.

Hobo S, Takayama H. Effect of canine guidance on working condylar path. Int J Prosthodont 1989;2:73–79.

Hobo S, Takayama H. Reevaluation of the condylar path as the reference for occlusion. J Gnathol 1995;14:31–40.

Hobo S, Takayama H. Twin-stage procedure. Part 1: A new method to reproduce precise eccentric occlusal relations. Int J Periodont Rest Dent 1997;17:113–123.

Hobo S, Takayama H. Twin stage procedure. Part 2: A clinical evaluation test. J Prosthet Dent 1997;17:457–463.

Katana TR. The effects of cusp and jaw morphology on the forces on teeth and the temporomandibular joint. J Oral Rehabil 1989;16:211–219.

Kawamura Y. Neurophysiologic background in occlusion. Periodont 1967;5:175.

Kelly JE, Sanchez M, Van Kirk LE. An assessment of the occlusion of teeth of children. (Data from the National Health Survey: DHEW Publication no. (HRA) 74–1612.) National Center for Health Statistics, US Public Health Service, 1973.

Keough B. Occlusal considerations on periodontal prosthetics. Int J Periodont Rest Dent 1992;12:359–370.

Kornfeld M. Mouth Rehabilitation, ed 2. Vols 1–2. St Louis: Mosby, 1974.

Lee RL. Anterior guidance. In: Lundeen AL, Cills CH (eds). Advances in Occlusion. Postgraduate Dental Handbook Series, Vol 14. Boston: J. Wright, 1982.

Lous I. Treatment of TMJ syndrome by pivots. J Prosthet Dent 1978;40:179–182.

Lundeen HC. Occlusal morphologic considerations for fixed restorations. Dent Clin North Am 1971;15:649–661.

Luschei ES, Goldberg LJ. Neural mechanisms of mandibular control: Mastication and voluntary liting. In: Handbook of physiology, sect 1, vol 2. Brooks (ed). Amer Physiol Doc. Bethesda, MD: 1984:1237–1274.

Lytle JD, The clinician's index of occlusal disease: Definition, recognition, and management. Int J Periodont Rest Dent 1990;10:103–123.

Mac Adam DB. Tooth loading and cuspid guidance in canine and group function occlusions. J Prosthet Dent 1976;35: 283–290.

Mac Donald JWC, Hannar AG. Relationships between occlusal contacts and jaw-closing muscle activity during tooth clenching. J Prosthet Dent 1984;52:862–867.

Mack MR. Vertical dimension: A dynamic concept based on facial form and oropharyngeal function. J Prosthet Dent 1991:66(4):478–485.

Mann AV, Pankey LD. Concepts of occlusion: The Pankey-Mann philosophy of occlusal rehabilitation. Dent Clin North Am 1963;Nov:621–636.

Manus A, Miralles R, Guerrero F. The changes in electrical activity of postural muscles of the mandible upon varying the vertical dimension. J Prosthet Dent 1981;45: 438–445.

McHorris WH. Occlusal adjustment via cutting of natural teeth. Int J Periodont Rest Dent 1985;5:9–25.

McHorris WH. Occlusion: With particular emphasis on the functional and parafunctional role of the anterior teeth. Part II. Int J Periodont Rest Dent 1985;53:692–696.

McNeill C. The optimum temporomandibular joint condyle position in clinical practice. Int J Periodont Rest Dent 1985;5:53–76.

Okeson JP. Fundamentals of Occlusion and Temporomandibular Disorders. St. Louis: Mosby, 1985.

Pelletier LB, Campbell SD. Evaluation of the relationship between anterior and posterior functionally disclusive angles. Part II. Study of a population. J Prosthet Dent 1990;63:536–540.

Posselt U. Recent trends in the concept of occlusal relationship. Int Dent J 1961;11:331–342.

Ramfjord SP, Ash M. Occlusion. Philadelphia: Saunders, 1966.

Romerowski J, Bresson G. The influence of mandibular lateral translation. Int J Prosthodont 1990;3:185–201.

Romerowski J, Bresson M. Changing the teaching of dental anatomy to change the mental habits of dental practitioners. Int J Periodont Rest Dent 1985;5:53–67.

Rosenberg MM, Kay HB, Keough BE, et al. Periodontal and Prosthetic Management for Advanced Cases. Chicago: Quintessence, 1988.

Rugh JD, Drago LJ. Vertical dimension: A study of clinical rest position and jaw muscle activity. J Prosthet Dent 1981; 45:670–675.

Schuyler CH. An evaluation of incisal guidance and its influence in restorative dentistry. J Prosthet Dent 1959;9: 374–378.

Schuyler CH. Correction of occlusal disharmony of the natural dentition. NY State Dent J 1947;13:445–462.

Schuyler CH. Factors contributing to traumatic occlusion. J Prosthet Dent 1961;11:708–717.

Schuyler CH. Factors of occlusion applicable to restorative dentistry. J Prosthet Dent 1953;3:772—782.

Schuyler CH. Freedom in centric. Dent Clin North Am 1969;13:681–686.

Schuyler CH. The function and importance of incisal guidance in oral rehabilitation. J Prosthet Dent 1963;13:1011–1029.

Schweitzer JM. Oral Rehabilitation: Problem Cases. Vols 1–2. St Louis: Mosby, 1964.

Shanahan TEJ. Physiologic vertical dimension and centric relation. J Prosthet Dent 1956;6:741–747.

Slavicek R. Die funktionellen Determinanten des Kauorgans. Munich: Verlag Zahnärzt-medizinisches Schrift, 1984.

Takayama H, Hobo S. The derivation of kinematic formulae for mandibular movement. Int J Prosthodont 1989;2: 285–295.

Tanaka A. Functional and precision occlusion with porcelain technics: Recovery of occlusal surface with one-bake techniques. Quintessence Dent Technol 1984;8:61–73.

Toolson LB, Smith DE. Clinical measurement and evaluation of vertical dimension. J Prosthet Dent 1982;47:236–247.

Turrel AJW. Clinical assessment of vertical dimension. J Prosthet Dent 1972;28:238-244.

Wheeler RC. Dental Anatomy. Physiology and Occlusion, ed 5. Philadelphia: Saunders, 1972.

Williamson EH, Lundquist DD. Anterior guidance. Its effect on EMG activity of the temporal and masseter muscles. J Prosthet Dent 1983;49:816–823.

Zwemer TJ (ed). Boucher's Clinical Dental Terminology, ed 3. St Louis: Mosby, 1982.

CHAPTER 5

Principles of Esthetic Setup

The principles ruling the integration of dental elements into the frame of the facial and dentofacial composition depend on the observation and application of the esthetic and functional factors developed in the preceding chapters. This process, which requires a systematic analysis of dentofacial particulars, an objective synthesis of information, and a consequential material realization of the restoration, is aimed at achieving three objectives:

(1) Restoration of facial and dentofacial harmony,
(2) Maintenance of morphopsychological profile, and
(3) Improvement of facial and dentofacial esthetic appeal.

Despite these ambitious objectives, which replace the reliable notion of dental rehabilitation, we should avoid any excess of pretension.

The restoration of facial harmony and morphopsychological profile manifesting the successful integration of dental elements into the facial composition may remain perfectly realistic objectives, even if the number of possible errors appears to increase progressively with the repetition of investigations or with the increase of personal visual perceptive capabilities. However, planned improvement of dentofacial and facial esthetic appeal, though an incredibly fascinating objective, must remain purely theoretical as long as the nature of the contact between individuals, shapes, and colors at the origin of esthetic taste defies explanation.

In practice, these objectives leave the esthetic clinician with exclusive responsibility for connecting dentofacial linear systems; reading the static and dynamic appearance of facial structures; and selecting, adapting, and modulating the architectural aspects of dental elements accordingly. This constructivist approach will give the esthetic clinician a unique opportunity to construct a realistic clinical simulation of a future restoration that will include tooth length, tooth width, tooth shape, tooth spatial location, and the arrangement of the whole anterior dental segment; to solicit the patient's suggestions and agreement; and to evaluate the therapeutic measures associated with the restoration. This approach will naturally determine the specific task assigned to each member of the dental team and the limits within which competent creativity can take place. It also confronts the dental technician with the challenge of duplicating and improving the intrinsic characteristics of the proposed restoration, using creative skills to achieve technical perfection in the manipulation of restorative materials.

Specific environmental conditions of work impose a selective division of labor among the dental team: for the dentist, macro-esthetic arrangement of the pieces constituting the puzzle of the facial map, and for the dental technician, microesthetic finalization of these elements. In other words, the dentist designs, the patient decides, and the technician executes.

The application of this rule of order stresses the importance of the initial esthetic evaluation and consequent architectural simulation. It takes into account the complementary competencies of the dental team and contains all the elements necessary for the esthetic integration of dental restorations into complex facial compositions.

Facial Analysis

In dentistry, the study of the facial map has always been approached from a polite distance since investigation of this area can hardly be advocated in usual dental health care. With the development of esthetic demand, however, the importance of the relationships with tooth-surrounding structures has received more recognition. Descriptive analyses of the anatomy of the smile have been published and a classification of the different types of smiles according to their spatial extension established. This classification includes three types of smile, which differ in lip position: Mona Lisa, canine, and posterior.

These elements have demonstrated that the esthetic quality of the smile depends not only on the esthetic quality of the dental arrangement but also on the esthetic quality of the lip-frame design, whose muscular dynamic, ruling its development, eludes conscious control. Therefore, when deviations affecting the basic types of smile generate an important decrease in the esthetic value of the dentofacial composition, a surgical displacement of muscle attachment, combined with a specific training of the deficient musculature, can be considered—a therapeutic possibility that until now has been rarely used.

However, at the dental consultation the anatomical design of the smile is far from being the first of a patient's preoccupations; the clinician is left with the task of adapting dental restorations to existing facial environmental conditions.

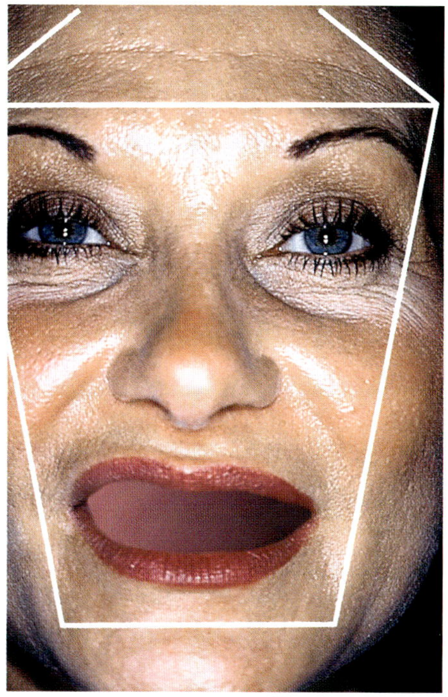

Fig 5-1 Schematic definition of the vestibular frame or plane support.

The evaluation of the facial environmental conditions has to follow a rule of order involving generalities and details constantly renewed and repeated. This progressive evaluation will involve elements described in the first chapter, such as the particulars of the lower lip and upper lip, both in smiling and rest position, and the appreciation of some morphological components such as the protuberance of the forehead, the zygomatic process, and mandibular angle, parameters that apply to tooth shape design and tooth spatial location. It must be stressed that most of these elements of interest seldom reveal their detailed characteristics on the first investigation. In esthetics, the more one looks the more one sees, and this applies as well to the esthetic evaluation of the elements of the dentofacial and facial composition. The progressive setup of a restoration will provide multiple opportunities to investigate detailed characteristics. In the initial phase of treatment only the facial linear tracings, both vertical and horizontal, that will serve as elements of anchorage of the anterior and posterior dental segments require immediate definition (Fig 5-1).

It has been proposed that the esthetic quality of the face could rest on craniofacial balance, identified in both vertical and horizontal facial segmentation, that is to say, on ideal proportional relationships between different segments of the face. If this hypothesis of ideal facial beauty based on mathematical order has valuable didactic uses, it ignores ethnic disparities, fashion variabilities, and individual differences, and finally, it condemns the majority of individuals to ugliness.

Although each segment may take up one third of the ideally proportioned face, both in the vertical and horizontal planes, this is merely an attractive archi-

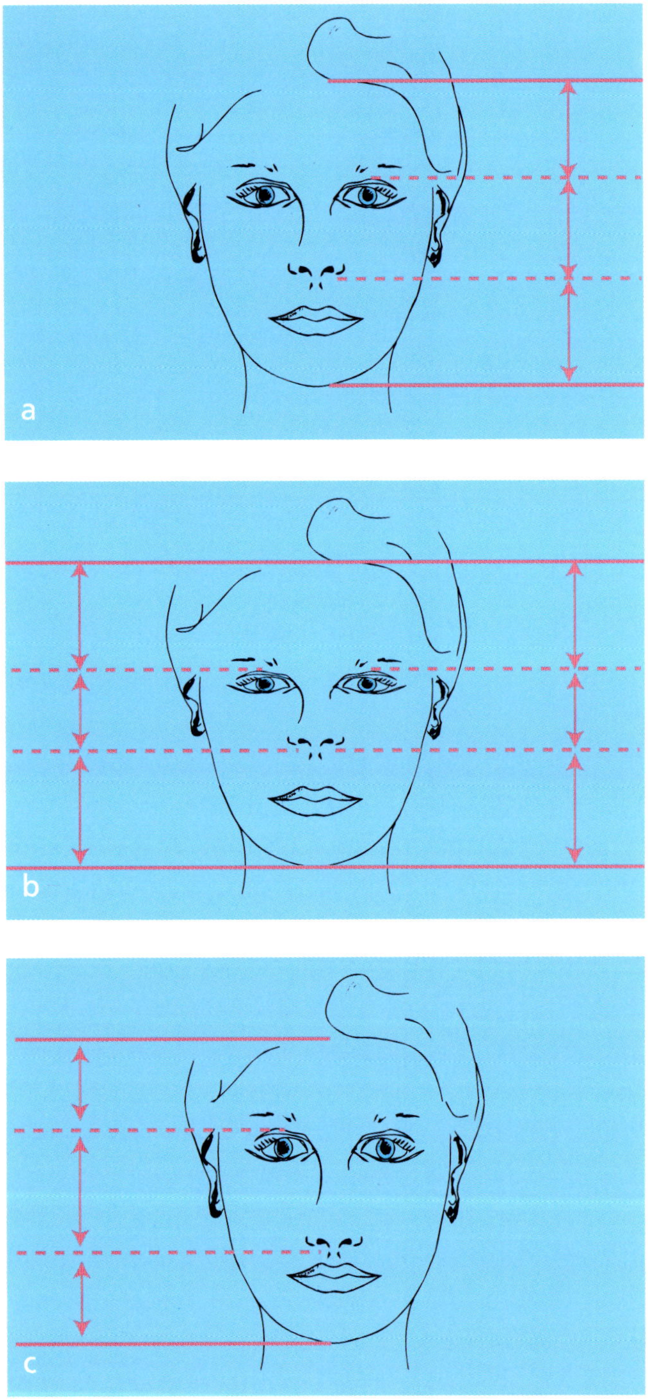

Figs 5-2a to 5-2c (a) This sketch of the facial proportions according to Leonardo da Vinci, ideally dividing the facial composition into three equal parts with ideally sized and located facial receptors, rests on a mathematical concept of human beauty. But human beauty rests on the perception of multiple parameters of an esthetic and psychological nature, among which the influence of an individual's personality requires particular attention. (b) A reduction of the middle facial third generates a comparative expansion of both upper and lower facial zones promoting the perceptive preponderance of complementary qualities of intellectual conception and material realization. (c) A quantitative expansion of the middle facial third, location of social and sentimental predispositions, institutes a qualitative hierarchical dominance of the individual's life tendencies and involves an active and nonconflicting participation of the two others.

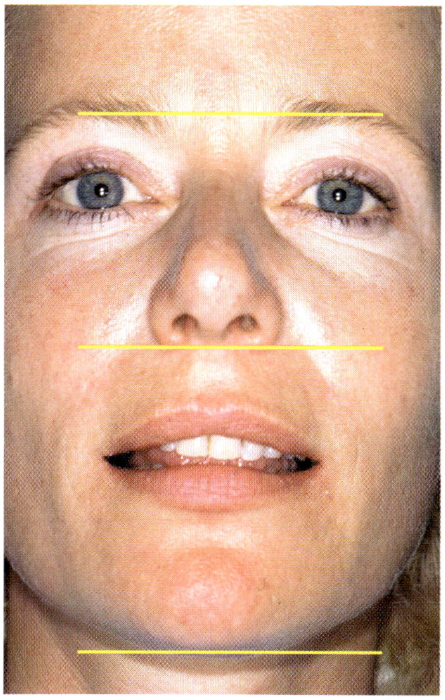

Fig 5-3 Interesting facial composition characterized by a strong reduction of the middle facial third and a controlled expansion affecting each upper subdivision of the three facial zones. This means that the intellectual elaboration is often idealized or realized more with love than obligation. It can be foreseen that the restoration of the dental composition, affected by an important abrasion, will give strength to the middle part of the lower facial third and may provide an element of qualitative and quantitative balance to the reduced middle facial third, which generates a sensation of too-strong disequilibrium.

tectural scheme to which the qualitative nature and expressivity of the receptors, eyes, mouth, and nose, have to give life (Fig 5-2). Facial evaluation is best attained through a morpho-psychological approach based on this segmentation but involving for each basic facial zone a specific qualitative significance linked to its development. These zones, together with the opening and closing of the receptors, constitute the essence of the morpho-psychological science and lay down well-defined parameters of esthetic quality according to a statement quoted in a previous chapter: "There exists no shape that says nothing" (Fig 5-2).

The facial zones, reflecting the profound tendencies of personality, may only express character tendencies and differences in the relative extension or retraction of one of these zones, modulated or accentuated by the retraction or opening of the receptors. This means that beyond the notion of facial architectural balance, which through the centuries has been a priority of philosophers, there arises the more complex and subtle notion of facial imbalance, in which an element of dominance is a necessary condition of esthetic quality (Fig 5-3).

Though the balance of facial zones may well constitute an element of architectural stability, esthetic appeal will predominantly originate in the sensation of a disequilibrium between these zones or between facial receptors, which expresses psychological significance, a characteristic of human beauty.

What matters in the initial facial approach is therefore less the appreciation of the quantitative and qualitative value of the facial zones than the sensitive understanding of imbalances between these zones, as they represent not only the decisive elements of esthetic quality but also of character individualization.

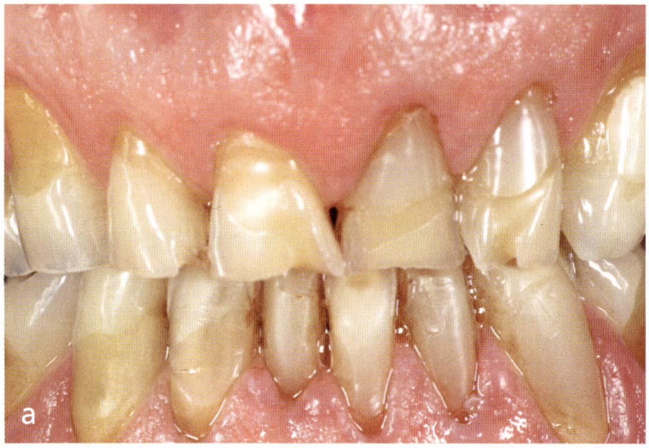

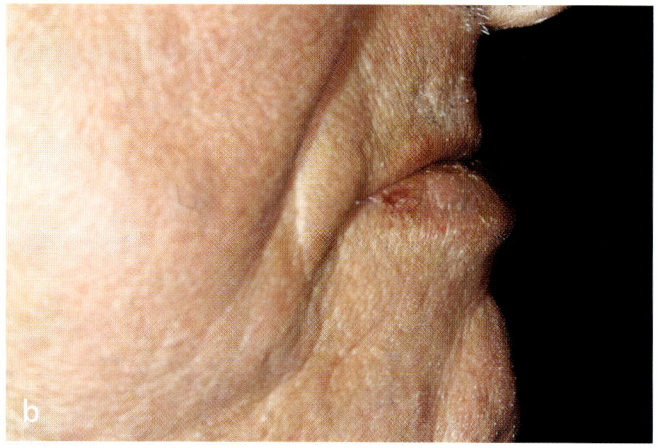

Figs 5-4a and 5-4b (a) Anterior relationships in a totally worn-out dentition. The restoration of tooth morphological normality requires an increase of VDO that will help reduce facial muscle laxness, (b) characterized by deepening of grooves and wrinkles. (See Rufenacht, *Fundamentals of Esthetics*, pp 67–74.)

Facial Evolution and VDO

One must keep in mind that of the three facial zones, the lower facial third remains unique in the sense that over the years it can be exposed to substantial modifications. The increase of infraorbital muscle laxness with the advancement of age strongly marks features, generates wrinkles, and affects the spatial position of the mouth pulled down by gravity. This situation, combined with the devastating action of dental pathologies such as tooth wear or loss of posterior tooth support, may lead to a decrease in facial height. In losing facial height, perioral grooves and wrinkles deepen, lip design fades away, facial appearance ages and loses its qualities synonymous with will, efficiency, and with the capacity for engagement and realization.

Where dental pathologies (Fig 5-4) are involved in this debilitating process it becomes imperative to restore the loss of the vertical dimension of occlusion so as to restore facial height and related facial soft tissue tone before planning anterior tooth placement and arrangement. It should be remembered that facial height is understood in two different positions: vertical dimension of occlusion and vertical dimension of rest. VDO and VDR differ in specific positions of the mandible and generate significant differences in facial height, muscle tensions, and soft tissue form. If VDO can be considered a more objective dimension of facial height, based on interocclusal contacts in centric occlusion, VDR, more subjective and influenced by posture and tension, involves a longer facial height and an absence of interocclusal contacts and is established by neuromuscular posturing.

We know that these two positions are intimately related since variations in VDO generate immediate adaptations of VDR by neuromuscular response. Therefore VDO must be considered a transitory mandibular position and at the same time an unavoidable point of clinical reference, while VDR can be considered a key functional parameter since all the movements of the mandible originate from this position and return to it, thus determining lip and facial position that in turn serve as points of esthetic relational reference. From an esthetic point of view, VDO and VDR are closely related, presenting facial characteristics of different natures requiring simultaneous evaluation.

Clinical Approaches to the Restoration of VDO

There is no specific or determined method to temporarily restore VDO. We find this restoration is best accomplished with the polymerization of a composite jig on the lingual aspect of the maxillary central incisors, which is no more nor less than the well-known "Lucia jig" (Fig 5-5), whose impact may be immediately appreciated on lip design and facial muscle ten-

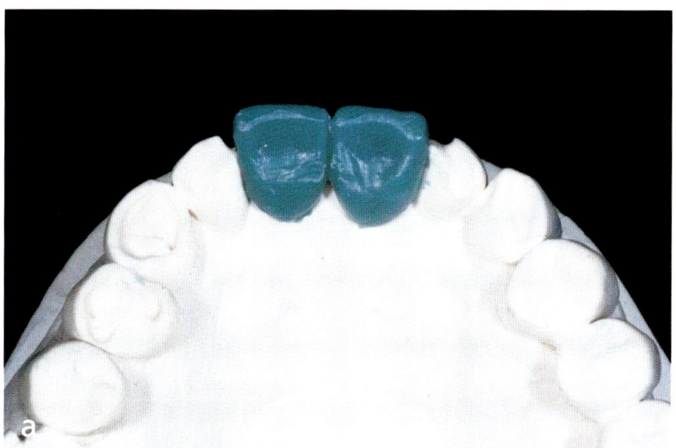

a

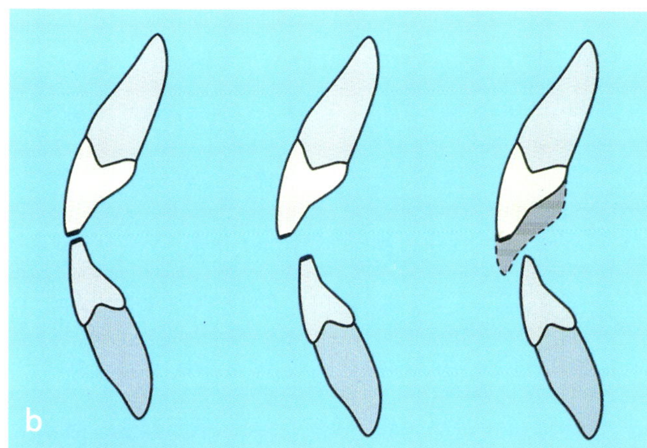

b

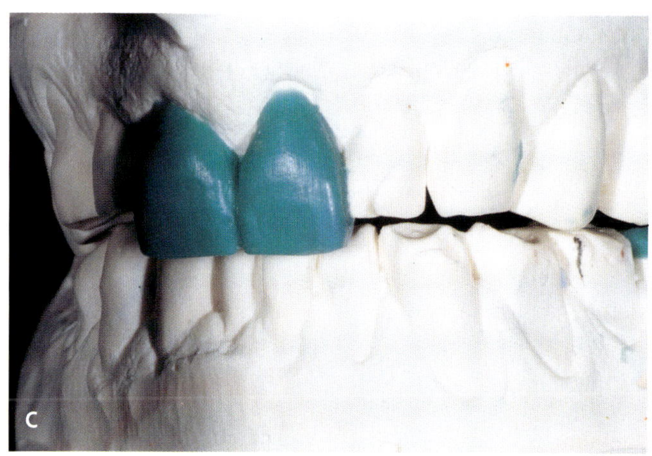

c

Figs 5-5a to 5-5c (a) This schematic representation shows that in the clinical approach to the increase of VDO the maxillary jig should be planned with a sufficient amount of anterior guidance to effect comfort and repeatable tooth closure patterns. (b,c) A preliminary laboratory waxup simulation will help in controlling the morphological and interocclusal limitations in the increase of VDO, which means a normal anterior tooth length, an adequate vertical and horizontal overbite, and possibilities of posterior intercuspation.

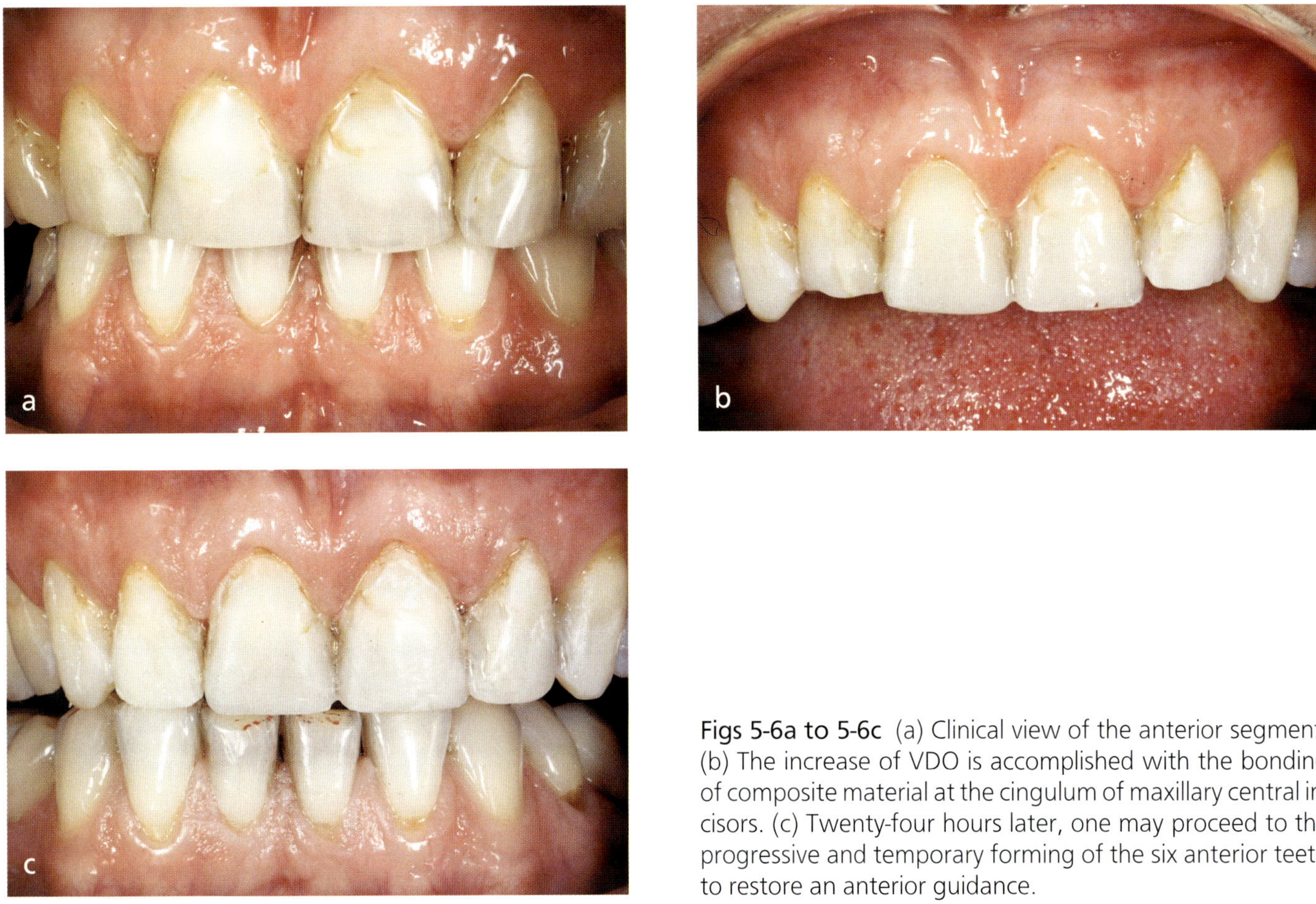

Figs 5-6a to 5-6c (a) Clinical view of the anterior segment. (b) The increase of VDO is accomplished with the bonding of composite material at the cingulum of maxillary central incisors. (c) Twenty-four hours later, one may proceed to the progressive and temporary forming of the six anterior teeth to restore an anterior guidance.

sion. This approach rests not only on the arbitrary compensation of structural tooth loss but also on the sensitive appreciation of a well-designed lip contour and a more tonic lower facial third, characterized by an imperceptible effacement of the mental groove and the labial groove and usually by a more pronounced effacement of the nasolabial ridge, while the inward roll of the upper lip toward mouth corners tends to lose its importance.

Though this approach to the restoration of VDO enables one to control facial form with no more reliable standard than the arbitrary sensibility of the operator, the increase of VDO remains subjected to solidly restrictive occlusal, morphological, and physiological conditions and must be submitted to reevaluation before or following jig placement.

Clinically, when the sensibility of the operator shows some inclination for an extension or reduction of facial height, the clinical procedure consists in adding material to the maxillary jig or in grinding off the occlusal thickness that has been shaped to meet the requirements of function. Interocclusal relation-

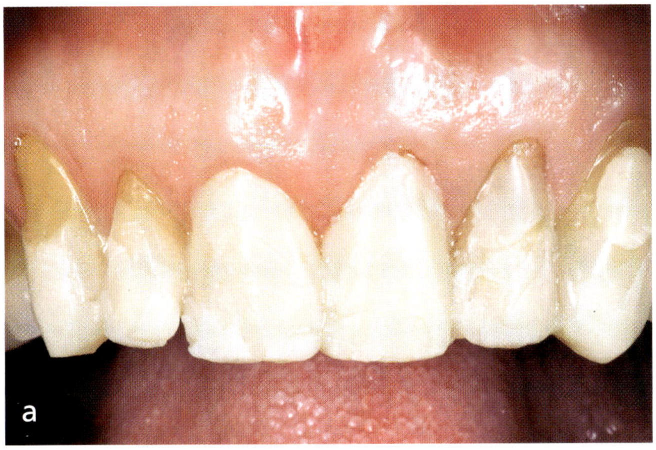

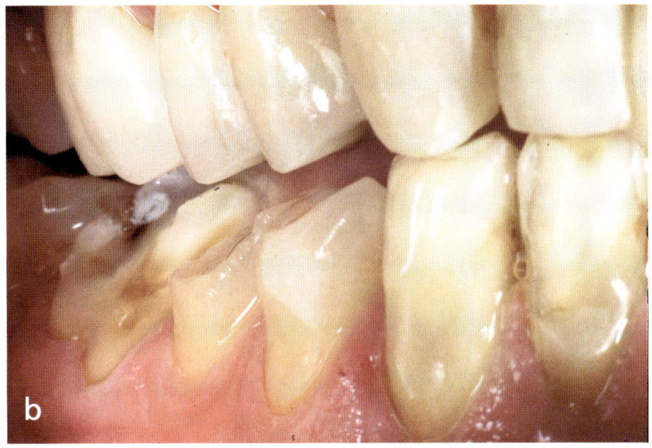

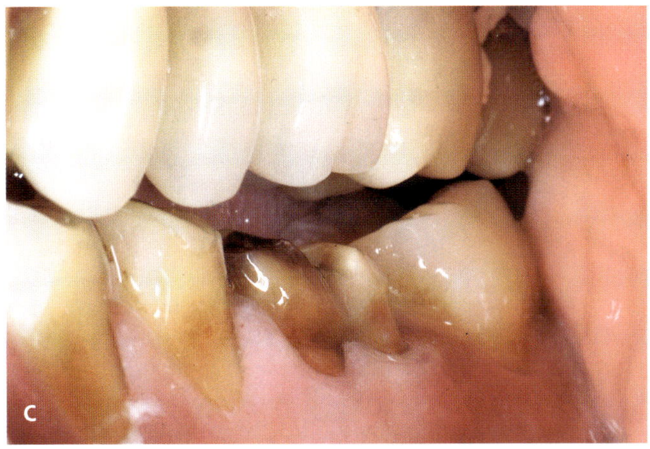

Figs 5-7a to 5-7c (a,b) Once VDO increase has been achieved and the temporary forming of the maxillary anterior segment completed, (c) one can proceed to the provisional restoration of posterior interocclusal relationships. Undesirable protrusive-retrusive interferences are eliminated 1 day later and anterior tooth shape refined and provisionalized.

ships should be reduced to a unique and minimal interincisal contact. This bonded anterior jig not only restores facial height but also reestablishes muscle balance, which should occur within 24 to 48 hours (Figs 5-6 and 5-7). The process leading to muscle balance, with unique interocclusal contact in the interincisal area and an absence of harmful posterior contacts, allows for a rapid seating of the condyle in its most anterosuperior position. This modification of the condyle position appears in the reduction of the posterior interocclusal void, which usually takes place after 1 or 2 days, demanding a rapid provisional restoration of posterior interocclusal contacts to prevent posterior tooth eruption. At the same time the anterior segment is temporarily built to fulfill the requirements of esthetics and function (Fig 5-6).

At this stage of the setup, it can be stated that the restoration of VDO has permitted the realization of safe biological occlusal relationships. This means that neuromuscular feedback becomes constant and interocclusal relationships repeatable and stable. At the same time, the neuromuscular reposturing of the

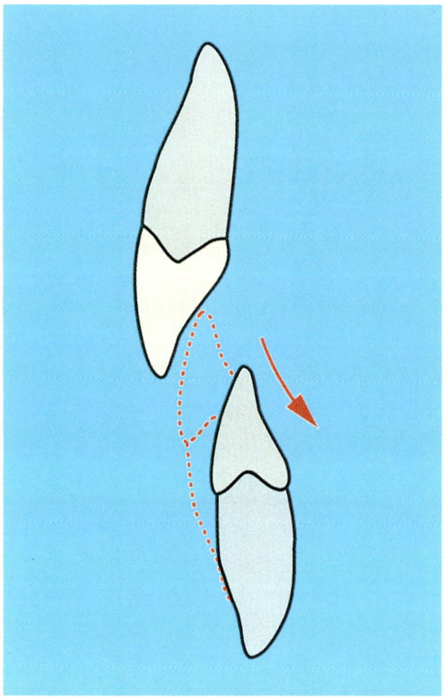

Fig 5-8 Schematic representation of anterior relationships related to Class II, division 2 interocclusal relationships characterized by upright antagonist tooth direction. In increasing VDO, the mandibular incisor loses contact with maxillary incisors in such a way that the restoration of interocclusal contacts requires a modification of the axial inclination of the mandibular segment or generates an unrealistic maxillary incisor width.

mandible has established a greater measure of facial height, restoring tone in perioral soft tissue morphology.

In deep Class II, division 2 situations, most often associated with lower facial third deficiencies, the increase of vertical dimension undergoes even more restrictive morphological and occlusal limitations (Fig 5-8). The introduction of an anterior jig will certainly reduce the amount of vertical overbite, but it will also destroy anterior interocclusal relationships, thus jeopardizing occlusal stability. In the slight opening movement of the mandible required by jig placement, the tips of the mandibular incisors follow a pathway that will bring them into a more retruded position, creating a horizontal overbite that would be clinically difficult to correct as it would implicate both a modification of the sagittal axial inclination of the mandibular anterior segment and an increase of maxillary anterior tooth width to realize interocclusal contacts. This would be too tortuous to meet the requirements of both esthetics and function.

In such a situation, a pivoting of the mandible around two artificial obstacles sealed at the level of the second molar will offer an interesting alternative to the Lucia jig procedure for increasing the VDO. Clinically, these two obstacles will act as interferences in

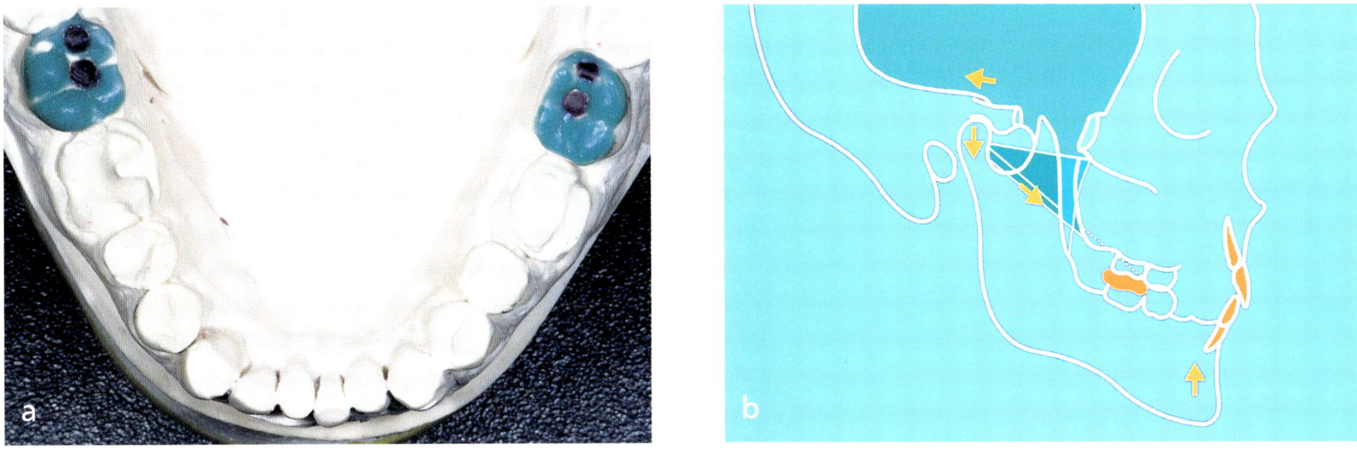

Figs 5-9a and 5-9b Two gold overlays of 0.5-mm to 0.9-mm thickness are waxed, cast, cemented, or bonded on the second molar and provided with a depression adapted to the antagonist cuspid preventing mandibular forward projection. Perceived as interferences, they will, by neuromuscular response, produce avoidance patterns around these obstacles until the nature of these obstacles is registered and repeatable closure patterns take place in a more anterior mandibular position. This scheme summarizes the result of electromyographic registrations stating the action of the posterior fibers of the temporal muscle and the inferior bundle of the pterygoid muscle in the pivoting movement of the mandible around the bonded posterior obstacle until anterior contacts are registered. (Courtesy of J. Assal.)

tooth closure movement and generate avoidance patterns which can be understood as a progressive and synergetic muscular action to reach incisal contacts (Fig 5-9) in a controlled pivoting of the mandible.

Automatic functional adaptation proceeds to physiological adaptation within a short period of time, and stabilization requires the consequent obliteration of the posterior interocclusal void opened following the newly created anterior relationships (Fig 5-10). At this point in the procedure the condyle position has moved downward and backward, opening the upper anterior articular interface, most of the time alleviating the painful TMJ manifestations that usually underline the closure of this interface. Yet control of the condyle's location before entering into this clinical procedure and after the treatment has reached its stabilization phase is most advisable (Fig 5-11).

The restoration of facial height and associated perioral soft tissue tone is a necessary step in any oral rehabilitation, leading to the determination of the location of occlusal planes that will best respond to functional and esthetic requirements.

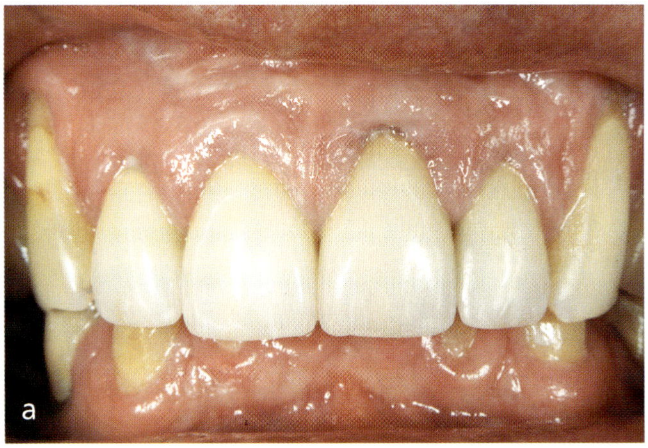

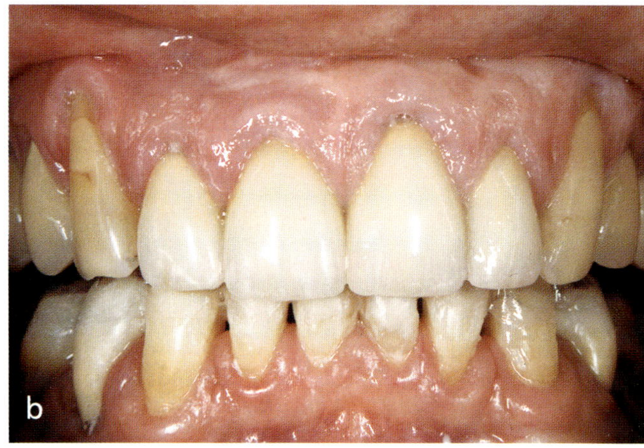

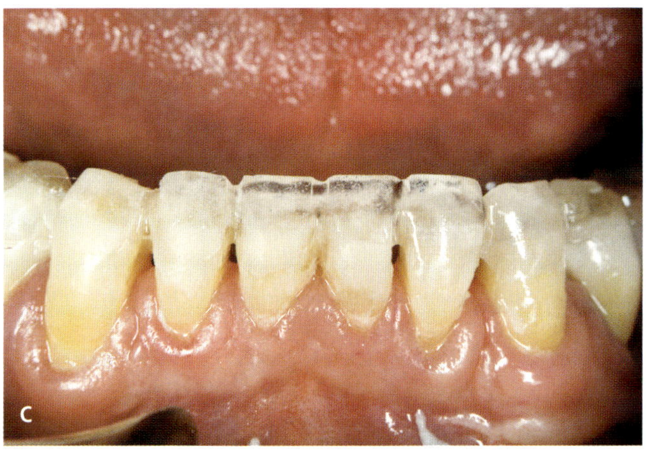

Figs 5-10a to 5-10c Clinical case with deep interocclusal relationships, centric protrusive-retrusive precontacts, and painful TMJ manifestations (a) before and (b) after mandibular pivoting and during the phase of stabilization, which in this case required a modification of mandibular anterior tooth shape (c) to restore sound anterior relationships and occlusal stability.

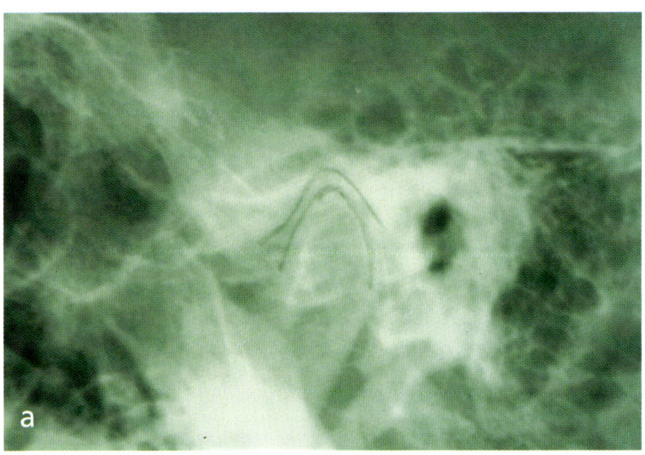

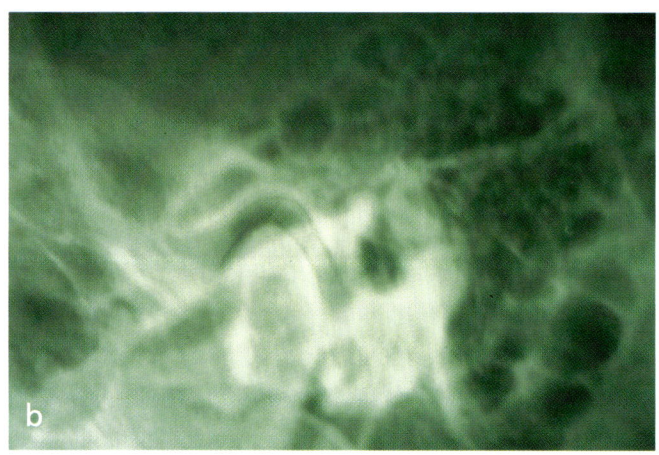

Figs 5-11a and 5-11b Control of condyle location (a) before and (b) after mandibular projection stating the downward-backward location of the condyle liberating the anterior articular interface.

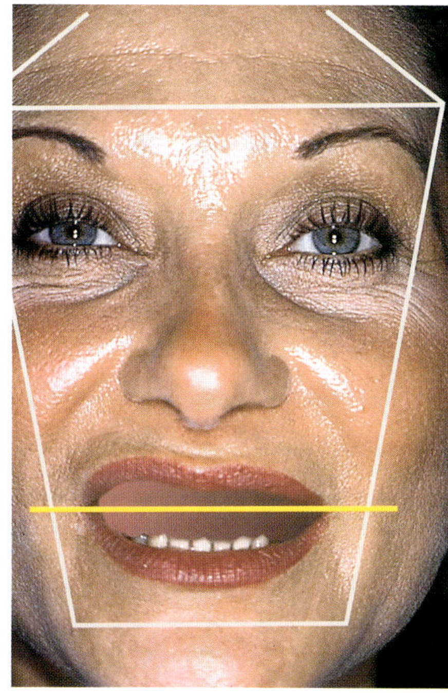

Fig 5-12 In the rehabilitative process, should it involve the whole dentition or be limited to the maxillary anterior segment and fixed or removable denture prosthesis, esthetics and function require one first to determine mandibular tooth visibility and the occlusal plane in relation to the constraints of the vestibular frame, with the purpose of providing the dentofacial composition with the most appealing rhythm of contradictory tensional strengths.

Integration of the Mandibular Anterior Segment

Tooth visibility in rest position, mouth slightly opened and lips relaxed, varies with age. Facial esthetic quality depends greatly on tooth display in the vertical dimension of rest, which can be most easily observed during speech. According to the degree of muscle laxness and the level of the lower frontal plane, one will see either maxillary teeth, a characteristic of youth, or the mandibular anterior segment which, by loading the lower facial third, suggests age and disdain.

It is mandatory before any restorative process, from a full-mouth restoration to one limited to the anterior segment, to appreciate this parameter of tooth visibility and to adopt appropriate corrective measures in consequence, which usually involve, when dealing with aging individuals, a systematic reduction of mandibular tooth display (Fig 5-12), because though increased infraorbital muscle laxness and the impact of gravity may strike with various degrees of intensity, no one escapes this phenomenon. Grinding and recontouring of the mandibular anterior teeth, combined or not with resective periodontal therapies, constitute the most usual therapeutic approaches for a mandibular tooth display, which should not extend beyond 1.5 mm in rest position and which should present a sharp incisal design to increase upward tensional strengths. This approach is valid provided anterior guidance can be reconstituted (Figs 5-13 to 5-15).

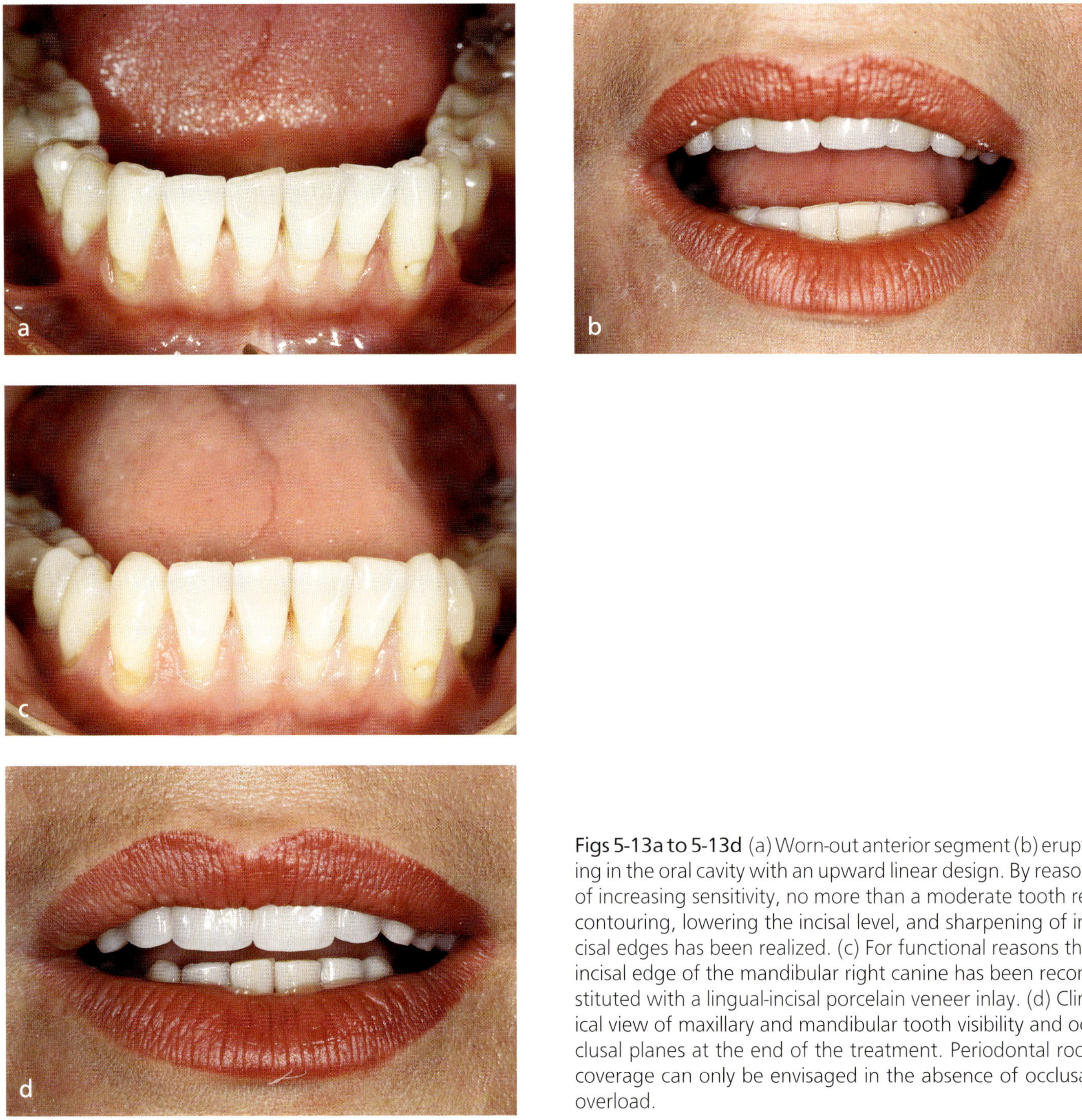

Figs 5-13a to 5-13d (a) Worn-out anterior segment (b) erupting in the oral cavity with an upward linear design. By reason of increasing sensitivity, no more than a moderate tooth recontouring, lowering the incisal level, and sharpening of incisal edges has been realized. (c) For functional reasons the incisal edge of the mandibular right canine has been reconstituted with a lingual-incisal porcelain veneer inlay. (d) Clinical view of maxillary and mandibular tooth visibility and occlusal planes at the end of the treatment. Periodontal root coverage can only be envisaged in the absence of occlusal overload.

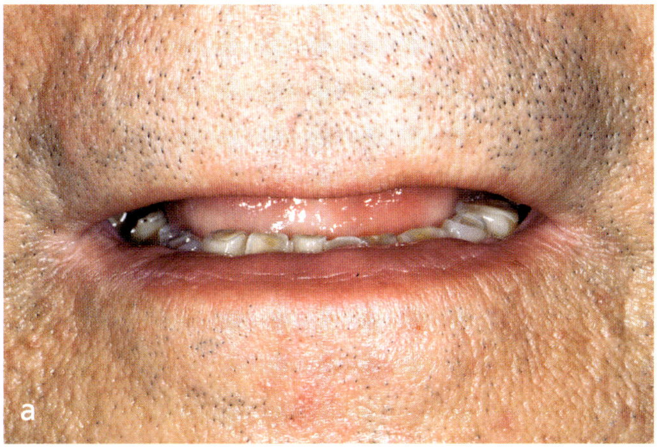

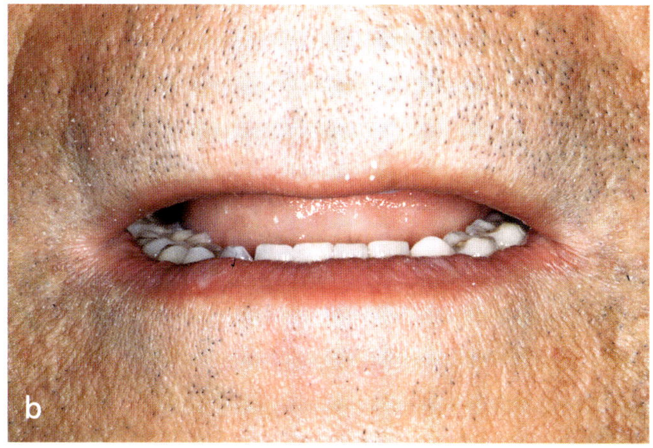

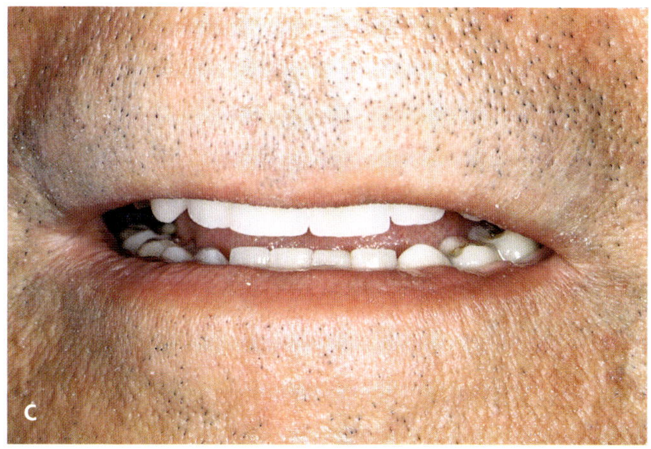

Figs 5-14a to 5-14c (a) Barely visible mandibular dental segment at rest position yet displaying large surfaces of wear (see Fig 5-4). The reconstitution of sharp mandibular incisal elements, producing an upward tensional strength, has to participate in the play of opposed tensions (b) displayed by the dentofacial composition and (c) realized in the final restoration.

The initial setup of the mandibular anterior segment should provide the dentofacial composition with the most appealing rhythmic qualities. In a number of cases where the mandibular anterior segment has dramatically erupted into the oral cavity, good function and dentofacial rhythmic qualities can hardly be advocated. A removal of mandibular anterior incisors and consequent crest reduction may sometimes necessitate repositioning the lower incisal edges of the new restorations slightly higher than lower lip level at the vertical dimension of rest. Identical objectives dictate treatment modalities in totally abraded dentitions, where an increase of morphological tooth length is necessary to introduce the most appealing play of tensions in the dentofacial composition (Fig 5-14).

Dentofacial esthetic requirements justify these clinical efforts focused on the determination of the mandibular anterior occlusal plane as the initial clinical measure of any type of rehabilitation. Yet such rehabilitation involves a simultaneous appreciation of the maxillary anterior occlusal plane, including tooth

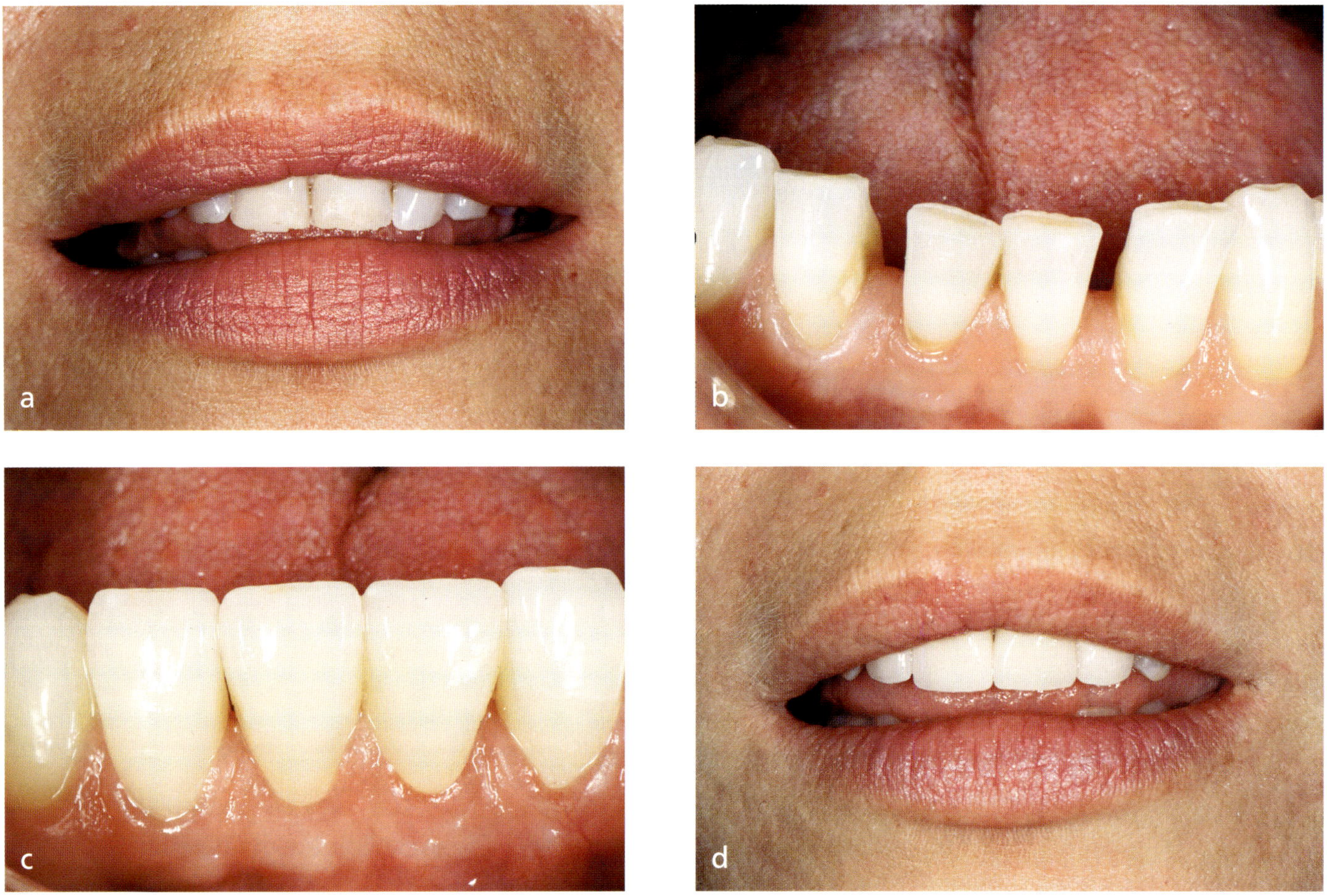

Figs 5-15a to 5-15d (a,b) Young woman in her 30s with lower lip design preventing malposed mandibular tooth display. (c) Restoration and elongation of mandibular anterior segment, (d) allowing for a moderate but favorable mandibular tooth display, improving interocclusal relationships and anterior guidance.

length and vertical overbite, and an appreciative adaptation of maxillary lingual tooth contour and morphology to the static and dynamic requirements of function.

The preliminary determination of the level of the lower frontal plane and its coordination with the horizontal constraints of the vestibular frame represents a necessary step in any esthetic restorative procedure. It will reveal the key esthetic elements of the future reconstruction aimed at promoting a rhythmic equilibrium in the dentofacial composition, according to a parameter that has been previously defined as the visual weight factor.

Integration of Posterior Segments

In a logical esthetic setup, the restoration of the posterior segments immediately follows that of the mandibular anterior segment. Most of the time this restoration consists of a more or less important tooth recontouring; once in a while it consists of a tooth restoration following periodontal tooth lengthening. Appropriate modification of the lingual surface of opposing maxillary teeth by means of temporary restorations such as composite bonding or a provisionalization of the maxillary antagonist segment is mandatory to temporarily ascertain interocclusal contacts, stability, and function. However, the final determination of the spatial position and the esthetic nature of the anterior elements should be postponed until the final phase of the esthetic setup.

The reconstructive restoration of posterior occlusal surfaces will require consideration not only of static interocclusal relationships and dynamic functions but also of a pure esthetics. The integration of the maxillary canines into the reconstruction of the posterior segments should respond not only to clinical necessity but also to esthetics since the spatial location of the canine is a privileged and unavoidable point of anchorage of the restoration in the framework of the facial geometry.

Prosthetic dentistry has long accepted the idea that the constraints of facial geometry should dictate the placement of a tooth, or even that of a whole dental segment. The facial plane, or more precisely the vestibular plane, a reduced geometric figure of

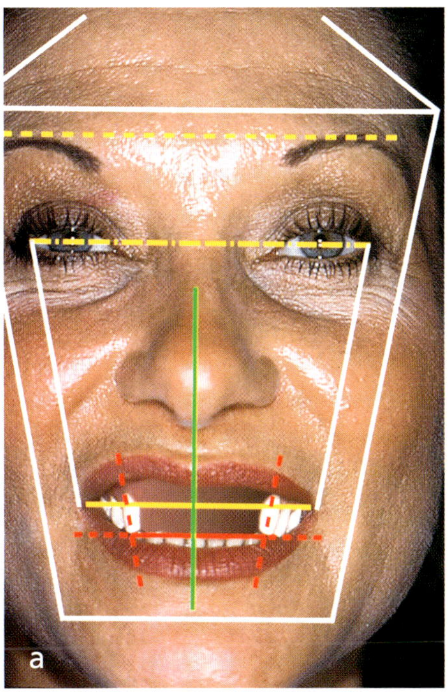

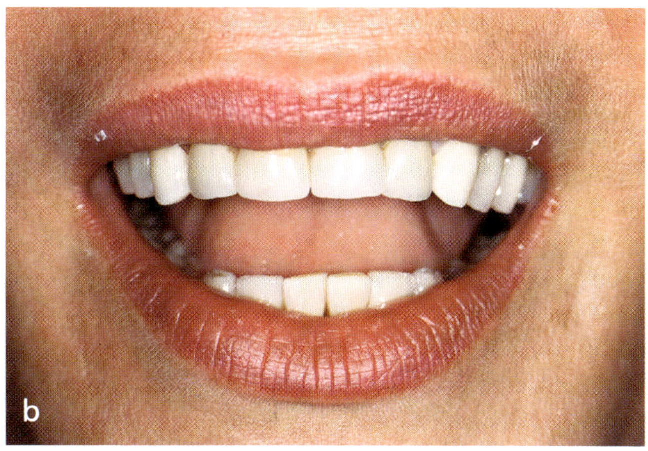

Figs 5-16a and 5-16b (a) Preparation for the restoration of the posterior segments, which involves the integration of the maxillary canine-canine line and canine axial direction into the facial linear system, (b) stressing the importance of a correct placement of the maxillary canine for the integration of the rehabilitation.

the facial pentagon described by Leonardo da Vinci, represents an essential basis for every dental reconstruction. As a matter of fact, the lines of tension generated by the vestibular plane should determine not only the placement of dental elements but also the location of all the other structures contained in this plane. Its lines of tension should make up a collective sensibility.

Facial receptors are naturally placed along characteristic horizontal and vertical lines of tension. In full smile an oblique line running from the corner of the eye to the corner of the mouth will not only run parallel to the vertical side of the vestibular plane but also dictate the axial direction of the canine, which in turn dictates the axial inclination of the whole posterior segment (Fig 5-16).

The horizontal parallelism between the bipupillary line, the commissural line, and many other lines naturally dictates the direction of the mandibular occlusal plane, which in turn dictates the direction of the maxillary anterior occlusal plane running from one canine to the other and gives a first indication of the spatial location of the tips of the canine. The determination of these elements imposed by the constraints of the vestibular plane, which allows for the material tracing of the anterior occlusal plane, has long been favored by prosthodontists seeking to integrate restorations naturally into the scheme of facial geometry. It pinpoints the canine as a key element of dentofacial esthetics.

Canine placement

Proper canine placement is critical as it determines how the anterior and posterior segments will be integrated into the facial scheme. But canine placement cannot rely only on the evaluation of single parameters to attain this integration. Fortunately, information relative to the spatial location of the canines is various and complementary. The study casts reveal that the base of the canine is located 1.5 mm to 2 mm buccal to the first palatal ruga, a morphological constant imposing an implant placement 4.5 to 5.0 mm buccal to this ruga to duplicate the conditions of original tooth placement, sometimes more buccally when overlying soft tissue thickness is reduced. Migratory movements of the canine forward or laterally are likely when this specific distance is substantially increased.

Study casts also show that a line drawn from the tip of one canine to the other crosses the palatal papilla right in its middle (Fig 5-17). This represents a second means of fixing the spatial location of the canine, whereas frontal facial evaluation provides a third in that the canine tip should fall on a line drawn vertically from the inner corner of the eye (Fig 5-18). The determination of its length according to the facial parameters of tooth visibility and functional requirements completes its spatial location.

Strongly anchored into the vertical and horizontal lines of constraints of the vestibular frame (Fig 5-18), controlled in its spatial location by purely visual and anatomical parameters, proper canine placement represents a key factor of dentofacial esthetics in dictating the location of anterior and posterior occlusal planes.

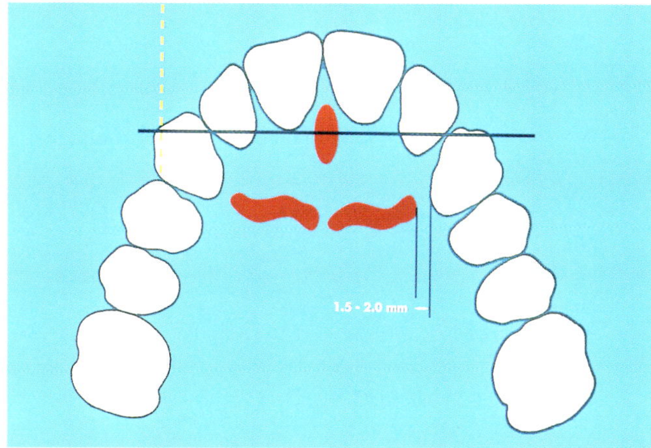

Fig 5-17 In the average case, a line drawn from the tip of one canine to the other, or CPC line, crosses the interdental papilla in its middle, whereas the base of the canine is usually located 1.5 to 2 mm away from the tip of the first palatal ruga. Facial frontal examination shows that a line drawn from the tip of the canine crosses the inner corner of the eye.

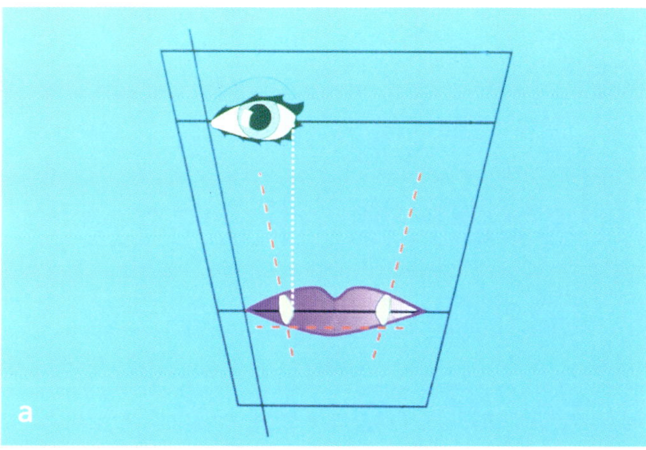

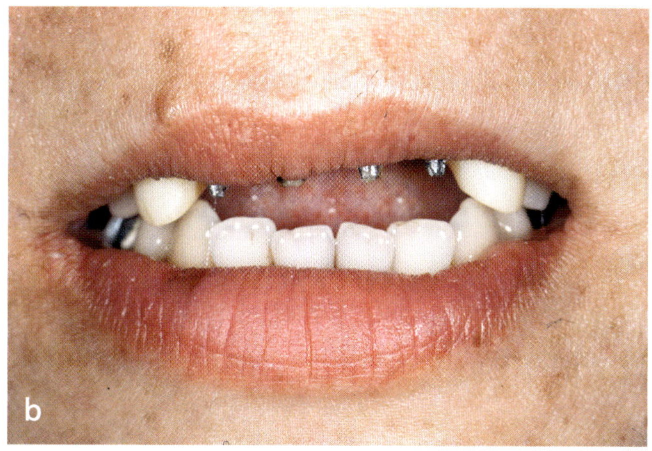

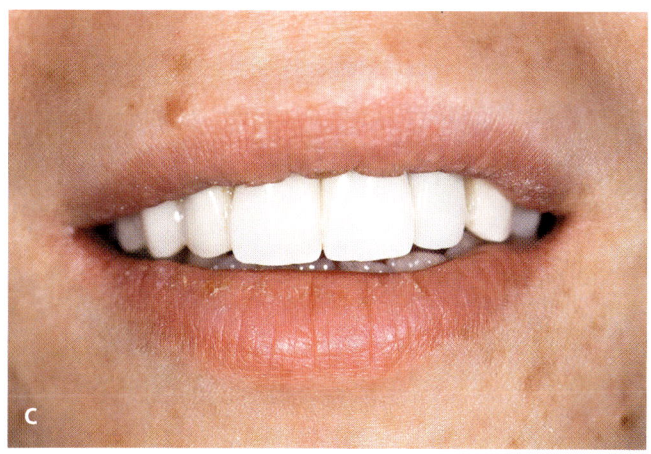

Figs 5-18a to 5-18c (a) Schematic representation of the line drawn vertically from the canine, (b,c) while canine-canine lines and the canine axial direction in any type of situation should integrate facial linear constraints, stressing the importance of a correct determination of the canine's spatial location to achieve a good esthetic result.

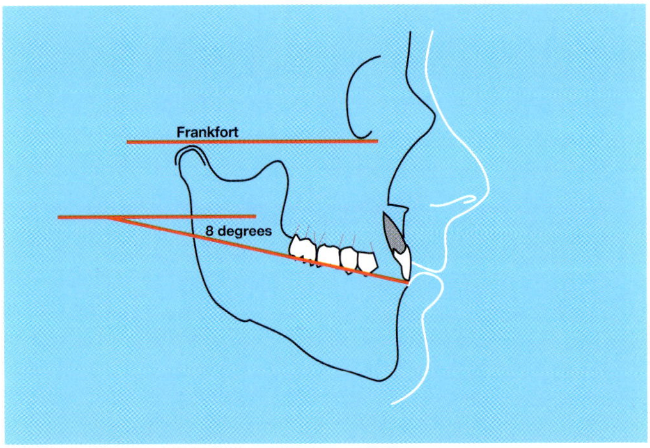

Fig 5-19 In natural dentitions, the sagittal inclination of the occlusal plane to the axio-orbital plane averages 8 degrees, so that during the development of a smile and from a frontal point of view, posterior maxillary teeth become progressively less visible during a smile the deeper they are placed in the oral cavity.

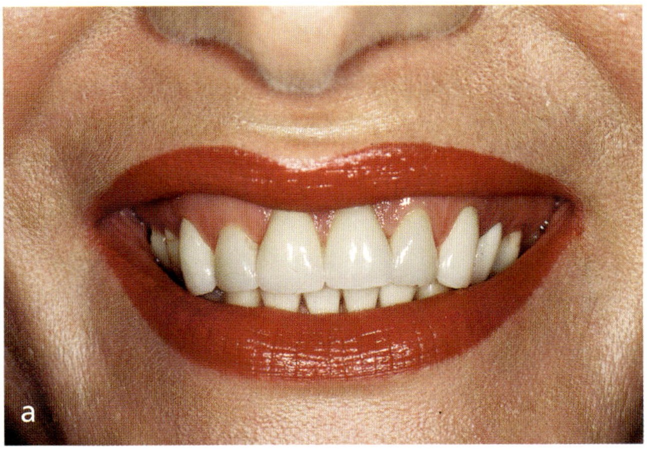

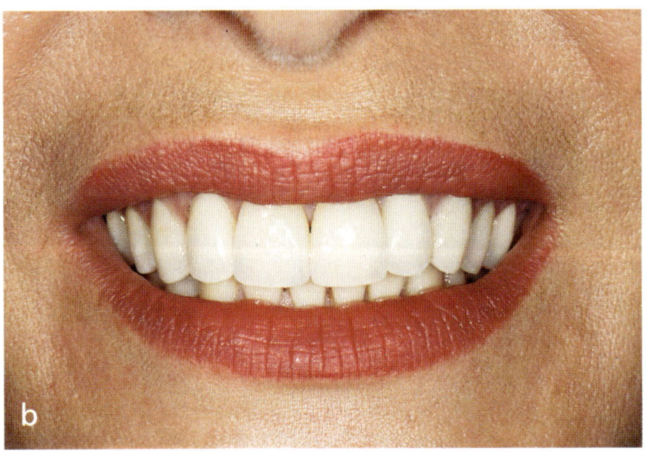

Figs 5-20a and 5-20b (a) The posterior soft tissue display detracting from the esthetic of the smile (b) has been corrected by means of a periodontal tooth elongation, leaving intact the molars' furcations. In Fig 5-19, morphological normality fixed at 8 degrees the sagittal inclination of the posterior planes by reference to the axio-orbital plane. The variation of the saggital inclination of the posterior occlusal planes, apprehended here according to esthetic considerations, raises questions relative to the impact of this inclination in functional tooth closure patterns.

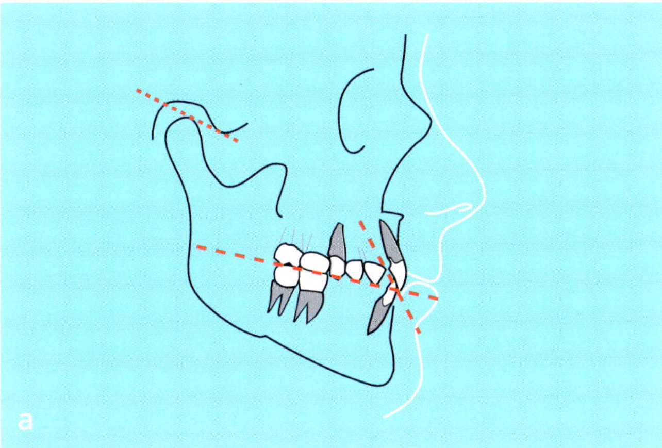

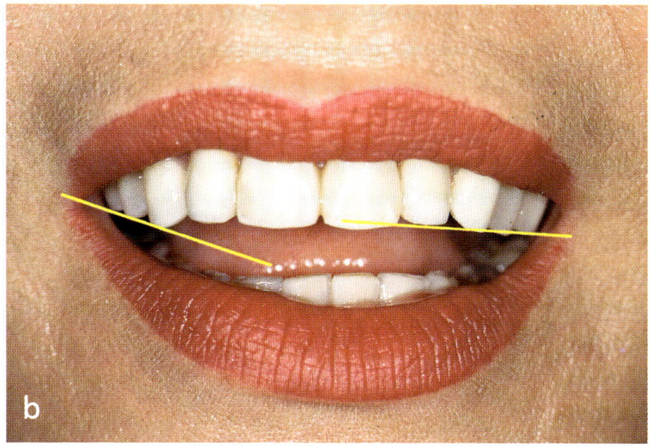

Figs 5-21a and 5-21b (a) Clinical reality shows that condylar guidance, incisal guidance, and the sagittal inclination of the occlusal plane control the mechanical pathway to tooth intercuspation. Given that condylar guidance escapes therapeutic manipulation and that the incisal guidance imposed by esthetic or morphological limitations may be insufficient, it remains to be known if a modification of the posterior sagittal occlusal plane can overcome this deficiency. In other words, what can be the impact of a modified plane inclination with reveals (b) to be flatter on the left side of this composition and steeper on the right side?

Posterior occlusal plane

In the dynamic of the smile that proceeds in the lateral elevation of the corners of the mouth, esthetic demand favors a front-back progression of the posterior segment, characterized by a progressive diminution of tooth visibility usually stressed by the natural sagittal inclination of the posterior occlusal plane. In a natural dentition, the sagittal inclination of the occlusal plane to the axio-orbital plane, or Frankfort plane, averages 8 degrees (Fig 5-19).

In extreme types of "posterior" smile, the perception of the whole molar crown length and sometimes of the supporting periodontal tissue may seriously negate esthetic value, calling for an increase of the mean sagittal inclination of the posterior occlusal plane (Fig 5-20). This involves a correction of posterior tooth visibility by means of orthodontic intrusion or periodontal tooth elongation, two different approaches with either clinical difficulties or counterindications.

The extrusion of maxillary posterior dental elements into edentulous areas of the mandibular arch can produce, whatever the type of smile, an identical inharmonious result, leaving the prosthodontist with no other option than providing correction to individual or collective tooth visibility by means of periodontal tooth lengthening and reduced artificial crown-length insertion. Yet posterior maxillary tooth visibility, generated by an inappropriate inclination of the posterior sagittal plane and detracting from the

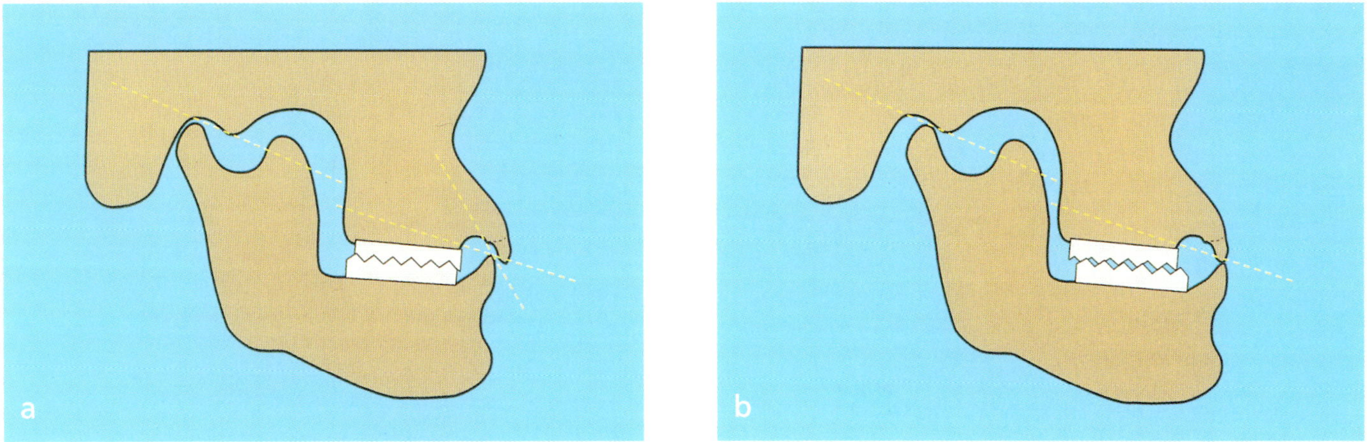

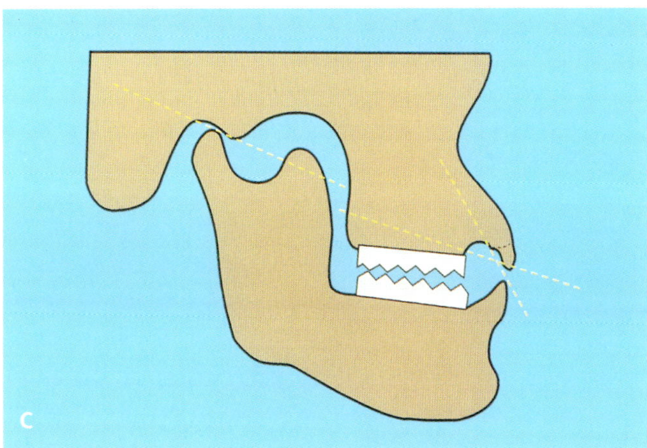

Figs 5-22a to 5-22c (a) For a given average inclination of the condylar pathway and an inclination of the occlusal plane close to the normality of 8 degrees (b) posterior tooth clush cannot be avoided with moderate incisal guidance. (c) Posterior tooth clush will probably take place with steep incisal guidance during tooth closure patterns.

esthetic of the smile, has never been one of a dentist's common preoccupations. In this area, functional preoccupations occupy front stage and impose an inclination of the posterior occlusal plane to prevent posterior tooth clush during tooth closure patterns.

Three factors control the path of intercuspation of posterior teeth (Fig 5-21): the anterior overbite, the condylar pathway, and the occlusal plane. These factors lead to the conclusion that the key to the posterior esthetic quality of the smile rests on an upward front-back progression and on anterior relationships generating a steep anterior pathway that permits, whatever the inclination of the condylar pathway, a good separation of posterior teeth during tooth closure patterns. However, in clinical reality these ideal conditions are far from being always realized.

In an occlusal scheme in which the incisal pathway runs parallel to the condylar pathway and an occlusal plane equals the condylar pathway, the way to posterior interferences during mandibular tooth clo-

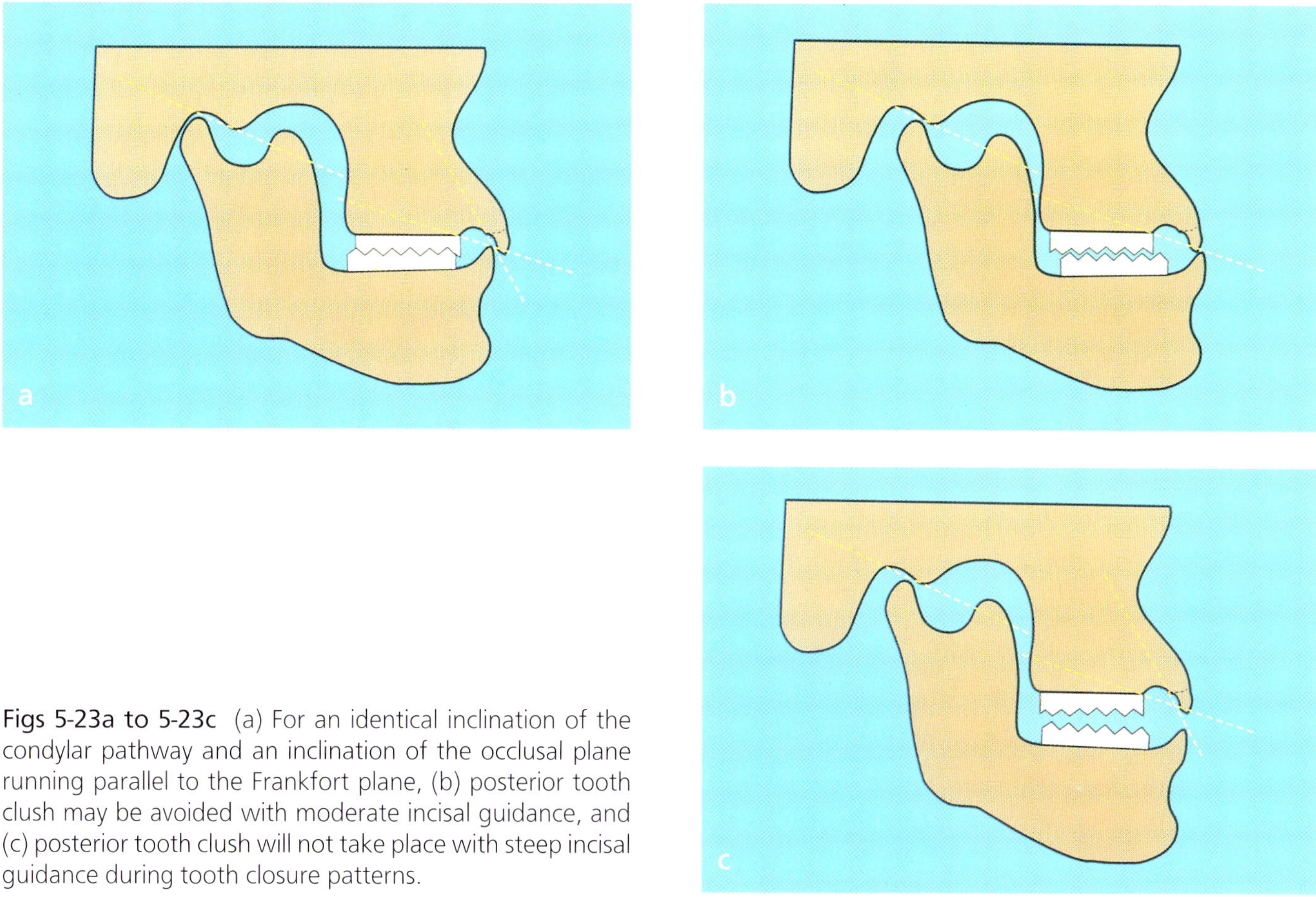

Figs 5-23a to 5-23c (a) For an identical inclination of the condylar pathway and an inclination of the occlusal plane running parallel to the Frankfort plane, (b) posterior tooth clush may be avoided with moderate incisal guidance, and (c) posterior tooth clush will not take place with steep incisal guidance during tooth closure patterns.

sure patterns is wide open, even if posterior teeth have been provided with shallow cusp angles (Fig 5-22). In contrast, with an identical condylar and incisal pathway and a flat occlusal plane approximating the axio-orbital plane, that is to say more obliquely positioned with reference to the condylar pathway, the possibility of posterior interference is greatly reduced, and greater posterior cusp angles are possible (Fig 5-23).

These statements demonstrate that it may become necessary to sacrifice the smile's posterior esthetics to the imperatives of good function in reducing posterior occlusal plane inclination so as to prevent posterior tooth clush in tooth closure patterns when anterior relationships are not sufficient to achieve a steep anterior guidance.

Posterior Occlusal Plane and Increase of VDO

The increase of VDO, which often accompanies the various manifestations of bite collapse and associated facial height collapse, usually affects the quality of anterior relationships. The appreciation of the functional impact of anterior relationships is critical in correctly restoring the posterior segments since these two elements are closely associated.

The irrepressible urge to restore sound anterior relationships by increasing maxillary tooth length morphology should be curbed by the observation that essentially, maxillary tooth length should not exceed morphological normality while mandibular anterior tooth length, if lengthened to achieve the same objectives, run an even more serious risk of interfering with the esthetic rhythm of the dentofacial composition.

Respect for morphological normality is deeply rooted in human sensibility and, rather than abandon the effort to restore facial height to full morphological normality in tooth length and anterior interocclusal relationships, one has to accept the idea of compensating for the reduced amount of anterior interocclusal relationships generated by the increase of VDO by a modification of posterior plane steepness to prevent posterior tooth clush in closure patterns. In such an event one should introduce a reduction of the inclination of the posterior occlusal planes into the treatment plan, which means the increase of maxillary posterior tooth length correlated with the reduction of posterior cusp angulation.

The posterior interocclusal void following the increase of VDO, therefore, is usually best filled by working on the maxillary posterior segment, even if periodontal support resistance would favor an increase of mandibular posterior tooth morphology. These treatment modalities, dictated by functional requirements, seem to be less compromising for dentofacial esthetics than modifications in anterior relationships. The increase of VDO remains a complicated treatment requiring experience, competence, and sensibility to keep control of all the parameters that participate in these compensatory measures and to fulfill esthetic needs without impairing functional requirements.

Integration of Anterior and Posterior Occlusal Planes

The restoration of the maxillary anterior segment represents for the practitioner routine work, most of the time understood in its technical aspects, which involve proper tissue management, adequate material and color selection, and a master technician's participation. These ingredients are perfectly suited to achieving a high quality of esthetics both dental and dentofacial when the clinical situation shows an absence of functional pathology and when original infraorbital muscles seem to have maintained their tensional strength.

Unfortunately, with age few people escape the increase of facial muscle laxness and therefore of mandibular tooth visibility, and debilitating toothwear patterns, not necessarily linked to the aging process, may strike at very young ages. These mani-

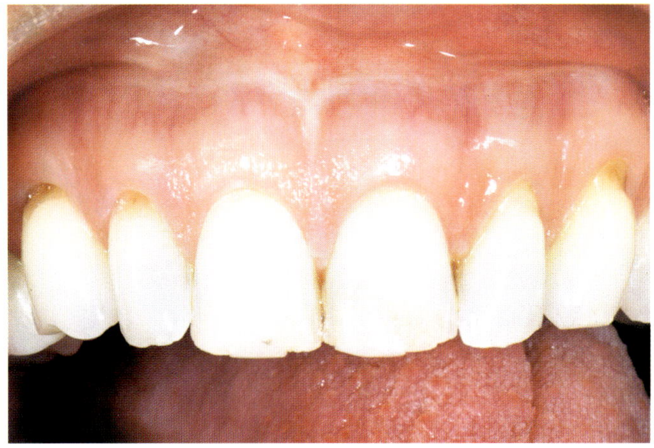

Fig 5-24 Manifestations of anterior wear with reduced implication of the posterior segment.

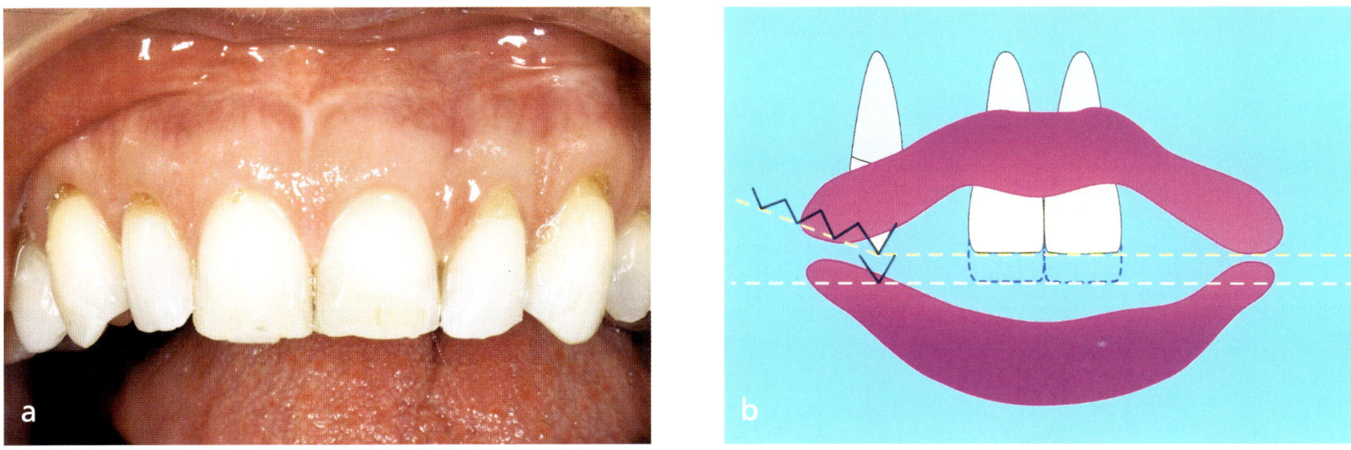

Figs 5-25a and 5-25b The restoration of canine morphology and spatial location, key factors in the determination of the anterior occlusal plane, introduces in the canine–first premolar area an element of rupture requiring correction.

festations of biological and accidental aging make the restoration of the six maxillary anterior teeth an extremely delicate clinical procedure when it has for its objective esthetics and the patient's satisfaction. Both full-mouth rehabilitation and the restoration of the maxillary anterior segment require a sensitive and careful appreciation and relocation of the anterior occlusal planes.

An abrasion limited to the six anterior teeth and leaving intact the morphology of the mandibular antagonist segment creates an ideally simple but purely hypothetical situation (Fig 5-24). Basic functional knowledge indicates that the simple restoration of the original clinical parameters, which include identical maxillary tooth length and anterior guidance, will prove unable to prevent the recurrence of tooth-wear symptoms that will eventually affect the mandibular anterior segment.

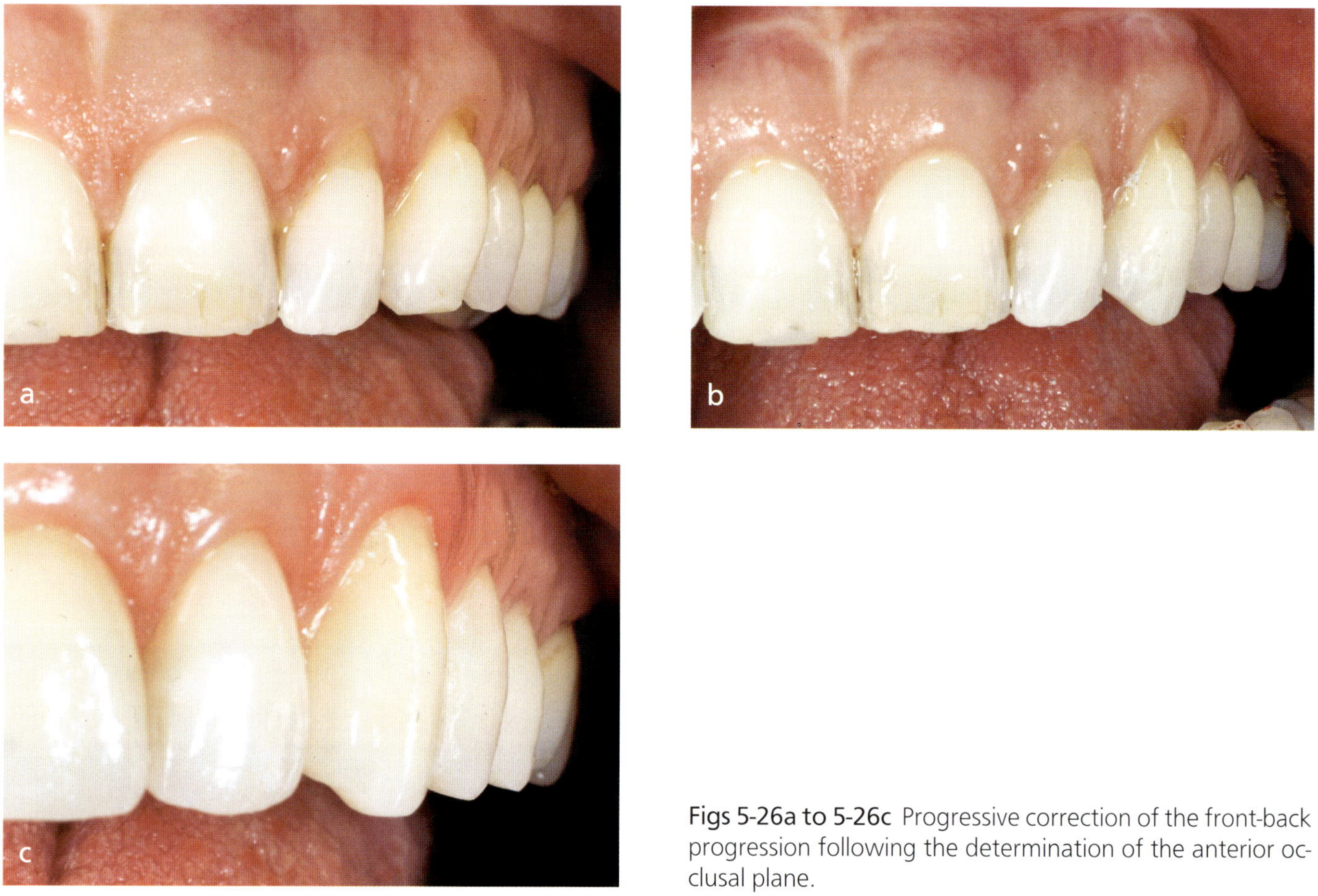

Figs 5-26a to 5-26c Progressive correction of the front-back progression following the determination of the anterior occlusal plane.

In such a case the restoration of good function will require an increase of maxillary tooth length and lead to an increase of anterior interocclusal vertical parameters, which can be interpreted as a lowering of the maxillary anterior occlusal plane. Yet this relocation of the occlusal plane introduces, at the level of the first premolar–second premolar area, an element of rupture between anterior and posterior occlusal planes (Fig 5-25). This element of rupture will be increased whenever tooth-wear patterns have reached and erased the buccal cusp of the first premolar and even the second premolar, or, to refer to a more usual clinical situation, whenever wear patterns have affected both maxillary and mandibular anterior segments.

The extension of the restorative process up to the first and second premolars is prerequisite to achieving a smooth connection between anterior and posterior occlusal planes (Fig 5-26) and preventing a patient's complaint of a "reduced mouth width" and

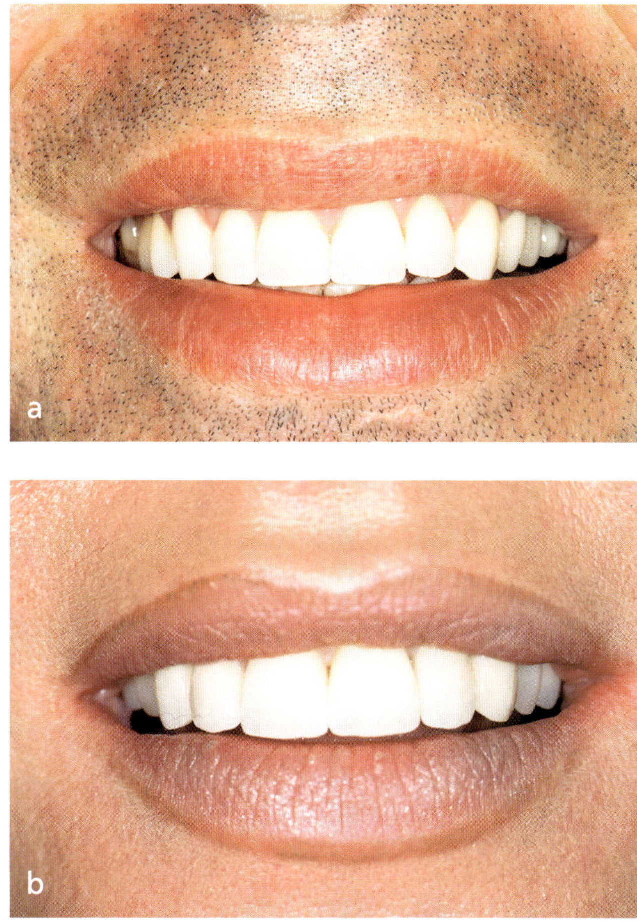

Figs 5-27a and 5-27b The absence of correction of this element of rupture between anterior and posterior occlusal planes is perceived by the patient as a reduction of mouth width. Seen at a certain distance of focus it will appear as a sudden shadow in the reading of the front-back progression, moderate in the upper left segment of (a) and important in the upper right segment of (b).

unsuccessful treatment. This unesthetic parameter never appears at close view but becomes apparent during the development of a smile seen from a distance at which perspective effects produce their impact (Fig 5-27).

Whatever the therapeutic measures to restore function in the maxillary anterior segment, the appreciation of dentofacial balance or the weight factor of the dentofacial composition is always the first thing that will be perceived. As a matter of fact, the indications for the recontouring or, more precisely, the lowering of the mandibular anterior dental elements invading the lower part of the dentofacial plane and made necessary with the increase of muscle laxness remain valid whatever the extension of the restorative process. Yet this corrective approach systematically implies a lateral extension of the planned partial restoration of the maxillary anterior segment to harmoniously connect anterior and posterior planes (Fig 5-28). However, this approach of

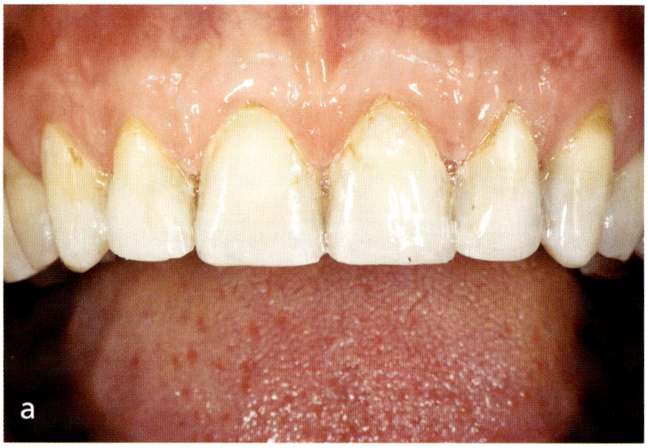

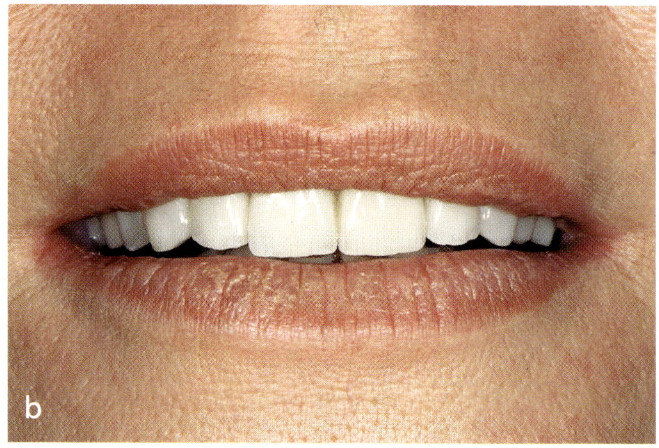

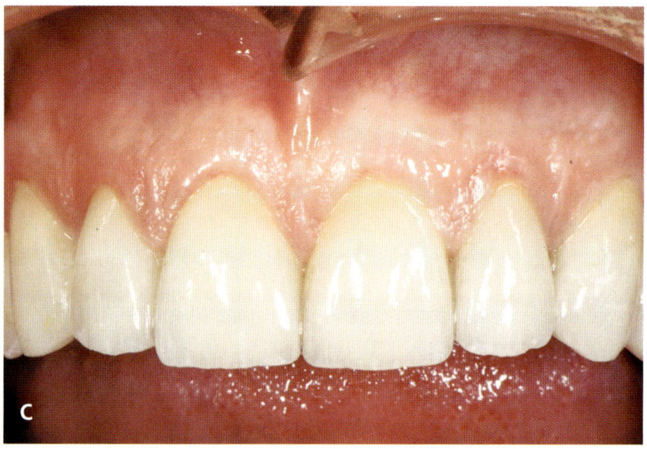

Figs 5-28a to 5-28c (a) A temporarily restored anterior segment clearly showing that elements of rupture at the canine-premolar area (b) have received perfect correction on the right segment in the final composition, (c) permitting a good and fluent visual reading of the front-back progression from any distance of focus.

mandibular anterior tooth recontouring is acutely restricted by the ethical concept of tissue maintenance when dealing with sound structures.

By starting rehabilitation with the appreciation of the dentofacial plane equilibrium, one may induce rhythmic esthetic qualities and integrate dental elements into the framework of the facial composition. As seen previously, this setup of the mandibular anterior occlusal plane requires a coincidental setup of the static and dynamic parameters associated with good function, for in the evaluation of a treatment plan, functional requirements should always take priority over esthetic ones. In this constructivist approach, which provides a feeling of solidity and satisfies the human inclination for mathematical order, one now needs to prepare the elements of the anterior segment, providing them with the characteristics necessary to create esthetic appeal (Fig 5-29).

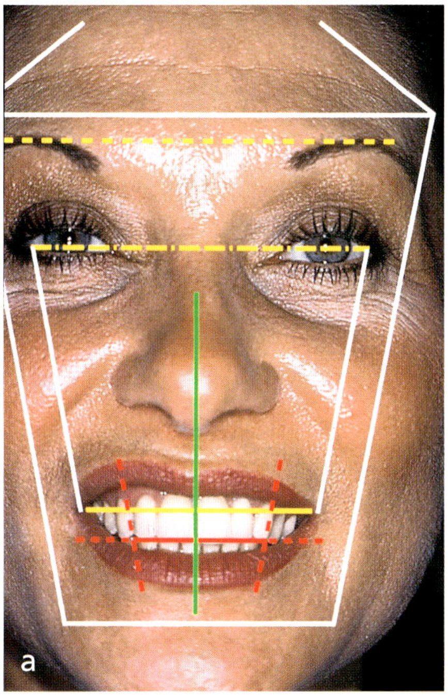

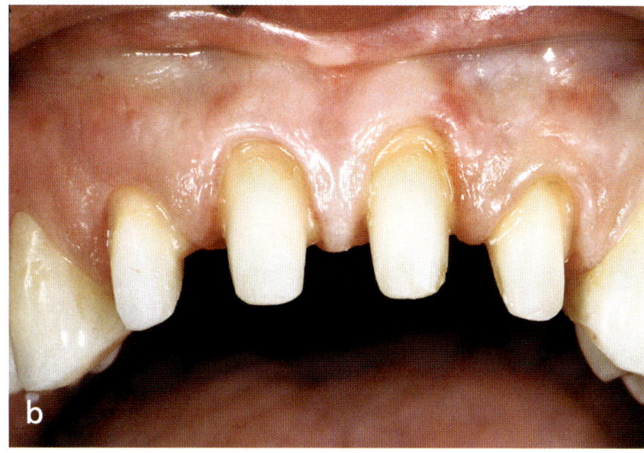

Figs 5-29a and 5-29b Once the mandibular anterior segment and the maxillary and mandibular posterior segments have been restored, it remains to prepare anterior dental elements whose morphological characteristics and spatial location have received successive esthetic refinements during provisionalization and need only to be duplicated at the laboratory level.

Esthetic Integration of the Maxillary Anterior Segment

Tooth shape determination

In esthetic dentistry we not only restore a tooth but also integrate it naturally into environmental conditions that involve periodontal support, interocclusal relationships, and perioral structures. Clinicians engaged in esthetic restorations have to understand the esthetic nature of these structures in selecting tooth shapes because it naturally dictates the character of the tooth or of the dental arrangement.

The correlation between these different elements rests on an esthetic logic expressed by the precept, "Shapes create relations as relations create shapes." This means that the definition of tooth shape, an integral part of a relational system, is naturally pre-established. The particular design of the periodontal support is dictated by and dictates the nature and design of tooth-gingival relationships that in turn dictate individual tooth form at the cementoenamel junction.

At the stage of the clinical preparation of the central incisor that will focus our attention, the definition of tooth contour is restricted to a linear design, resulting from the tracing of periodontal and interocclusal relationships (Fig 5-30). On the frontal and sagittal planes this tracing follows the gingival contour

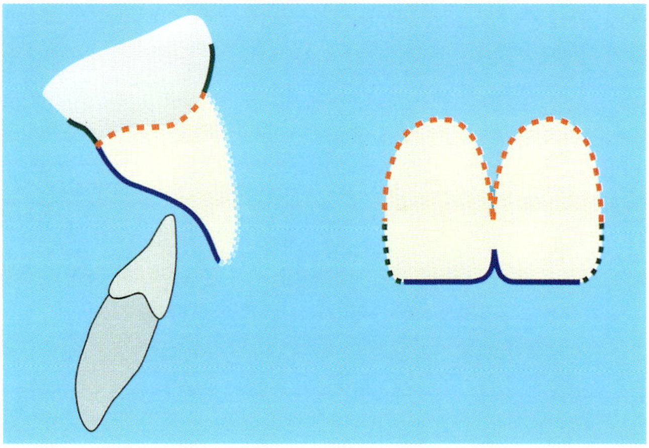

Fig 5-30 Maxillary tooth design is dictated both by functional and esthetic parameters of a periodontal, dentofacial, and facial nature. The gingival and functional relational tracings produce the first participating elements to the future maxillary incisor morphological design. Incisal edge and mesial angle characteristics will be modeled by the close relation of lower lip design, while the distal curvature and tooth angle will reproduce the character and esthetic correspondence of facial structures.

extending up to the tips of the interdental papilla marking the overhanging location of the contact point, whereas the dynamic and static aspects of tooth closure patterns delineate, in the sagittal plane, the lingual tooth morphology. At this point of advancement of tooth contour tracing, one must examine perioral and facial structures to complete a design left incomplete by intraoral referential elements.

The reading of the lower lip anatomy, especially the variations of its vertical width and the characteristics of its upper border line, will provide us with elements of interest not only in the spatial location of the elements of the maxillary anterior segment but also in the design of the incisal edge and interincisal angles. Clinically, the particulars of lower lip design are best examined in a mandibular rest position when soft tissues are subjected to a slight pull at the corner of the mouth, simulating what has been described as a quarter of a smile. In this dynamic position, delicate anatomical particulars located in the center of the upper border lip line may suggest the characteristics of the interdental incisal space and angles and of the incisal line design.

The determination of the incisal edge, whether straight or convex, of the nature of the mesial incisal angle and of interdental space, whether more or less open, does not complete the whole tooth contour tracing. One must then determine the characteristics of the distal tooth angle and complete its distal contour.

Given the lack of distinct elements of close proximity, specific landmarks of the facial composition are extremely useful since they establish obvious relations of correspondence with natural teeth. It has been observed that a line drawn from the lateral protuberance of the forehead to the side of the zygomatic process and the mandibular angle could, in a reduced dimension and reversed position, foreshadow the tracing of the distal contour of the central incisor and its distal angle (Fig 5-30).

This means that a line drawn from the protuberance of the forehead to the zygomatic process around more or less opened or closed eyes determines the distal angle of the maxillary central incisor; a straight line determines a square angle while an increase in curvature determines a rounder angle. The line from the zygomatic process to the mandibular angle as seen from a frontal point of view reflects more moderate variations and curvatures on the distal contour of the tooth.

These elements of character correspondence are easily verified in the majority of individuals, and if dissimilarities can sometimes be noted they are far from calling into question the pertinence of these observations.

Tooth spatial location

When the mouth is slightly opened in a mandibular rest position and there is a slight lateral pull of lip soft tissue, this position, called a quarter of a smile, will display variations in lower lip width or thickness, basic elements of information fixing specific tooth position in the sagittal and frontal planes. This point of anchorage, which has been called a "knot of tension," completes the esthetic qualification of tooth position along with tooth-gingival and interocclusal relationships.

The importance of the relation of tooth-perioral structures in dentofacial esthetics is based on the nature of lip structures that over the years have resisted progressive and debilitating modifications affecting the nature of facial soft tissues. Most often when original occlusal and periodontal relationships have been altered by destructive oral pathologies, lip design constitutes the only available referential element in the determination of tooth spatial location. Nevertheless it must be stressed that the exact determination of these referential elements for the constitution of natural tooth-perioral relationships requires patient and repetitive investigation.

Such investigations show that localized prominences in lip width, or "bumps," raising the upper border of the lower lip are always correlated with a longer or more buccally inclined tooth position, while a reduced lower lip width indicates a lingual inclination of the related dental element or a reduction of its length. And what is true for a maxillary central incisor is no less true for a lateral incisor. The correlation between tooth sagittal inclination and tooth-gingival relational level follows a rule of order that can be expressed as follows: the higher the tooth-gingival level, the more pronounced the tooth buccal inclination and the shorter it appears in the vertical plane. As a corollary, the longer it appears in the vertical plane, the lower its tooth-gingival level location and the more lingual its sagittal inclination. This means that for a given tooth length, tooth-gingival location, tooth position, and tooth-lip relationships are inseparable parameters of dentofacial esthetics.

The idea has been advanced that good esthetics could only be achieved for the anterior segment when tooth-gingival relationships present a gingival level located high for the central incisors and canines and low for the lateral incisors. This, however, should be regarded with some suspicion and qualified with regard to natural tooth arrangement. Good esthetics for the anterior segment can also be achieved when the gingival level on the lateral incisors is located higher than that of the central incisors and canines or when other related tooth-gingival levels are correlated to tooth-sagittal inclination and tooth-lip relationships. This underlines the importance of a sound clin-

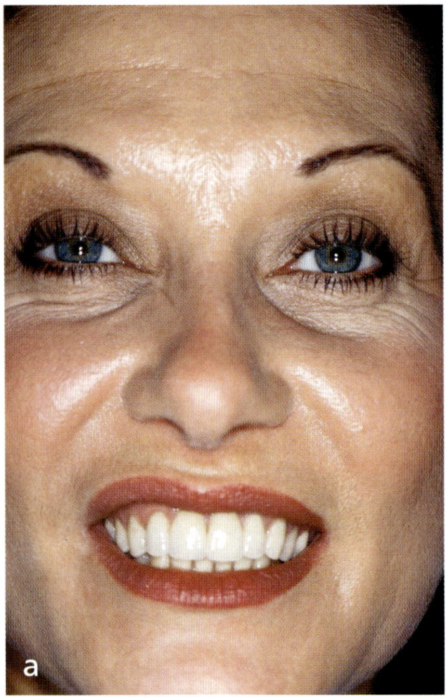

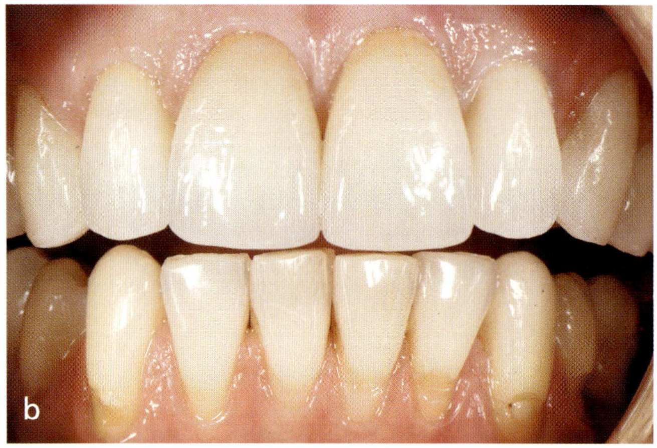

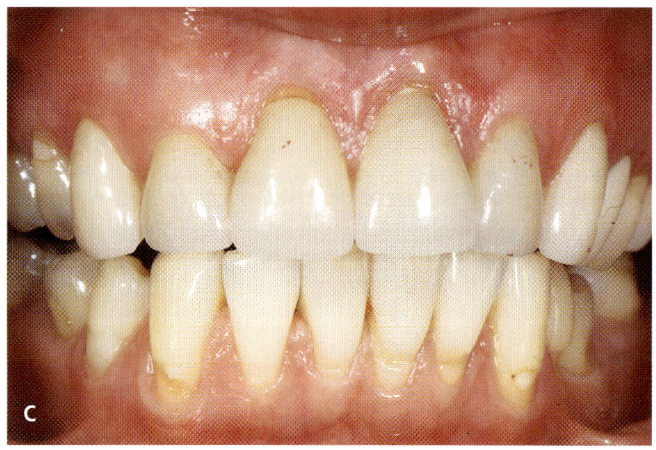

Figs 5-31a to 5-31c (a) Final facial composition (b) following the setup of the maxillary anterior segment (c) restoring a morphological design and tooth location more compatible to related facial structures than the previous restoration.

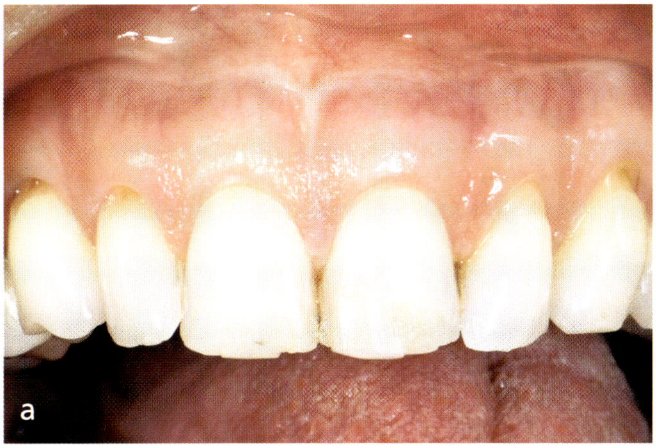
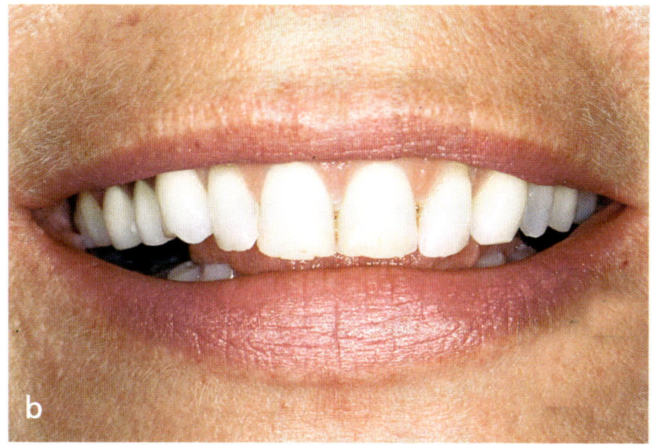
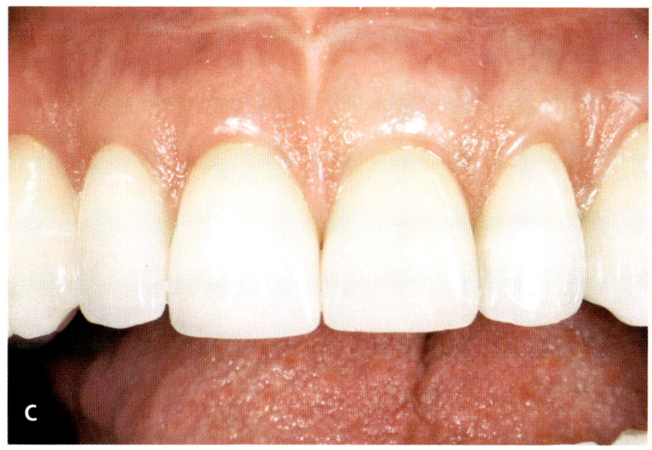
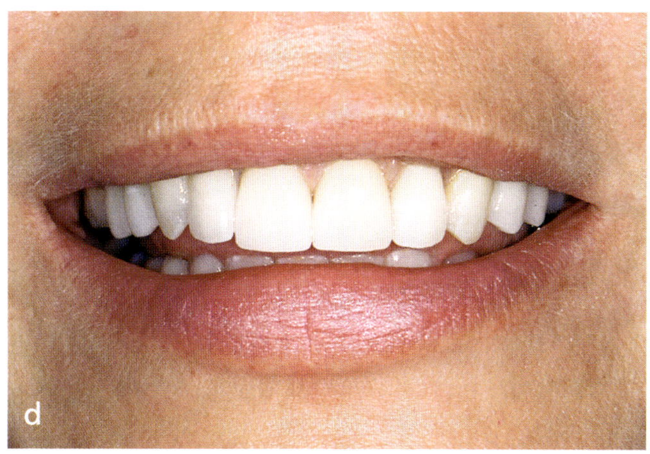

Figs 5-32a to 5-32d (a) Dental composition characterized by an advanced stage of wear. (b) In smiling, the composition presents disturbances in tooth arrangement and unesthetic gingival tissue display. (c) Maxillary teeth have been restored according to facial parameters (distal angle and curvature) adapted to the gingival contour resulting from periodontal elongation and related to lower lip design with the elongation of the maxillary right central incisor, which will constitute, along with lower lip increase, a "knot" of attention. (d) In smiling, the composition reflects the natural integrity of its elements: "unity in variety."

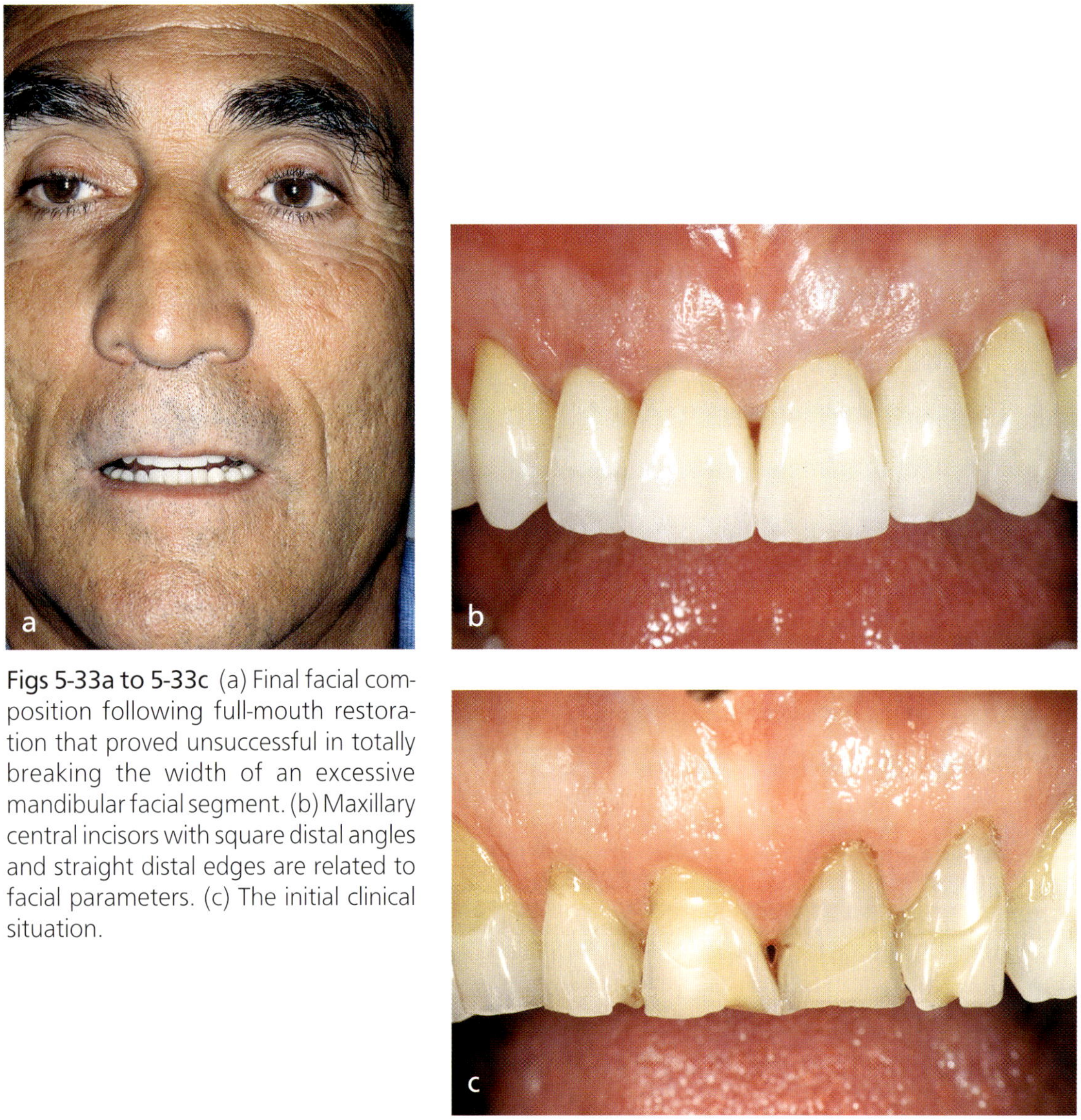

Figs 5-33a to 5-33c (a) Final facial composition following full-mouth restoration that proved unsuccessful in totally breaking the width of an excessive mandibular facial segment. (b) Maxillary central incisors with square distal angles and straight distal edges are related to facial parameters. (c) The initial clinical situation.

ical analysis of these parameters, one that will find in the observation of study casts crucial information relative to arch form and space availability, basic factors dictating tooth position or malposition.

Yet whatever the arch forms for a given tooth width, space availability is a key determining factor in tooth spatial location, for a tooth entertains specific esthetic relationships with lip morphological particulars. The appreciation and application of the multiplicity and variety of these parameters represents an ongoing challenge for the restorative dentist seeking esthetic perfection (Figs 5-31 to 5-33).

Functional Integration of the Maxillary Anterior Segment

The esthetic setup of the four maxillary anterior teeth should establish the esthetic correlation between elements of different natures such as periodontal support, antagonist dental elements, and perioral structures and should restore the parameters constituting the esthetic chain of reaction: "Shapes create relations and relations create shapes." The final esthetic setup of the four maxillary anterior teeth cannot precede but always concludes a rehabilitation, when its integration into facial geometry and the linear system has been achieved and once the elements susceptible to displaying the most interesting rhythmic properties generated by the visual weight factor have been organized.

It must be remembered that, at the stage where maxillary anterior teeth have to be prepared, the mandibular anterior occlusal plane, mandibular anterior dental elements' posterior interocclusal rela-

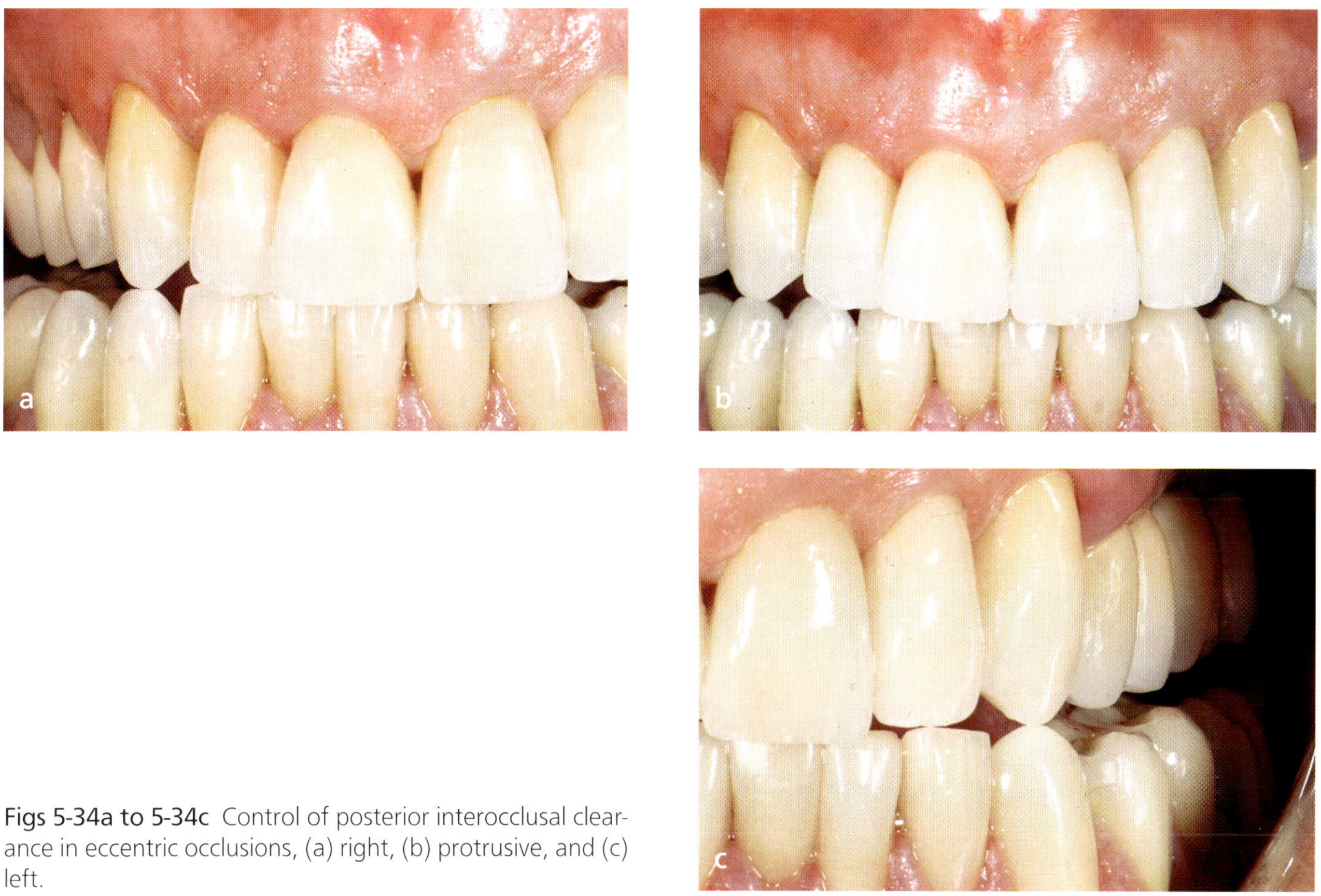

Figs 5-34a to 5-34c Control of posterior interocclusal clearance in eccentric occlusions, (a) right, (b) protrusive, and (c) left.

tionships and posterior occlusal planes, and maxillary anterior occlusal planes or canine-canine lines have already been restored. On the other hand, anterior elements have long been subjected in the course of the development of the treatment's modalities to repetitive adaptations of form and position to conform to the esthetic requirements of related environmental structures.

One must now simply but precisely duplicate these conditions and focus the technician's artistic creativity on the elaboration of the material aspect of the restoration and on the steepest possible incisal guidance without interfering with tooth engagement and disengagement. The concave maxillary lingual tooth surface should be sculpted in harmony with existing antagonist tooth surface, avoiding flattened areas that invite deflective interferences and favoring parabolic designs that naturally appear in occluding areas.

Because of the reduced resistance of most modern esthetic materials, one should proceed to the control of possible deflective interferences in tooth engagement and disengagement after the bonding of porcelain restoration and control of posterior interocclusal clearance in eccentric occlusion (Fig 5-34). This will finalize a setup whose sequential development has been intended to correlate and unify the requirement of esthetics and function.

Final Considerations

Shapes only exist by and for the creation of relationships. The esthetic science consists in apprehending the nature of these relationships and in instituting a network of tensional relationships between straight lines and curved lines and shapes that can be considered infinite and generators of a specific resonance.

A conscious esthetic setup is based on the institution of tensional points covering an ordered geometric canvas. This establishes, between the variety of forms and between each of them and the esthetic support, a rhythm of mutual relations requiring a continual action of the eyes and mind which can be defined as a dynamic equilibrium. The involvement of dentistry in dentofacial esthetics and patients' well-being requires the perception and application of this dynamic.

Esthetic creativity induces the transmission of an emotion through the perception of the resonance displayed by the nature of forms and relationships. Dentofacial esthetics embraces these definitions and responds to the same principles. In proposing the examination of some elements of tensional resonance and a sequential esthetic setup of these elements in a routine daily practice, we have tried to break the barriers that have obstructed comprehensive esthetic knowledge in dentistry.

Bibliography

Ackerman F. Le Mécanisme des Mâchoires. Paris: Masson & Cie, 1933.

Bauer A, Gutowski A. Gnathologie. Einführung in Theorie und Praxis. Berlin: Quintessenz, 1975.

Fradeani M, Bottachian R, Tracey T, Parma-Benfenati S, Stein J, de Paoli S. The restoration of functional occlusion and esthetics. Int J Periodontics Restorative Dent 1992;12: 63–71.

Goldstein RE. Change Your Smile. Chicago: Quintessence, 1984.

Hulsey CM. An esthetic evaluation of lip-teeth relationships present in the smile. Am J Orthod 1970;57:132–144.

Lorgnes C. Les proportions du corps humain d'après les traités du Moyen Age et de la Renaissance. L'Information d'Histoire de l'Art Mai-Juin 1968.

Lucia VO. Modern Gnathological Concepts. St Louis: Mosby, 1961.

Lucia VO. Principles of Articulation. Dent Clin North Am 1979;23:199–211.

Mack MR. Vertical dimension: dynamic concept. J Prosthet Dent 1991;68:479–486.

Magne P, Magne M, Belser U. The diagnostic template: A key element to the comprehensive esthetic treatment concept. Int J Periodontics Restorative Dent 1996;16: 561–569.

Martone AL, Edwards LF. Anatomy of the mouth and related structures. Part I. The face. J Prosthet Dent 1961;11: 1009–1018.

Matthews. The anatomy of a smile. J Prosthet Dent 1978; 39:128–134.

Monteith BD. Evaluation of a cephalometric method of occlusal plane orientation for complete dentures. J Prosthet Dent 1986;55:64–70.

Morchio S. Choix des dents artificielles: Les cinq composantes de l'harmonie. Prosth Dent 1996;116:29–35.

Peck S, Peck H. A concept of facial esthetics. Angle Orthod 1970;40:284–318.

Schäffer H, Richter M. Functional preprosthetic orthodontic and prosthetic reconstruction with resin-bonded fixed partial dentures. Int J Periodontics Restorative Dent 1991;11:127–148.

Shawell HM. The art and science of complete-mouth occlusal reconstruction: A case report. Int J Periodontics Restorative Dent 1991;11:439–458.

Shawell HM. The bioesthetics of complete porcelain occlusal rehabilitation. Int J Periodontics Restorative Dent 1990; 10:257–279.

Sicher H. Temporomandibular articulation in mandibular overclosure. J Am Dent Assoc 1948;36:131–137.

Silverman MM. Occlusion in Prosthodontics and in the Natural Dentition. Washington: Mutual, 1962.

Stewart Bruce. Restoration of the severely worn dentition using a systematized approach for a predictable prognosis. Int J Periodontics Restorative Dent 1998;18: 47–56.

Tjan AHL, Miller GD. Some esthetic factors in smile. J Prosthet Dent 1984;51:24–28.

Tweed CH. The diagnostic facial triangle in the control of treatment objectives. Am J Orthod 1969;55:651–657.

Zaffagnini I. Saggi di Estetica. Parma: Pratiche, 1999.

Zide MF. Evaluation of facial esthetics. JDC Dent Soc 1981; 55:27–40.

Index

D

E

F

K

L

M

N

O

P

Q

R

S

T

U

V

W

Z